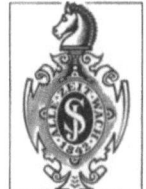

H. Menge   M. Gregor   G. N. J. Tytgat
B. J. Marshall (Eds.)

Campylobacter pylori

Proceedings of the First International
Symposium on Campylobacter pylori
Kronberg, June 12 – 13th, 1987

With 46 Figures and 33 Tables

Springer-Verlag Berlin Heidelberg New York
London Paris Tokyo

Professor Dr. H. Menge
Medizinische Klinik II, Krankenanstalten der Stadt Remscheid,
Akademisches Lehrkrankenhaus der Universität Bonn,
Hans-Potyka-Straße 28, 5630 Remscheid 11, FRG

Privat-Dozent Dr. M. Gregor
Universitätsklinikum Steglitz, Freie Universität Berlin,
Hindenburgdamm 30, 1000 Berlin 45, FRG

Professor Dr. G. N. J. Tytgat
Department of Gastroentero-Hepatology,
Academisch Ziekenhuis bij de Universiteit van Amsterdam,
Academisch Medisch Centrum, Meibergdreef 9,
1105 AZ Amsterdam, The Netherlands

Dr. B. J. Marshall
Division of Gastroenterology, Department of Internal Medicine,
University of Virginia, Box 145,
Charlottesville, VA 22908, USA

ISBN-13: 978-3-642-83324-3   eISBN-13: 978-3-642-83322-9
DOI: 10.1007/978-3-642-83322-9

Library of Congress Cataloging-in-Publication Data
International Symposium on Campylobacter pylori (1st : 1987 ; Kronberg im Taunus,
Germany)
Campylobacter pylori : proceedings of the First International Symposium on Cam-
pylobacter pylori ; [held in Kronberg, Germany on June 12–13, 1987] / H. Menge . . . [et
al.], editors. p. cm. Bibliography: p. Includes index.

1. Campylobacter pylori infections—Congresses. 2. Campylobacter pylori—Congresses.
I. Menge, H., 1939–   . II. Title.
QR201.C26I56 1987   616.3′3–dc 19   88-12392

The use of registered names, trademarks, etc. in this publication does not imply, even in
the absence of a specific statement, that such names are exempt from the relevant protective laws and regulations and therefore free for general use.

Product Liability: The publisher can give no guarantee for information about drug dosage and application thereof contained in this book. In every individual case the respective user must check its accuracy by consulting other pharmaceutical literature.

Preface

Campylobacter pylori was described for the first time in 1983. Up to now more than 100 papers have been published dealing with its microbiological properties and its clinical implications.

The time has come to survey the field, to evaluate the hitherto accumulated information, and to discuss the questions that should be answered in the future. It was for these purposes that the First International Symposium on *Campylobacter pylori* was held, bringing together specialists from a variety of disciplines, including basic scientists as well as clinicians. This book is based on papers given at the symposium.

We are very grateful to Röhm-Pharma for undertaking to sponsor this meeting, and to Mrs. C. J. Klein and her staff for the impeccable organisation which permitted us to work in such a pleasant environment.

In the interest of rapidity of publication, we have reduced the amount of editing to a minimum and have not, in any sense, "refereed" the discussions, which were written by the contributors at the time of the question-and-answer session. They were also vetted by their authors at the proof stage, and we have done our best to retain their original spontaneous flavour. We hope, in this way, to have produced a satisfactory record of the events and an up-to-date overview of research on *Campylobacter pylori*.

H. Menge
M. Gregor
G. N. J. Tytgat
B. J. Marshall

Table of Contents

Section 6   State of the Art Lecture

Chairmen and Senior Authors

AXON, A. T. R.
Gastroenterology Unit, General Infirmary, Great George Street,
Leeds LS1 3EX, Great Britain

CADRANEL, S.
Hôpital Universitaire des Enfants Reine Fabiola,
Avenue Jean Cocq 15, 1020 Bruxelles, Belgium

CLASSEN, M.
2. Medizinische Klinik und Poliklinik rechts der Isar,
TU München, Ismaninger Straße 22, 8000 München, FRG

DELTENRE, M.
Clinique de Gastro-Entérologie, Hôpital Brugman,
Place van Gehuchten 4, 1020 Bruxelles, Belgium

ENGSTRAND, L.
Institute of Bacteriology, University of Uppsala, 75123 Uppsala,
Sweden

FLEMSTRÖM, G.
Department of Physiology and Medical Biophysics,
Biomedical Center, Uppsala University, Post Box 572,
75123 Uppsala, Sweden

GOODWIN, C. S.
Microbiology Department, Royal Perth Hospital,
Box X 2213, GPO, Perth,
Western Australia 6001, Australia

GREGOR, M.
Universitätsklinikum Steglitz, Freie Universität Berlin,
Hindenburgdamm 30, 1000 Berlin 45, FRG

HAHN, H.
Institut für Medizinische Mikrobiologie,
Freie Universität Berlin, Hindenburgdamm 27, 1000 Berlin 45,
FRG

HALTER, F.
Abteilung für Gastroenterologie, Inselspital Bern, 3010 Bern,
Switzerland

HOUTHOFF, H. J.
Department of Pathology, Academisch Ziekenhuis bij de
Universiteit van Amsterdam, Academisch Medisch Centrum,
Meibergdreef 9, 1105 AZ Amsterdam, The Netherlands

KIST, M.
Institut für Medizinische Mikrobiologie und Hygiene,
Universität Freiburg, Hermann-Herder-Straße 11,
7800 Freiburg, FRG

KONTUREK, S. J.
Institute of Physiology, Medical Academy, Krakow,
Grezegorzecka, Poland

KRAFT, W. G.
Norwich Eaton, Pharmaceuticals Inc., Procter & Gamble Comp.
Post Box 191, Norwich, N.Y. 13815, USA

LANGENBERG, W.
Department of Medical Microbiology, Academisch Ziekenhuis
bij de Universiteit van Amsterdam, Academisch Medisch
Centrum, Meibergdreef 9, 1105 AZ Amsterdam,
The Netherlands

MARSHALL, B. J.
Division of Gastroenterology, Department of Internal Medicine,
University of Virginia, Box 145, Charlottesville, VA 22908, USA

McNULTY, C. A. M.
Public Health Laboratory, Gloucestershire Royal Hospital,
Great Western Road, Gloucester GL1 3NN, Great Britain

MÉGRAUD, F.
Laboratoire de Bactériologie, Hôpital des Enfants,
168 Cours de l'Argonne, 33077 Bordeaux, France

MENGE, H.
Medizinische Klinik II, Krankenanstalten der Stadt Remscheid,
Akademisches Lehrkrankenhaus der Universität Bonn,
Hans-Potyka-Straße 28, 5630 Remscheid 11, FRG

Ó'MORÀIN, C.
Consultant Gastroenterologist, 35 Charlemont Street, Dublin 2,
Ireland

OTTENJANN, R.
Städtisches Krankenhaus München-Neuperlach,
Oskar-Maria-Graf-Ring, 8000 München 83, FRG

RATHBONE, B. J.
Department of Medicine, St. James' University Hospital,
Leeds LS9 7TF, Great Britain

RAUWS, E. A. J.
Department of Gastroentero-Hepatology,
Academisch Ziekenhuis bij de Universiteit van Amsterdam,
Academisch Medisch Centrum, Meibergdreef 9,
1105 AZ Amsterdam, The Netherlands

RIECKEN, E. O.
Universitätsklinikum Steglitz, Freie Universität Berlin,
Hindenburgdamm 30, 1000 Berlin 45, FRG

RÖSCH, W.
Medizinische Klinik, Nordwest-Krankenhaus,
Steinbacher Hohl 2 – 26, 6000 Frankfurt 90, FRG

STROHMEYER, G.
Medizinische Universitätsklinik und Poliklinik D,
Moorenstraße 5, 4000 Düsseldorf 1, FRG

TYTGAT, G. N. J.
Department of Gastroentero-Hepatology,
Academisch Ziekenhuis bij de Universiteit van Amsterdam,
Academisch Medisch Centrum, Meibergdreef 9,
1105 AZ Amsterdam, The Netherlands

WARRELMANN, M.
Institut für Medizinische Mikrobiologie,
Freie Universität Berlin, Hindenburgdamm 27, 1000 Berlin 45,
FRG

VON WULFFEN, H.
Institut für Medizinische Mikrobiologie und Immunologie,
Universitätskrankenhaus Eppendorf, Martinistraße 52,
2000 Hamburg 20, FRG

WYATT, J. I.
Department of Pathology, St. James' Hospital, Leeds LS9 7TF,
Great Britain

Section 1

Microbiology and Biochemistry of *Campylobacter pylori*

Morphological and Biochemical Characterization of *Campylobacter pylori*

F. Mégraud

Culturing of this "new" organism named *Campylobacter pylori* has been one of the major advances in bacteriology in the 1980s. This bacterium still has many secrets left to be revealed, but several special features have already been discovered. In this review we would like to emphasize the morphological and biochemical characteristics of *C. pylori*.

Morphology

C. pylori was observed in gastric mucosa, in fact, a long time ago. At that time, when microscopy was the essential tool for a bacteriological diagnosis, some observers noticed the presence of a spiral-shaped bacterium in close contact with the mucosa in autopsy and surgical specimens removed from the stomach [8, 14, 23]. These aspects were rediscovered by Fung et al. [15], Steer and Colin-Jones [58], and Warren [61]. Warren was the only researcher interested in further investigating the findings which eventually led to the discovery of *C. pylori*.

Morphology in Biopsy Specimens

The spiral or kidney shape of *C. pylori* makes it easily recognizable. The examination can be performed on tissue smears, disrupted material, or the biopsy itself.

Pinkard et al. proposed to examine minced biopsy specimens using phase-contrast microscopy [53]. *C. pylori* appeared as a typically black, well defined, curved rod. The sensitivity of this technique was found to be as good as that of silver staining, considered as the reference technique. Many stains used in bacteriology have been applied to gastric biopsies. We found that Gram's stain is a very quick and reliable technique (Fig. 1). Others have used acridine orange [60], Giemsa stain [5], and recently ethidium bromide [32]. Immunological techniques have also been applied using monoclonal antibodies in a fluorescence test and immunoperoxidase test with very encouraging results [10].

For histological identification the Warthin and Starry (W&S) technique gives the best contrast and is the most likely to lead to a good result [61]. The

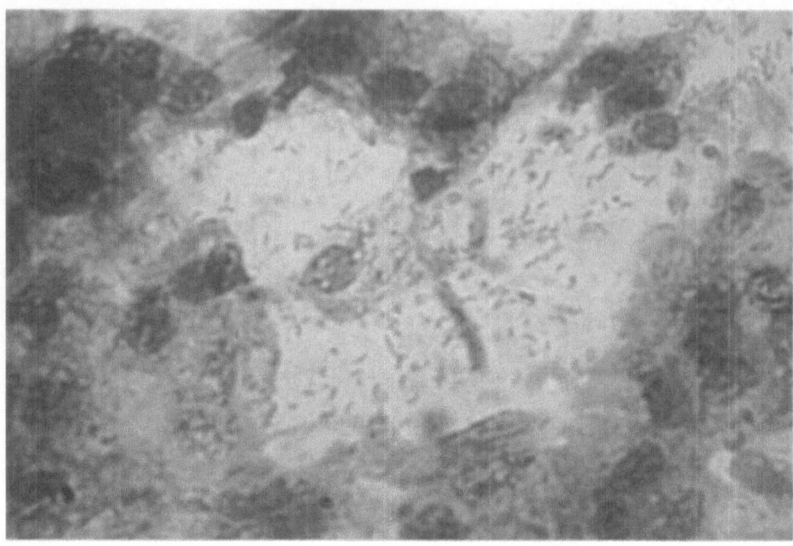

Fig. 1. Biopsy smear specimen stained with Gram (× 1000)

interest in haematoxylin and eosin (H&E) staining is more controversial. One could ask why, when pathologists have been using this technique for decades, no mention of this bacterium was ever made. In fact, it was not a conventional procedure either to observe specimens under high field power microscopy or to study the mucus surface layer and mucous glands. Since these advances we have had excellent results with H&E staining [25]. The most obvious advantage compared to W&S staining is that pathological and bacteriological observations can be made on the same preparation.

Other techniques have also been applied, such as the Gimenez technique [41] used to detect *Rickettsia* and *Legionella*, and acridine orange [60]. Fluorescence using polyclonal antibodies can also be used [59].

Using any one of these techniques, *C. pylori* shows a typical morphology. Some elements are S-shaped, similar to the classical *Campylobacter* but differing in their larger size, while others are kidney shaped. The bacteria are always found in close association with cells in the mucus layer or in the mucous glands. On smears a patchy distribution is usually observed.

Electron microscopy has been used to look at the association of these microorganisms to the mucosa. Their typically S-shaped and kidney-shaped morphology is also observed at the intercellular junctions [52, 54, 57] (Fig. 2).

Morphology in Culture

A unique feature of *C. pylori* is that its aspect observed after culture on agar is quite different from that in vivo. *C. pylori* can be grown on blood agar or choc-

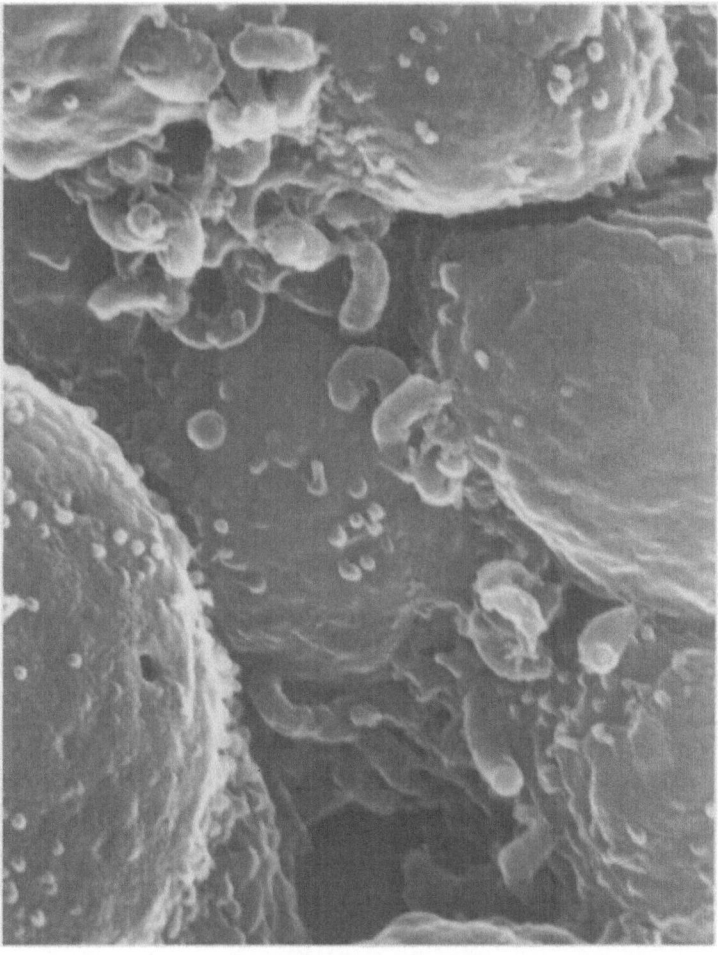

Fig. 2. Scanning electron microscopy of *Campylobacter pylori* at intercellular cell junctions of human gastric mucosa (× 6000)

olate agar at 37 °C in a microaerobic atmosphere. The colonies appear after 3–4 days of incubation. The microscopic appearance is more diversified, and S-shaped bacteria are seldom found. In young cultures most of the cells are rod-shaped, ring-shaped, or "ox-bow" shaped (Fig. 3). Mobility is rarely observed after culture. However, the flagella arrangement has been shown to be especially efficient in mucus [20]. As is the case in several *Campylobacter* species such as *C. jejuni, C. coli, C. laridis, "C. upsaliensis"*, and *C. cinaedi", C. pylori* evolves rapidly toward coccoidal forms which are considered as degenerated, non-cultivable microorganisms (Fig. 3). The cause of this transformation could be linked to a lack of nutrients in the medium. The occurrence of such forms constitutes the difficulty in culturing these organisms. The reality of the non-cultivable state is debatable.

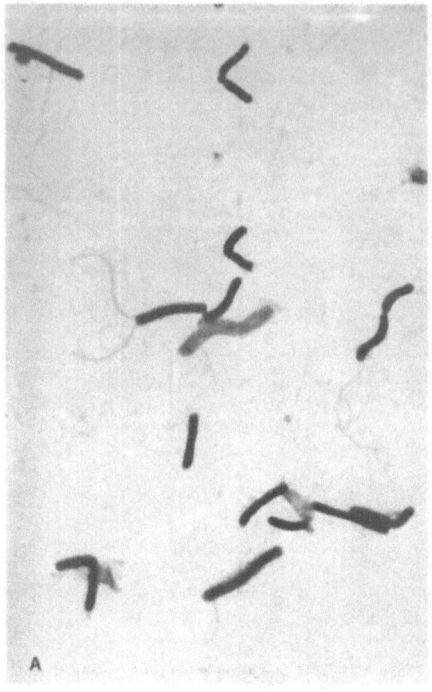
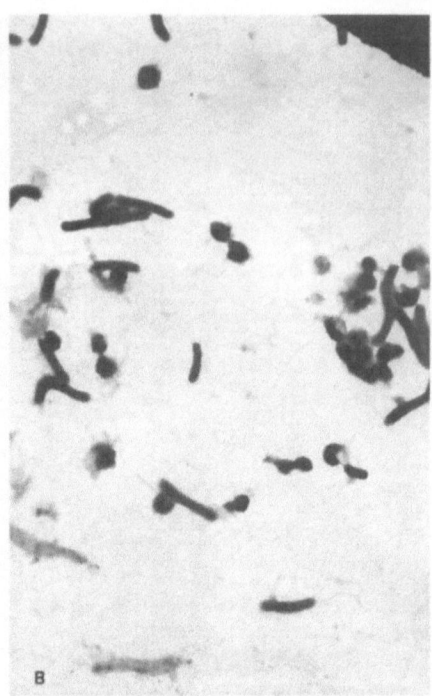
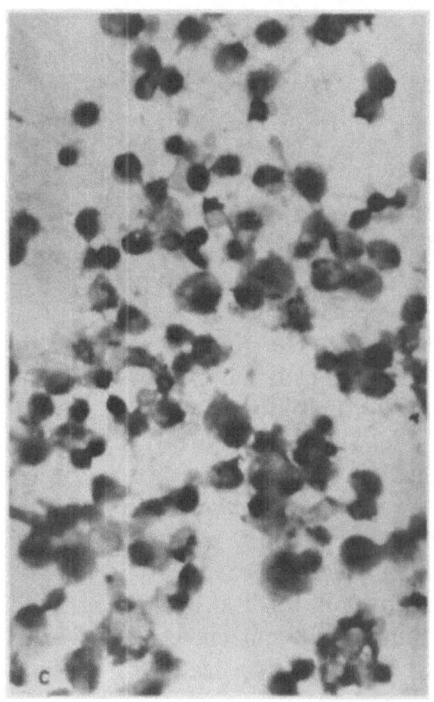

Fig. 3. Electron microscopy of *Campylobacter pylori* grown on agar (transfer technique (× 4000) **A** after 2 days' culture, **B** after 3 days' culture, **C** after 5 days' culture

Ultrastructure

The ultrastructure of *C. pylori* has been studied by Goodwin et al. [19] and Jones et al. [22]. The organisms are 0.5 – 1.0 μm wide and approximately 3 μm or greater long. In thin sections the cell wall has a double membrane. The external cell wall is smooth in contrast to the rugose surface of *C. jejuni*. A honeycomb-like thickening or submembranous complex is present beneath the cytoplasmic membrane on each side of the flagellar attachment site [19]. This was described by Jones as an electron-lucent zone [22]. The terminal region is different in shape from that of *C. jejuni* (dome-shaped versus conical-shaped).

In negatively stained preparations *C. pylori* shows one or multiple flagella (up to 5) at one pole. When the cell divides, a bipolar flagellation occurs. Occasionally some elements can be found without flagella. An ovoid terminal bulb is present at each flagellar extremity [19].

The flagella are sheathed, in contrast to that observed with other *Campylobacter* species [50], but similar to that of the genus *Vibrio* [12]. The flagellar sheath is approximately 15 nm wide. In sarcosinate-treated cell suspensions basal discs similar to those observed in other *Campylobacter* species have been seen. These basal discs are approximately 90 nm in diameter and have a central hole surrounded by a more densely stained inner annular zone. They are sensitive to trypsin treatment [22].

Other structures described as "doughnut" structures (12 nm in diameter) were present in large numbers and were probably associated with the cell surface [22]. These structures also exist in *Aquaspirillum serpens*.

Biochemical Characterization

Characterization in Biopsy Specimens

The major feature of *C. pylori* is the production of a strong urease [27]. This property is seldom found in *Campylobacter* species; *C. nitrofigilis*, an environmental bacterium, can harbour this enzyme [45] as well as the organisms described as urease-positive *Campylobacter* organisms (UPTC) [1]. UPTC isolates have been found in human faeces [46] but never in the stomach.

It was first noted in 1924 that a urease is present in gastric tissues of animals. The initial work here was carried out by Luck, who observed marked ammonia production in vitro in mixtures of gastric mucosa from dogs [33]. The enzyme responsible was found to have the same properties as soybean urease [34] and also to be present in vivo [35].

In 1936 Linderstrom-Land and Ohlsen studied the distribution of urease in the stomach [31]. They found that the urease activity varied extremely from stomach to stomach and was present in the pyloric and fundic regions. The enzyme was concentrated in the surface layers of the mucosa. Other authors have shown that not only dogs but also cats, rabbits, rats, pigs, and man harbour the enzyme in their stomach [11]. The first experimental results implying that urease was of bacterial origin were published in 1968 [7].

Since the discovery of Marshall [36] we can postulate that this unique feature of the stomach is indeed a property due to the presence of microorganisms. This is especially true for humans, where *C. pylori* is found in the stomach, and may be the case for pigs where Jones et al. have isolated a very closely related organism [21]. In dog stomach, a spiral organism different from *C. pylori* has been observed [62] but has yet to be cultured. It has urease activity like *C. pylori*.

The strong urease activity of *C. pylori* can easily be detected using a rapid diagnostic test [43]. The test consists of incubating a biopsy specimen in 0.5 ml of urease medium, such as Christensen medium, for 24 h at 37°C. It is possible to quantitate the magnitude of *C. pylori* colonization by taking readings after 1 h, 4 h, and 24 h. Presence of a large number of bacterial cells will lead to a colour change after 1 h. McNulty et al. found this test positive for 80 specimens (as opposed to 85 using Gram's stain) among 86 biopsies [44]. In general, its sensitivity is not as good as that of Gram's stain [4]. The specificity is excellent. However, if *Pseudomonas aeruginosa* (35% of which are urease producers) is present as a contaminant, a falsely positive reaction will most likely be observed.

A marketed preparation (CLO test, Delta West, Western Australia) is now available for detecting urease. A biopsy specimen is inserted into a small piece of agar and the preformed urease of *C. pylori* acts on the substrate, increasing the pH to produce a colour change from yellow to red-violet. This test was positive in 77% (1 h) and 96% (24 h) of the cases positive by culture in one study [49], and in 72% and 92%, respectively, in another study [2]. Its high sensitivity and specificity have subsequently been proven [38, 40]. Nevertheless, a controversy exists concerning its sensitivity compared to the conventional urease test. The CLO test has the advantage of being very easy to use by physicians in endoscopic wards.

The availability of such tests is very important for patient inclusion in clinical trials. However, a biopsy specimen is necessary, and the need for non-invasive tests has prompted some researchers to use ^{13}C-labelled urease as a substrate for urease activity [16].

After a test meal in which ^{13}C urea is administered orally, urea-derived $^{13}CO_2$ appears in the respiratory CO_2 of infected individuals at a constant rate for a period of more than 100 minutes. At the lowest level urease levels are two-fold higher than the highest level in a negative subject. The breath test seems reproducible and is not affected by meal consumption. The test has the advantage of not using radioactive material, ^{13}C being a stable, non-radioactive isotope; however, a gas-isotope ratio mass spectrometer must be available for measuring the urease levels. A test using ^{14}C urea has also been described.

Another possibility, described by Marshall and Langton [37], consists of measuring the gastric juice urea level. *C. pylori* positive patients have a urea level significantly lower than *C. pylori* negative patients (0.45 ± 0.05 mmol/l versus 2.9 ± 0.98 mmol/l in a series of 48 consecutive patients). This finding offers a simple diagnostic method for patients for whom a gastroscopy is contraindicated. It can be performed on vomitus or on samples from patients with nasogastric tubes in situ.

Characterization after Culture

This organism has been characterized by all the techniques used in modern bacteriology, including DNA studies, protein profile, gas-liquid chromatography, and enzymatic content.

DNA Studies

The DNA base composition of *C. pylori* NCTC 11637 (type strain) has been found to be 37.1 mol% guanosine plus cytosine [39]. Clinical isolates of *C. pylori* were also found to have a value similar to the other *Campylobacter* species (29–36 mol%) in another study [56].

Presently we have no knowledge concerning quantitative hybridization studies which would clarify the exact relationship between *C. pylori* and the other *Campylobacter* species. We have prepared a non-radioactive probe labelled with 2-acetylaminofluorene using whole *C. pylori* DNA [6]. This probe was used in a semiquantitative hybridization dot blot assay and did not hybridize with DNA from 16 *Campylobacter* species and subspecies.

The restriction endonuclease pattern of *C. pylori* DNA has been found to be an interesting tool for epidemiology. The serotyping schema is still at an early stage of development [29], and no other possibilities exist at the moment. By using a unique enzyme, Hind III, Langenberg et al. were able to distinguish between recrudescence and reinfection in relapses following apparently successful antibacterial treatment and were able to show the persistence in the stomach of the same *C. pylori* strains during a period of 2 years [26].

Recently in a study by Penfold et al. [51] *C. pylori* was found to possess plasmids; 13 of 27 isolates examined contained between two and six plasmids. They could not allocate any function to these plasmids.

Gas-Liquid Chromatography

Gas-liquid chromatography of fatty acids is an interesting tool for taxonomy and identification. Four fatty acids have been found to be common to all *Campylobacter* species: tetradecanoic acid (14:0), hexadecanoic acid (16:0), hexadecenoic acid (16:1), and octadecenoic acid (18:1) [24]. *C. pylori* can be characterized by the presence of a large amount of tetradecanoic acid (14:0), the absence of 3-hydroxytetradecanoic acid (3-OH-14:0), and the presence of *cis*-9,10-methylene octadecanoic acid (19:0 cyc) (Fig. 4). A large homogeneity has been found between the strains tested.

Thermoplasmaquinones are not present in *C. pylori* in contrast to all other known *Campylobacter* species [17].

Enzymatic Content

Urease. Probably the most interesting enzyme to study is *C. pylori* urease. We have studied its properties after culture with and without 1% urea (Babin and

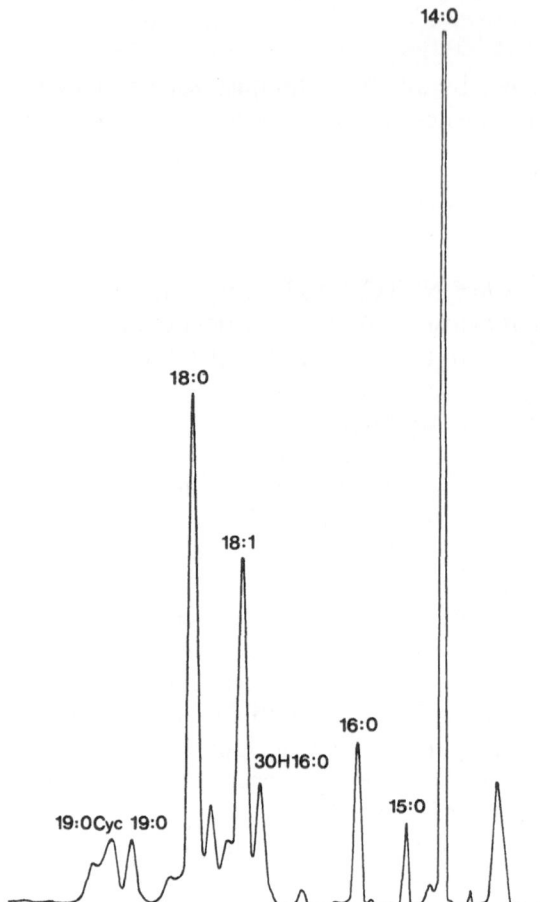

Fig. 4. Gas chromatogram of methylated fatty acids of *Campylobacter pylori* CIP 101260 analyzed on an Supelco SPB1 fused-silica capillary column (15 m by 0.53 mm. Temperature range 140° C to 220° C (increase of 4° C/min).

Megraud, unpublished observations). Using polyacrylamide gel electrophoresis (PAGE) without sodium dodecyl sulfate (SDS) treatment, its molecular weight was found to be 480000 daltons; and using SDS-PAGE, subunits were found to have a molecular weight of 30000 and multiples of 30000, with the major band at 120000 daltons.

The urease concentration was higher in urea-containing medium. The pH was 4.78 when measured by isoelectrofocusing, which is very close to the figure for jack bean urease.

The conventional methods for detecting urease, e.g. Christensen urea medium and urea-indole medium, can be used to detect *C. pylori* urease in culture for identification purposes. Urease-negative strains are seldom found but can occur after subculture [48].

Other Enzymes. On the oxidase and catalase tests *C. pylori* is positive. The extracellular catalase has a highly specific activity compared to its intracellular activity, suggesting a very efficient transport system. The catalase values are

Table 1. Important biochemical tests to identify *Campylobacter pylori*

Oxidase	+
Catalase	+
Urease	+
γ-Glutamyltransferase	+
Alkaline phosphatase	+
DNAse (toluidine blue medium)	+
Hippuricase	−
Indole production	−
H_2S production (TSI and FBP media)	−
Nitrate reductase	v

v: variable

Table 2. Enzymes found in 20 *C. pylori* strains [48]

Enzyme	Number of positive strains
Arylamidase of:	
L-Tyrosine	5
L-Pyrrodidonyl	6
L-Lysyl	14
L-Arginyl	14
L-Alanyl	2
N-Benzoyl-leucine[a]	20
S-Benzyl-cysteine[a]	20
DL-Methionine	17
Glycyl-phenylalanine	2
Glycyl-proline	14
L-Glutamine	13
α-L-Glutamate	2
L-Tryptophane	10
L-Alanyl-L-arginine	17
L-Alanyl-L-phenylalanyl-L-proline[a]	19
L-Argininyl-L-arginine	3
L-Phenylalanyl-L-arginine	4
L-Phenylalanine-proline[a]	20
L-Prolyl-L-arginine	3
L-Seryl-L-methionine	8
Esterase of:	
Butyrate (C_4)	20
Valerate (C_5)[a]	20
Caproate (C_6)[a]	20
Caprylate (C_8)[a]	20
Nonanoate (C_9)[a]	20
Caprate (C_{10})	20
Laurate (C_{12})[a]	19
Acid phosphatase[a]	20
Phosphoamidase[a]	20

[a] Strong activity

higher at pH 10.5 than at pH 7.0. Superoxide dismutase activity is also important in extracellular preparations [28].

The presence of a nitrate reductase is controversial. Generally this enzyme
is cited as being absent; however, Buck et al. found two positive strains among
19 [3], and our results confirm their findings. *C. pylori* contains neither hippuricase to hydrolyze hippuric acid nor tryptophanase to convert tryptophane to in-
dole. The metabolic pathway needed to produce H_2S in TSI medium, as well as
in sensitized FBP medium, is not present, but the blackening of a lead acetate
strip can be observed.

In addition to urease the most interesting enzymes for identification are
γ-glutamyltransferase and alkaline phosphatase. These two enzymes can be detected by using the kits available for blood analysis (Boehringer, Mannheim,
FRG). A colour change (from colourless to yellow) occurs in less than 2 h at
37 °C. These enzymes were found consistently in *C. pylori* strains. γ-glutamyltransferase has a narrow distribution among *Campylobacter* species. Only
C. jejuni biotype 2 and some strains of biotype 1 are positive [9]. Alkaline phosphatase is more widely distributed. Another enzyme, leucine aminopeptidase,
is also present in *C. pylori* but not in *C. jejuni* and, therefore, is of diagnostic
value [42]. DNAse activity can be detected on the toluidine blue agar described
by Lior and is present in all strains [30]. The main tests to be used for diagnosis
are shown in Table 1.

Other enzymes, arylamidases and esterases, have also been detected
(Table 2) [48].

We have developed a micromethod using API strips for the rapid identification of *Campylobacter* species [47]. The strip contains tests for nitrate reductase,
hippuricase, urease, γ-glutamyltranspeptidase, alkaline phosphatase, and five
arylamidases. It allows a good identification of *C. pylori*.

Comparison to Other Bacteria Isolated from the Stomach

Human

In some rare instances a *Campylobacter*-like organism different from *C. pylori*
can be isolated from human stomach specimens. The first strain described was
named GCLO-2 and is now known to be a variant of *C. jejuni* [18]. GCLO-2
can easily be differentiated by its weak catalase activity and positive hippurate
hydrolysis. Other *Campylobacter* strains from the mouth, such as *C. sputorum*
and *C. concisus*, can also be recovered.

Contaminants can grow on non-selective media. One example is
Pseudomonas aeruginosa, which led to the misinterpretation of early microscopic observations of Steer and Colins-Jones in 1975 [58].

Animal

The spiral bacteria observed in dog and cat stomach [62] are very different from *C. pylori*. They have never been grown in artificial media and, thus, we are limited to morphological findings.

More recently, an organism similar to *C. pylori* has been cultivated from ferret stomach [13]. Morphologically it also has several sheathed polar flagella, a dome-shaped extremity, and a regular cell wall. It is a strong urease producer but consistently possesses a nitrate reductase. In contrast to *C. pylori* it is sensitive to cephalothin and is resistant to nalidixic acid.

A very important step has been made with the discovery by Jones et al. [21] of organisms similar if not identical to *C. pylori* in the gastric mucosa of pigs and baboons. The epidemiology of *C. pylori* will be considerably stimulated by these findings.

These organisms have many properties in common with the classical *Campylobacter* species in terms of morphology and biochemical characteristics, as well as in culturing techniques. However, their unique features concerning flagellar arrangement, strong urease production, and ecological niche, raise the question of their classification in a new genus. Recently published studies of the ribosomal RNA cistrons have shown that *C. pylori* is probably the first of a new genus.

Acknowledgments

We acknowledge the help of M. T. Droy-Lefaix (Institut Beaufour, Paris, France) for the scanning electron microscopy photograph, M. Garnier (INRA, Bordeaux, France) for the transfer electron microscopy photograph, and M. Capdepuy (Université de Bordeaux 2, Bordeaux, France) for the gas-liquid chromatography.

References

1. Bolton FJ, Holt AV, Hutchinson DN (1985) Urease-positive thermophilic Campylobacters. Lancet i:1217–1218
2. Borromeo M, Lambert JR, Pinkard KJ (1987) Evaluation of "CLO-test" to detect *Campylobacter pyloridis* in gastric mucosa. J Clin Pathol 40:462–468
3. Buck GE, Gourley WK, Lee WK, Subramanyam K, Latimer JM, DiNuzzo AR (1986) Relation of *Campylobacter pyloridis* to gastritis and peptic ulcer. J Inf Dis 153:664–669
4. Burette A, Glupczynski Y, Jonas C, DeReuck M, Van Gossum M, Deprez C, Tielemans C, Deltenre M (1986) Signification de la présence du *Campylobacter pyloridis* dans l'antre gastrique. Résultats d'une étude prospective chez 212 patients. Acta Gastroent Belg 49:70–84
5. Caselli M, Trevisani P, Pazzi P, Stabellini G (1987) Diagnostic rapide de la présence d'organismes de type Campylobacter. Presse Med 16:966
6. Chevrier D, Larzul D, Mégraud F, Guesdon JL (1987) Non-radioactive DNA probe for identification of *Campylobacter species* (Abst 179). IV Int Workshop on Campylobacter infection, June 1987. Goteborg
7. Delluva AM, Markley K, Davies RE (1968) The absence of gastric urease in germ-free animals. Biochim Biophys Acta 151:646–650

8. Doenges JL (1939) Spirochetes in the gastric glands of Macacus Rhesus and of man without related disease. Arch Pathol 27:469–477

9. Elharrif Z, Mégraud F (1986) Characterization of thermophilic Campylobacters: II. Enzymatic profile. Curr Microbiol 13:317–322

10. Engstrand L, Pahlson C, Gustavsson S, Schwan A (1986) Monoclonal antibodies for rapid identification of Campylobacter pyloridis. Lancet ii:1402–1403

11. Fitzgerald O (1946) Urease in the gastric mucosa and its increase after a meat diet, soy bean flour diet or urogastrone injections. Nature 158:305

12. Follet EAC, Gordon J (1963) An electron microscopic study of vibrio flagella. J Gen Microbiol 32:235–239

13. Fox JG, Edrise BM, Cabot EB, Beaucoge C, Murphy JC, Prostack KS (1986) Campylobacter-like organisms isolated from gastric mucosa of ferrets. Am J Vet Res 47:236–239

14. Freedberg AS, Barron LE (1940) The presence of Spirochetes in human gastric mucosa. Am J Dig Dis 7:443–445

15. Fung WP, Papadimitrious JM, Matz LR (1979) Endoscopic, histological and ultrastructural correlations in chronic gastritis. Am J Gastroenterol 71:269–279

16. Graham DY, Klein PD, Evans DJ, Evans DG, Alpert LC, Opekun AR, Boutton TW (1987) Campylobacter pylori detected noninvasively by the ^{13}C-urea breath test. Lancet i:1174–1177

17. Goodwin CS, Collins MD, Blincow E (1986) The absence of thermoplasma quinones in Campylobacter pyloridis and its temperature and pH growth range. Microbios Letters 32:137–140

18. Goodwin CS, Blincow E, Armstrong J, McCulloch R (1985) Campylobacter pyloridis is unique: GCLO-2 is an ordinary Campylobacter. Lancet II:38–39

19. Goodwin CS, McCulloch RK, Armstrong JA, Wee SH (1985) Unusual cellular fatty acids and distinctive ultrastructure in a new spiral bacterium (Campylobacter pyloridis). J Med Microbiol 19:257–267

20. Hazell SL, Lee A, Brady L, Hennessy W (1986) Campylobacter pyloridis and gastritis: association with intercellular spaces and adaptation to an environment of mucus as important factors in colonization of the gastric epithelium. J Inf Dis 153:658–663

21. Jones DM, Eldridge J (1987) Gastric Campylobacter-like organisms (GCLO) from man ("C. pyloridis") compared with GCLO strains from the pig, baboon and ferret (Abst 72). IV Int Workshop on Campylobacter infection, June 1987. Goteborg

22. Jones DM, Curry A, Fox AJ (1985) An ultrastructural study of the gastric Campylobacter-like organism "Campylobacter pyloridis". J Gen Microbiol 131:2335–2341

23. Krienitz W (1906) Über das Auftreten von Spirochäten verschiedener Form im Mageninhalt bei Carcinoma ventriculi. Deutsch Medizin Woch 28:872

24. Lambert MA, Patton CM, Barret TJ, Moss CW (1987) Differentiation of Campylobacter and Campylobacter-like organisms by cellular fatty acid composition. J Clin Microbiol 25:706–713

25. Lamouliatte H, Mégraud F, De Mascarel A, Roux D, Quinton A (1987) Campylobacter pyloridis and epigastric pain: endoscopic, histological, and bacteriological correlations. Gastroenterol Clin Biol 11:212–216

26. Langenberg W, Rauws EAJ, Widjojokusumo A, Tytgat GNJ, Zanen HC (1986) Identification of Campylobacter pyloridis isolates by restriction endonuclease DNA analysis. J Clin Microbiol 24:414–417

27. Langenberg ML, Tytgat GNJ, Schipper ME, Rietra PJG, Zanen HC (1984) Campylobacter-like organisms in the stomach of patients and healthy individuals. Lancet I:1348

28. Lior H, Johnson WM (1985) Catalase, peroxidase and superoxide dismutase activities in Campylobacter spp. In: Pearson AD, Skirrow MB, Lior H, Rowe B (eds) Campylobacter III, PHLS, London, pp 226–227

29. Lior H, Pearson AD, Woodward DL, Hawtin P (1985) Biochemical and serological characteristics of Campylobacter pyloridis. In: Pearson AD, Skirrow MB, Lior H, Rowe B (eds) Campylobacter III, PHLS, London, pp 196–197

30. Lior H, Patel A (1987) Improved Toluidine blue-DNA agar for detection of DNA hydrolysis by campylobacters. J Clin Microbiol 25:2030—2031

30a. Lior H, Patel A, Larose M, Winter WP, Lammerding AM, Woodward DL (1985) Evaluation of media for testing DNA hydrolysis by Campylobacters. In: Pearson AD, Skirrow MB, Lior H, Rowe B (eds) Campylobacter III, PHLS, London, pp 225—226

31. Linderstrom-Lang K, Ohlsen AS (1936) Distribution of urease in dog stomach (XX. Studies on enzymatic histochemistry). Enzymologia 1:92—95

32. Lopez-Brea M, Pajares JM, Blanco M, Jimenez ML (1987) Ethidium bromide stain to identify *Campylobacter pyloridis* in gastric biopsies (Abst 98). IV Int Workshop on Campylobacter infection, June 1987. Goteborg

33. Luck JM (1924) Ammonia production by animal tissues in vitro. I. The use of mixed tissue extracts. Biochem J 18:814—825

34. Luck JM, Seth TN (1924) Gastric urease. Biochem J 18:1227—1231

35. Luck JM, Seth TN (1925) The physiology of gastric urease. Biochem J 19:357—365

36. Marshall BJ (1983) Unidentified curved bacilli on gastric epithelium in active chronic gastritis. Lancet i:1273—1275

37. Marshall BJ, Langton SR (1986) Urea hydrolysis in patients with *Campylobacter pyloridis* infection. Lancet I:965—966

38. Marshall BJ, Francis GJ, Langton SR, Warren JR, Goodwin CS, Blincow ED (1986) CLO test. A rapid urease test for the detection of *Campylobacter pyloridis* infection in gastric mucosal biopsies (abst). Dig Dis Sci 31:152S

39. Marshall BJ, Royce H, Annear DI, Goodwin CS, Pearman JW, Warren JR, Armstrong JA (1984) Original isolation of *Campylobacter pyloridis* from human gastric mucosa. Microbios Letters 25:83—88

40. McCarthy PG, Kronborg NL, Dudley FJ, Davidson W, Spicer WJ, McLean AJ (1986) A rapid enzyme based, screening test for the presence of *Campylobacter pyloridis* in endoscopic antral biopsies (abst). Aust NZ J Med 16:608

41. McMullen L, Walker MM, Bain LA, Karim QN, Baron JH (1987) Histological identification of Campylobacter using Gimenez technique in gastric antral mucosa. J Clin Pathol 40:464—465

42. McNulty CAM, Dent JC (1986) Characterisation of *Campylobacter pyloridis* (Abst B8-4). XIV Int Congress of Microbiol, Sept 1986. Manchester

43. McNulty CAM, Wise R (1985) Rapid diagnosis of Campylobacter-associated gastritis. Lancet i:1443—1444

44. McNulty CAM, Gearty JC, Crump B, Davis M, Donovan IA, Melikian V, Lister DM, Wise R (1986) *Campylobacter pyloridis* and associated gastritis: investigator blind, placebo controlled trial of bismuth salicylate and erythromycin ethyl-succinate. Brit Med J 293:645—649

45. McClung CR, Patriquin DG, Davis RE (1983) *Campylobacter nitrofigilis* sp. nov. a nitrogen-fixing bacterium associated with roots of *Spartina alterniflora* Loisel. Int J Syst Bacteriol 33:605—612

46. Mégraud F, Chevrier D, Desplaces N, Sedallian A, Guesdon JL (1988) Urease positive thermophilic campylobacter (*Campylobacter laridis* variant) isolated from appendix and from humen feces. J Clin Microbiol 26:(in press)

47. Mégraud F, Belbouri A, Monget D, Gayral JP (1987) A micromethod to identify *Campylobacter* species. Preliminary results (Abst 197). IV Int Workshop on Campylobacter infection, June 1987. Goteborg

48. Mégraud F, Bonnet F, Garnier M, Lamouliatte H (1985) Characterization of *"Campylobacter pyloridis"* by culture, enzymatic profile and protein content. J Clin Microbiol 22:1007—1010

49. Morris A, McIntyre D, Rose T, Nicholson G (1986) Rapid diagnosis of *Campylobacter pyloridis* infection. Lancet i:149

50. Pead PJ (1979) Electron microscopy of *Campylobacter jejuni*. J Med Microbiol 12:383—385

51. Penfold SS, Lastovica AJ, Elisha BG (1987) Demonstration of plasmids in *Campylobacter pyloridis* (Abst 126), IV Int Workshop on Campylobacter infection, June 1987. Goteborg

52. Philipps AD, Hine KR, Holmes GKT, Woodings DF (1984) Gastric spiral bacteria. Lancet ii:100–101
53. Pinkard KJ, Harrison B, Capstick JA, Medley G, Lambert JR (1986) Detection of *Campylobacter pyloridis* in gastric mucosa by phase contrast microscopy. J Clin Pathol 39:112–113
54. Price AB, Levi J, Dolby JM, Dunscombe PL, Smith A, Clark J, Stephenson ML (1985) *Campylobacter pyloridis* in peptic ulcer disease: microbiology, pathology, and scanning electron microscopy. Gut 26:1183–1188
55. Roumaniuk PJ, Zoltowsak B, Trust T, Lane DJ, Olsen GJ, Pace NR, Stahl DA (1987) *Campylobacter pylori*, the spiral bacterium associated with human gastritis, is not a true *Campylobacter* sp. J Bacteriol 169:2137–2141
56. Smith JS, Buck GE, Niesel D (1986) Genetic relationship of *Campylobacter pyloridis* to other species of Campylobacter. D169. Abstracts Annual Meeting Am Soc for Microbiol, March 1986. Washington
57. Steer HW (1984) Surface morphology of the gastroduodenal mucosa in duodenal ulceration. Gut 25:1203–1210
58. Steer HW, Colin-Jones DG (1975) Mucosal changes in gastric ulceration and their response to carbenoxolone sodium. Gut 16:590–597
59. Steer HW, Newell DG (1985) Immunological identification of *Campylobacter pyloridis* in gastric biopsy tissue. Lancet ii:38
60. Walters LL, Budin RE, Paull G (1986) Acridine-orange to identify *Campylobacter pyloridis* in formalin fixed, paraffin-embedded gastric biopsies. Lancet i:42
61. Warren J (1983) Unidentified curved bacilli on gastric epithelium in active chronic gastritis. Lancet i:1273
62. Weber AF, Schmittdiel EF (1962) Electron microscopic and bacteriological studies of Spirilla isolated from the fundic stomachs of cats and dogs. Am J Vet Res 23:422–427

Discussion

von Wulffen: I have a question concerning the testing of the enzymes. You showed test strips; do you simply test these as preformed enzymes as with the urease test? Or do you incubate these strips in a microaerophilic atmosphere?

Mégraud: In fact we tested the preformed enzymes. The test was designed for the identification of all *Campylobacter* species and to be read at one time. This is the reason why we do not read it after 4 h which could be possible. The reading is done on the next day. We incubate at 37°C in air, but not in a microaerobic atmosphere. It could be read before, because these are preformed enzymes. For example, urease activity is usually positive after 5 min. But it is easier to read all the tests at the same time. For the growth tests the incubation is made in a microaerobic athmosphere.

Ober: Could you speculate on the reversibility of the shape changes. Is the spiral form transformed into cocci and cocci into spiral forms as the living conditions improve or worsen. I assume that this shape change is the main reason why the natural source for *Campylobacter pylori* has not yet been found.

Mégraud: I think this is a very important question. It is debated as to whether the coccoidal forms are still viable or are dead organisms. Some people think that they are not dead and are able to yield spiral forms if given good conditions. For example, not for *C. pylori* but for other *Campylobacter* species there was a study performed in the United States showing that coccoidal forms are still viable. I saw a picture by Dr. Jones showing a coccoidal form dividing. So there is some evidence that the coccoidal form is perhaps not degenerated, but can grow in some conditions. This was also shown a long time ago with *Aquaspirillum*. I think it is an open question.

Deltenre: You have told us Gram's staining was superior to the urease test in your experience. May I know your figures in percentage of sensitivity for both tests, and whether you used Gram's staining on biopsy or on cytology brush specimens.

Mégraud: In terms of sensitivity Gram's stain was about 90% and the corresponding feature for urease test after 24 h was 80%. But it depends upon how the test is done. Probably we used too much broth. If the test is performed with a few drops, the chance of obtaining a quicker result is better. Concerning the way we do Gram's staining, we just take the biopsy to make smears with it. As I told you, the problem with Gram's stain arises when there are very few organisms and when they do not have the typical shape. In these cases, it is difficult to conclude. But we can be helped in this field if we use monoclonal antibodies made by some of the contributors to this symposium.

O'Moráin: You mentioned that contamination with other *Campylobacter* may give you a falsely positive test. In your experience have you found this?

Mégraud: I had once isolated $GCLO_2$, as have some other researchers, the first being in Germany (Kasper and Dickissier). I know from the literature that Dr. Goodwin mentioned once the isolates *C. sputorum* in a biopsy. And I am aware that in the culture collection of Göteborg there are some *Campylobacter concisus* which were isolated from the gastric mucosa of humans.

Tytgat: I heard that some researchers in Ulm had the impression that the bacteria which they cultured from the bulb were somewhat different morphologically from those seen in the antrum. They were shorter and smaller. Have you any information in this regard?

Mégraud: I have no experience with this problem. We had some isolates from the bulb, but they did not look different from the others. So I think we should look carefully now. But I cannot give a response.

Protein Antigens of *Campylobacter pylori:* The Problem of Species Specificity

M. Kist, I. Apel, and E. Jacobs

Introduction

Since *Campylobacter pylori (C. pylori)* was first isolated and identified from gastric biopsies by Marshall [6], data have accumulated which indicate a strong association of *C. pylori* with gastritis and peptic ulcer disease [14]. Despite this fact the natural course of infection, the pathomechanisms, and the occurrence in the total population remain largely unclear.

Serological methods specific and sensitive enough to monitor a disease-related immune response could be helpful in answering such questions. In various studies significant antibody levels in patients' sera against *C. pylori* were demonstrated using various serological methods, such as the complement fixation test [2, 8, 17], passive hemagglutination [7], the enzyme-linked immunosorbent assay [1–4, 10, 12], and the Western immunoblotting technique [17]. Until now nearly all serologic investigations were done with whole-cell sonicates or rather crude antigenic preparations, i.e. acid extractions, which were not well defined and were therefore hampered, to a certain degree, by antigenic cross-reactions and a loss of specificity. Such problems could be overcome if species-specific and disease-related antigens exist and can be obtained as well-defined antigenic preparations.

The predominant aims of the present study were to analyze the protein profiles of *C. pylori* strains freshly isolated from acutely ill patients, to identify overlapping cross-reactivity between different species, to evaluate the immunological potency of protein bands of interest, and to search for species-specific, immunologically relevant microbial antigens.

Material and Methods

Origin of Strains and Sera. Patients who underwent gastroscopy in five centers involved in an epidemiological study, were selected randomly for the serological investigation. Of these, 63 had cultural proof of *C. pylori* infection, 31 were negative. Blood samples were drawn before gastroscopy and sera were stored at −20°C. Sera samples of patients with *Campylobacter* infections other than *C. pylori* were from the second to third week after onset of symptoms. *C. pylori* were grown from biopsies on yeast extract-cystein-blood agar (YCB agar) supplemented with vancomycin (3 mg/l) and nystatin (50000 I.U./l) in a microaerophilic atmosphere and stored in skim milk at −70 °C.

Preparation of Protein Samples. C. pylori was grown on YCB agar without antimicrobial agents and harvested in 1 ml PBS. After washing with PBS, bacteria were sonicated for 10 s, redissolved in 1 ml of protein sample buffer, and boiled for 5 min. For some experiments bacteria were pretreated for 30 min with 10 µg/ml trypsin at 37 °C.

SDS-PAGE and Immunoblotting Technique. Protein profiles of the strains (25 µg protein samples/lane) were studied by SDS-polyacrylamide gel electrophoresis (PAGE) using a 12% separating slab gel. The protein bands were then transferred to nitrocellulose by the Western blotting technique [16]. After incubation for 2 h in 10% skim milk to saturate nonspecific binding sites, the nitrocellulose strips were overlaid with patients' sera, diluted 1:100. After washing with PBS 0.05% Tween 20 the blots were incubated with rabbit antihuman Ig class specific antisera for detection of IgG, IgA, and IgM antibodies. Using swine antirabbit immunoglobulin as an amplifying system, the antigen-antibody complexes were finally stained with the peroxidase-antiperoxidase technique [15].

Detection of Cross-Reacting Antigens. Cross-reactions were examined by crossover-immunoblotting experiments of the various *Campylobacter* species with sera of patients with *C. coli, C. jejuni,* and *C. fetus* ssp. *fetus* infections.

Localization of Antigens. To differentiate between surface-exposed and cytoplasmatic *C. pylori* antigens, mild digestion with trypsin (10 µg/ml for 30 min at 37 °C) and absorption experiments with washed *C. pylori* (30 min at 37 °C; 30 min at 4 °C) were carried out. Both the trypsinized strain and the absorbed sera were examined by immunoblotting.

Results

After separation on SDS-PAGE all *C. pylori* strains tested exhibited similar protein patterns when stained with Coomassie blue. The protein profiles consisted predominantly of seven major bands with molecular weights of 88, 62, 59, 56, 45, 29, and 25 kDa (Fig. 1). Proteins banding in the 62-kDa, 29-kDa, or 25-kDa regions were detected almost constantly in all strains examined, while other major proteins (88 kDa, 59 kDa, 45 kDa) showed remarkable strain-dependent variations. Interestingly, a 120-kDa protein which elicited a strong antibody response in infected patients (Fig. 2) stained only very weakly with Coomassie blue.

To investigate the immune response of patients infected with *C. pylori* 63 sera were tested for IgG, IgA, and IgM antibody-recognizing *C. pylori* pro-

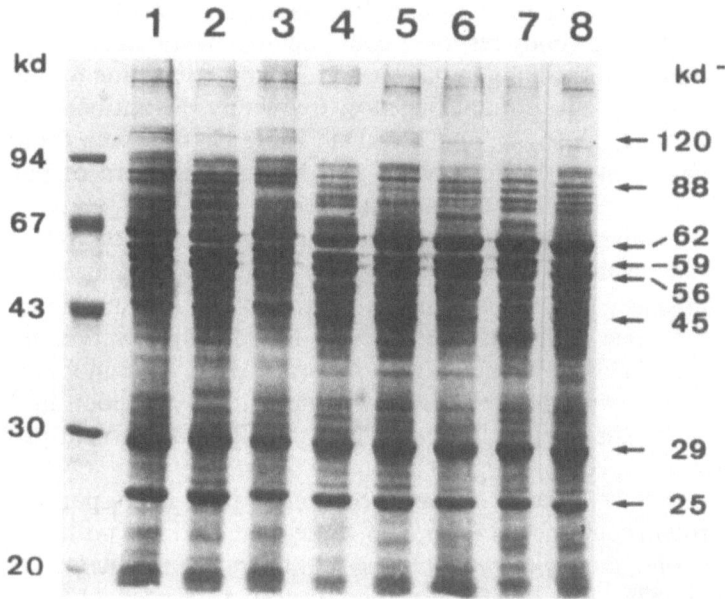

Fig. 1. Protein profiles of *C. pylori* strains, isolated from different patients, and analyzed by SDS-PAGE. *Lanes 1–8:* CP 123, CP 124, CP 128, CP 132, CP 133, CP 138, CP 139, CP 141. *Arrows* indicate major protein bands

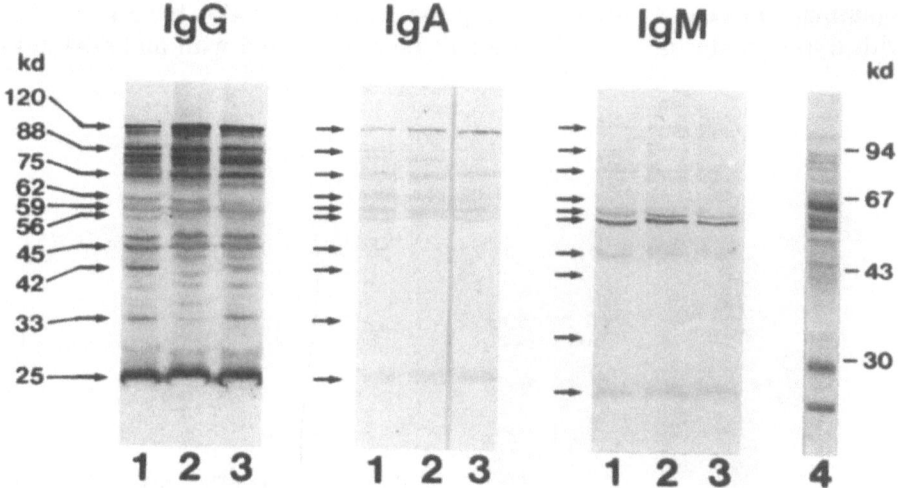

Fig. 2. Immunoblots of a patient's serum (S 141) for the presence of IgG, IgA, and IgM antibodies with the corresponding *C. pylori* strain (CP 141, *lane 1*), and with two other *C. pylori* strains (CP 123, *lane 2;* CP 149, *lane 3*). *Lane 4,* Amido black 10 B stain of *C. pylori* 141. *Arrows* indicate major antigens

teins. Applying the immunoblot technique, a prominent IgG and a minor IgA and IgM antibody response could be demonstrated (Fig. 2). Strain-specific differences in the antigen pattern were found, according to the variations detected in the protein profiles, but most frequently the antibodies recognized proteins of 75, 62, 59, 56, 45, and 120 kDa (Table 1). To search for species-specific antigens *C. pylori* proteins were also blotted with sera of patients infected with *C. jejuni, C. coli,* or *C. fetus* ssp. *fetus.*

While most of the major antigens showed marked cross-reactions with other *Campylobacter* species – probably indicating common *Campylobacter* group antigens – the 120-kDa protein and also 88-, 42-, and 33-kDa proteins did not cross-react with any control serum tested. Furthermore, anti-120-kDa positive sera of patients infected with *C. pylori* when immunoblotted with proteins of other *Campylobacter* spp. showed no antibody reaction in the 120-kDa region. These data support the view that the 120-kDa protein probably represents a species-specific, antigenic region of *C. pylori.*

In 82% of positive sera tested, an IgG immune response against the 120-kDa protein could be demonstrated while other antigens without detectable cross-reactions, namely the 88-, 42- and 33-kDa proteins, elicited antibody responses in only 57%, 49%, and 28% of the sera tested, respectively. Anti-120-kDa specific IgA antibodies were detected in 73%, and IgM response in 47% of the patients' sera tested. In the remaining 18% of the sera, without IgG antibodies against the 120-kDa protein, the corresponding strains could also be shown to lack this particular antigen when blotted with anti-120-kDa positive patients' sera (Fig. 3).

To determine whether the 120-kDa antigen is cell surface exposed or a cytoplasmatic protein, *C. pylori* strains possessing the 120-kDa band were treated with trypsin under mild conditions and immunoblotted with an anti-120-kDa

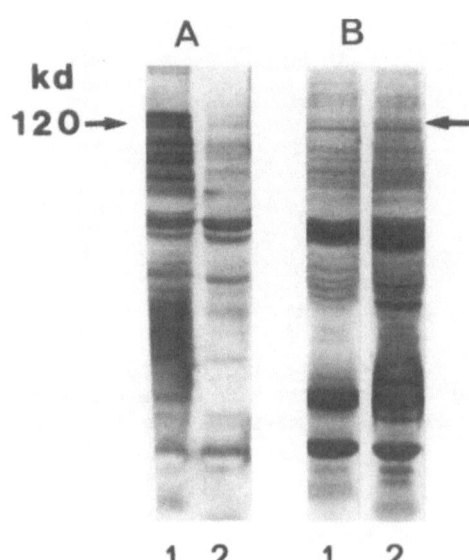

Fig. 3 a,b. Immunoblot of *C. pylori* strains possessing or lacking the 120-kDa antigen with sera and with or without the corresponding antibody. **A** serum S 151 (120 kDa+) blotted with *C. pylori* CP 149, possessing the 120-kDa antigen (*lane 1*), and with CP 132 (*lane 2*), lacking this protein. **B** serum S 132 (120 kDa−) blotted with CP 149 (*lane 1*) and with the corresponding strain CP 132 (*lane 2*)

Table 1. Distribution of the major *C. pylori* antigens detected by immunoblotting with sera of 61 patients with *C. pylori* infection and with control sera of patients infected with other *Campylobacter* species

Origin	n	Ig class	Molecular weights (kDa)							
			120	88	75	62	59	56	42	33
Patients[a] infected with *C. pylori*	63	IgG	52 (82)[b]	36 (57)	38 (60)	57 (90)	60 (95)	61 (96)	31 (49)	18 (28)
		IgA	46 (73)	16 (25)	45 (71)	42 (66)	53 (84)	58 (92)	9 (14)	7 (11)
		IgM	30 (47)	24 (38)	49 (77)	18 (28)	40 (63)	62 (98)	5 (7)	1 (1)
Patients with *C. jejuni*	2	IgG	–	–	2	2	2	2	–	–
Patients with *C. coli*	2	IgG	–	–	2	2	2	2	–	–
Patients with *C. fetus fetus*	1	IgG	–	–	1	1	1	1	–	–

[a] Patients who underwent gastroscopy; [b] Percentage of sera tested

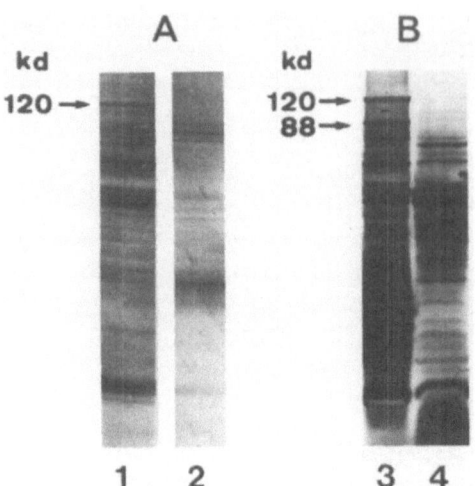

Fig. 4. A Absorption experiment of serum S 107 with the corresponding *C. pylori* strain CP 107. *Lane 1,* Immunoblot before absorption; *lane 2,* antibody pattern after 1 h absorption with washed CP 107 cells. **B** Enzymatic splitting of surface proteins of *C. pylori* CP 149 with trypsin (10 mg/ml). Immunoblot with serum S 151 before (*lane 1*) and after (*lane 2*) trypsinization of CP 149

positive serum before and after trypsinization (Fig. 4). Furthermore, an anti-120-kDa positive serum was absorbed with a suspension of a *C. pylori* strain possessing the antigen and then immunoblotted with the 120-kDa positive strain before and after the absorption experiment. In both cases after trypsinization as well as after absorption, the 120-kDa band was removed from the strain or the serum, respectively (Fig. 4). According to these preliminary results it can be concluded that the 120-kDa antigen probably is cell surface exposed and easily removable by trypsin digestion.

Discussion

A species-specific, disease-related serological assay would be helpful for the diagnosis of *C. pylori* infections. Furthermore it could be used to monitor the natural course of infection or to control success of therapy. The specificity of such an assay could be markedly hampered by antigens cross-reacting with other microorganisms, i.e. *Campylobacter* species, as seen by Goodwin et al. [1] applying the ELISA technique before and after absorption of *C. pylori* antisera with other *Campylobacter* spp. Also when the Western immunoblot method was applied, serological cross-reactions between *C. pylori* and other *Campylobacter* species especially for flagellar proteins of about 62 kDa were observed, as published by Lee et al. [5], Newell [10], and Perez-Perez and Blaser [12].

    In the present study we have also been able to identify antigens, especially in the regions of 75, 62, 59, and 56 kDa, which cross-react with various *Campylobacter* species. Furthermore, it was possible in our study to demonstrate, besides other proteins, an 120-kDa *C. pylori* antigen without cross-reactions with control sera. This 120-kDa region could be of interest because Wulffen et al. [17] have also shown that most of the sera of *C. pylori* patients tested exhibited antibody reactions with a comparable protein. But in contrast to our study, in which an IgM response to this antigen was demonstrated, these authors found IgM antibodies exclusively against a 60-kDa region.

Interestingly enough, other authors have not described the 120-kDa protein band when *C. pylori* strains were analyzed exclusively by SDS-PAGE [9, 11]. This may be due to the fact that the 120-kDa protein itself stained only very weakly with Coomassie-blue and may be easily detectable only when immunoblotted with antisera. One could therefore speculate whether this protein is predominantly a soluble, easily shedded antigen, eliciting a high antibody response, rather than a structural protein of importance. This possibility is underlined by the results of the preliminary attempts to localize the protein, where the 120-kDa protein was found to be probably surface-exposed and easily removable by mild trypsinization.

The fact that the 120-kDa protein was not found in 11 of 63 *C. pylori* isolates raises the question as to whether this is a strain or a host-dependent phenomenon. The first possibility is more probable because patients infected with such a strain did not develop an immune response against a protein of this molecular weight region. This finding indicates that the 120-kDa negative strains did not lose this structure during subculture in vitro. Further studies will have to clarify whether such strains also differ in other phenotypic characteristics or possibly in their pathogenic capacity.

The species specificity of the 120-kDa protein has not been definitively proven in our study. Despite the fact that no cross-reaction with other *Campylobacter* species antisera was found, cross-reactions with other bacteria species are not excluded. Furthermore the disease-related specificity has to be proven by testing larger, healthy population groups. Nevertheless, the 120-kDa protein is a promising candidate to be included in a set of specific antigens for serodiagnosis or therapy control of *C. pylori* infection.

Conclusion

A probably species-specific 120-kDa antigen, without detectable serological cross-reactivity with immune sera against other *Campylobacter* spp., was demonstrated in 82% of 63 sera of patients with *C. pylori* infection. This antigen obviously elicited an immune response of IgG, IgA, and IgM antibodies in infected patients when investigated with the immunoblotting technique. The corresponding *C. pylori* strains which were isolated from patients without antibodies against the 120-kDa proteins were shown not to possess this protein band. Preliminary experiments indicated the 120-kDa proteins to be probably cell surface exposed.

References

1. Goodwin CS, Blincow E, Peterson G, Sanderson C, Cheng W, Marshall B, Warren JR, McCulloch R (1987) Enzyme-linked immunosorbent assay for Campylobacter pyloridis: Correlation with presence of C. pyloridis in the gastric mucosa. J Inf Dis 155:488–494
2. Jones DM, Lessells AM, Eldridge J (1984) Campylobacter-like organisms on the gastric mucosa: Culture, histological and serological studies. J Clin Pathol 37:1002–1006
3. Jones DM, Eldridge J, Fox AJ, Sethi P, Whorwell PJ (1986) Antibody to the gastric campylobacter-like organism ("Campylobacter pyloridis"). Clinical correlations and distribution in the normal population. J Med Microbiol 22:57–62
4. Kaldor J, Tee W, McCarthy P, Watson J, Dwyer B (1985) Immune response to campylobacter pyloridis in patients with peptic ulceration. Lancet 1:921
5. Lee A, Logan SM, Trust TJ (1987) Demonstration of a flagellar antigen shared by a diverse group of spiral-shaped bacteria that colonize intestinal mucus. Infect Immun 55:828–831
6. Marshall B (1983) Unidentified curved bacilli on gastric epithelium in active chronic gastritis. Lancet 1:1273–1275
7. Marshall BJ, McGeckie DB, Francis GJ, Utley PJ (1984) Pyloric campylobacter serology. Lancet 2:281
8. McNulty CAM, Crump B, Gearty J, Lister DM, Davies M, Donovan IA, Melikian V, Wise R (1985) The distribution of and serological response to Campylobacter pyloridis in the stomach and duodenum. In: Campylobacter III: Proceedings of the Third International Workshop on Campylobacter infections. Public Health Laboratory Service, London, pp 174–175
9. Megraud F, Bonnet F, Garnier M, Lamouliatte H (1985) Characterization of "Campylobacter pyloridis" by culture, enzymatic profile, and protein content. J Clin Microbiol 22:1007–1010
10. Newell DG (1987) Identification of the outer membrane proteins of campylobacter pyloridis and antigenic cross-reactivity between C. pyloris and C. jejuni. J Gen Microbiol 133:163–170
11. Pearson AD, Bamforth J, Booth L, Holdstock G, Ireland A, Walker C, Hawtin P, Millward-Sadler H (1984) Polyacrylamide gel electrophoresis of spiral bacteria from the gastric antrum. Lancet 1:1349–1350
12. Perez-Perez GI, Blaser MJ (1987) Conservation and diversity of campylobacter pyloridis major antigens. Infect Immun 55:1256–1263
13. Rathbone BJ, Wyatt J, Worsley BW, Trejdosiewicz LK, Heatley RV, Losowsky MS (1985) Immune response to campylobacter pyloridis. Lancet 1:1217
14. Rathbone BJ, Wyatt JI, Heatly RV (1986) Campylobacter pyloridis – a new factor in peptic ulcer disease? Gut 27:635–641
15. Sternberger LA, Hardy PH, Cuculi JJ, Meyer HC (1970) The unlabeled antibody enzyme methods of immunohistochemistry. J Histochem Cytochem 18:315–333
16. Towbin H, Staehlin T, Gordon J (1979) Electrophoretic transfer of proteins from polyacrylamide gels to nitrocellulose sheets. Procedure and some applications. Proc Natl Acad Sci USA 76:4350–4354
17. Wulffen v H, Heesemann J, Bützow GH, Löning T, Laufs R (1986) Detection of Campylobacter pyloridis in patients with antrum gastritis and peptic ulcers by culture, complement fixation test and immunoblot. J Clin Microbiol 24:716–720

Discussion

Goodwin: Did you study sera after treatment and discover whether any bands disappeared?

Kist: We have not until now. We tested in this study only sera which were drawn immediately before gastroscopy and in the slides shown you could not see sera from follow-up or controls after therapy or after certain time periods after the first sera were drawn. But now we have drawn more sera from patients after some weeks or months since the first drawing of serum, but these have not yet been investigated.

von Wulffen: I would like to confirm this finding reported by Professor Kist; we have found the same thing. I have calculated a molecular weight of 110 kDa for the 120 kDa bands that Professor Kist described, but there are problems, as Dr. Pearson told us, in determining molecular weights in gels; so I think it is the same band. We also observed these strain differences, and, interestingly, I have one strain that is urease-negative and is apparently missing this 120-kDa band, but otherwise shows the same bands on the immunoblots with sera from patients who normally react with the 120-kDa band. We also found other strains that apparently lack the 120-kDa protein, but these were all urease-positive, so I cannot speculate that the lack of the 120-kDa protein is associated with urease-deficient *C. pylori* strains.

Kist: We saw 11 strains which were negative for this 120-kDa band, and we tested all these for urease: all were urease-positive. But we have not until now investigated these strains in DNA restriction tests or in broad panel enzyme tests.

Wyatt: May I ask whether there are any clinical or histological differences between the patients who have the 120-kDa protein positive strains of bacteria and those with the negative strains?

Kist: You ask for histopathological differences between patients with this 120-kDa band and other patients. We have not evaluated this question until now, but all the relevant data are on computer file, and we hope to get results in the near future.

O'Moráin: You mentioned that approximately 20% of students and children reacted with this 120-kDa protein. What do you think causes this cross-reaction?

Kist: It may be rather an immunoreaction than a cross-reaction, I think. We found this antigen in 23% of patients who underwent gastroscopy but in only 16% of students and 11% of children. This may indicate an increase in immunity in the population against this antigen with increasing age or an infection with the strain. On the other hand I think it is a very interesting point that we found this 120-kDa protein in about 80% of patients, because if you look at the latest publication of Dr. Goodwin about his ELISA test, he found that the specificity of the test was 81%, and I think one can speculate as to whether this may be due to the presence of this specific antigen.

Differences Between in Vitro and in Vivo Sensitivity of *Campylobacter pylori* to Antibacterials

C. S. GOODWIN, J. A. ARMSTRONG, and D. H. WILSON

The spiral bacteria isolated from the gastric mucosa in 1982 in Western Australia were originally called *Campylobacter pyloridis* [15] but this specific epithet was technically inappropriate, and the name has since been revised to *C. pylori* [12].

In Vitro Sensitivity of *C. pylori* to Antibiotics

Studies of the susceptibility of *C. pylori* to antibiotics have shown that it is higly sensitive to most antibiotics, except vancomycin, trimethoprim and sulphonamides [4, 7, 10, 16]. In a Canadian study 20 isolates were found to be sensitive to nalidixic acid 48 mg/L but resistant to 40 mg/L [18]. For two of 20 isolates in Western Australia the MIC of colistin was less than 5 mg/L [7]. About 20% of 100 isolates were resistant to metronidazole and tinidazole [8].

Failure of Single-Drug Therapies to Eliminate *C. pylori* from the Gastric Mucosa

Ofloxacin and erythromycin as single therapy failed to eliminate *C. pylori* from the gastric mucosa [5, 17], and in four of the five patients treated with ofloxacin *C. pylori* became resistant to this drug and to other quinolones. When metronidazole was given as sole antibacterial therapy, 70% of isolates became resistant, and in only 3% of patients was *C. pylori* eliminated [8]. Among eight patients given amoxycillin, *C. pylori* was eliminated from five, but among the others bacterial colonization returned [11]. However colloidal bismuth subcitrate (CBS) as single therapy had a moderate rate of elimination of *C. pylori;* after 8 weeks of treatment with CBS (one tablet every six hours) 36% of patients were cleared of *C. pylori* [8]. Physicians experienced in infectious diseases should not perhaps be surprised that single-drug therapy may be inadequate, in view of the peculiarly sheltered environment (under the gastric mucus and in the gastric pits) where morphological and ultrastructural studies have shown the organism to be sequestered [3, 6, 13, 19]. Dual therapy with CBS and amoxycillin eliminated *C. pylori* in only 47% of our patients [8].

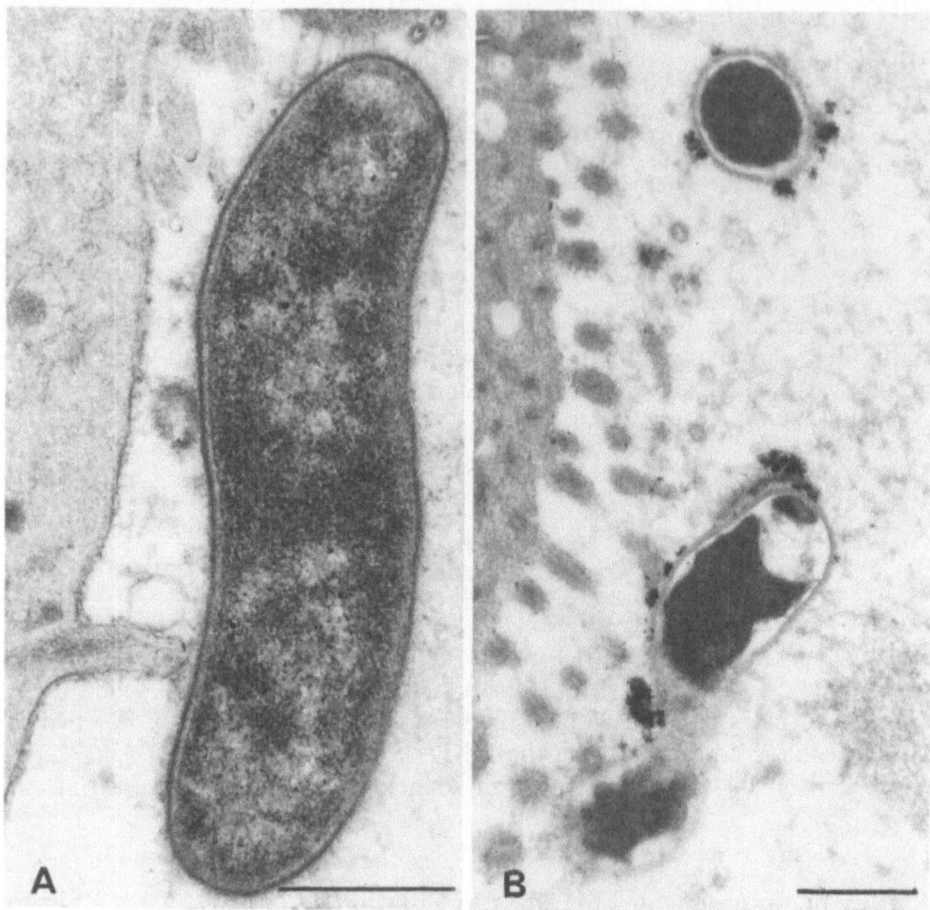

Fig. 1. A Typical appearance in vivo of *C. pylori*, in close proximity to the antral epithelium in a human gastric biopsy specimen. **B** Similar specimen obtained 70 min after administration of an initial single dose of liquid CBS (De-Nol), revealing bacterial degenerative changes and external dense deposits of bismuth complex (*bar* = 500 nm)

Not only does *C. pylori* colonize a unique organ, the stomach, but it exhibits a strong preferential affinity for the mucus-secreting cell type, to which it commonly attaches through adherence pedestals [6, 14, 15]. It is usually distributed most prolifically on the antral mucosa, but is also found to a variable extent in both the body and the fundic areas of the stomach. Systemic antibiotics such as amoxycillin probably have no action intraluminally in the stomach but are absorbed into the blood stream. However, bismuth compounds such as CBS (De-Nol) and Peptobismol can be expected to act in the stomach, but the dynamics of their topical interaction with *C. pylori* have not been studied. When gastric biopsy specimens were obtained from the antrum 1.0 – 1.5 h after ingestion of CBS in liquid or tablet form, the numerous *C. pylori* organisms seen on a pre-treatment biopsy specimen (Fig. 1 a) were found to be mostly detached from the surface and to exhibit gross degenerative changes including cell-wall separation and detachment (Fig. 1 b) [14]. Biopsy at similar short intervals after ingestion of Peptobismol showed less obvious signs of detachment and less severe bacterial degenerative changes than after CBS. It is not unreasonable to suppose that *C. pylori* in the fundus could be less effectively exposed to intraluminal bismuth than those in the antrum. Intragastric studies are required, possibly with radiopaque tracers, to determine the distribution patterns of oral bismuth compounds over the different areas of the gastric mucosa, and the levels of drug retention.

As viable *C. pylori* do not invade the gastric mucosa but colonize the luminal surface of the epithelium, they are presumably not readily accessible to the action of systemic antibiotics acting through the bloodstream. These antibiotics must diffuse through the mucosal cells or intercellular fluid and then penetrate to the surface to be effective against *C. pylori*. However, the organism is sensitive to even low concentrations of beta-lactam antibiotics, and amoxycillin may have a secondary but useful part to play in combination-drug therapy − for example in clearing residual organisms, perhaps within the gastric pits that have escaped exposure to effective concentrations of bismuth compounds in the stomach.

Ultrastructural Analysis of the Interaction in Vitro Between *C. pylori* and Antibacterial Agents

Exposure of *C. pylori* to CBS in vitro does not lead within 24 h to gross degeneration of the bacteria but results only in penetration of small amounts of particulate bismuth complex under the cell wall (Fig. 2a). This observation of the action of CBS in vitro is in sharp contrast to the marked effect observed in vivo (Fig. 1 b). Beta-lactam antibiotics such as amoxycillin and cephalexin cause classical spheroplast-like changes and disintegration of *C. pylori* after 24 h even at low concentrations such as 0.5 mg/L (Fig. 2b) [1]. Macrolide antibiotics, such as erythromycin at 1 mg/L, produce rather different degenerative changes including internal vacuolation, ribosomal coagulation and impaired cross-wall formation.

Recently we have extended the ultrastructural studies to include effects on *C. pylori* of exposure to different pH environments in vitro. At pH 5 very minor cell-wall changes were detectable; but at pH 4 after exposure for 10 min many of the bacteria were showing focal ballooning and detachment of the cell wall from the cell membrane and underlying cytoplasm. At pH 3 this became very marked and was accompanied by cytoplasmic coagulation and flagellar fragmentation (Fig. 3a). At pH 2, when CBS at 2000 mg/L was also introduced, deposits of bismuth were seen extracellularly (Fig. 3b), and the picture then closely resembled that found in vivo shortly after oral CBS administration (Fig. 1 b). Urea has been found to ameliorate these effects of acid on *C. pylori*, presumably by virtue of the powerful urease of *C. pylori* which results in the organism being surrounded by a protective "cloud" of ammonia.

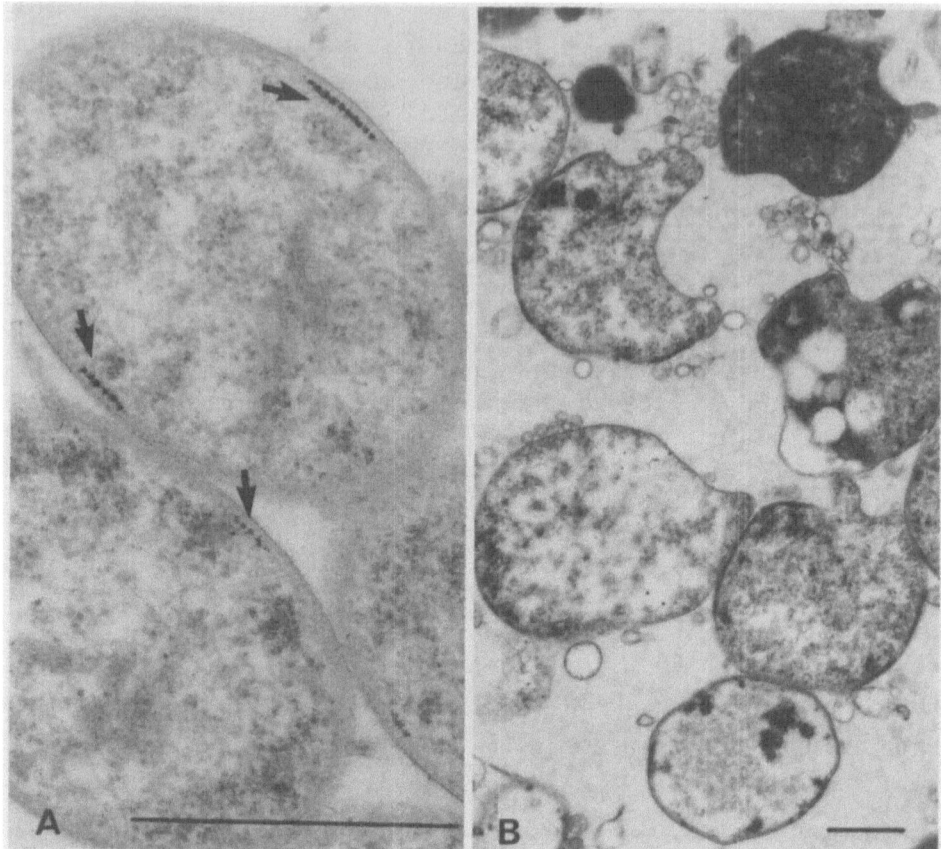

Fig. 2. A Sectioned *C. pylori* organisms in vitro after 8-h exposure to CBS (De-Nol, 1000 mg/
l). Discret plaque-like deposits of particulate bismuth complex (*arrows*) have penetrated under
the cell walls of the apparently intact bacteria (section viewed without staining). **B** Culture of
C. pylori exposed to amoxycillin (0.5 mg/l) for 24 h. Only degenerate spheroplast-like forms
remain (*bar* = 500 nm)

Viability of *C. pylori* After Exposure to Metronidazole and CBS in Vitro

Metronidazole, although producing no gross structural changes, exerted a pro-
gressive bactericidal effect against *C. pylori* in vitro; but in the first 8 h after exposure to CBS *C. pylori* showed no loss of viability. A marked fall in viable
count did however occur during the period from 8 to 24 h after exposure to
CBS (Fig. 4). Thus the rapid-onset antibacterial effect of bismuth against
C. pylori in vivo (Fig. 1b) is not reproduced by either the ultrastructural appearances or the viability counts in vitro. However, if the initial effect of bismuth against *C. pylori* in vivo is not one of bacterial killing, but rather of en-
zymic inactivation leading to detachment from the mucosal surfaces (possibly

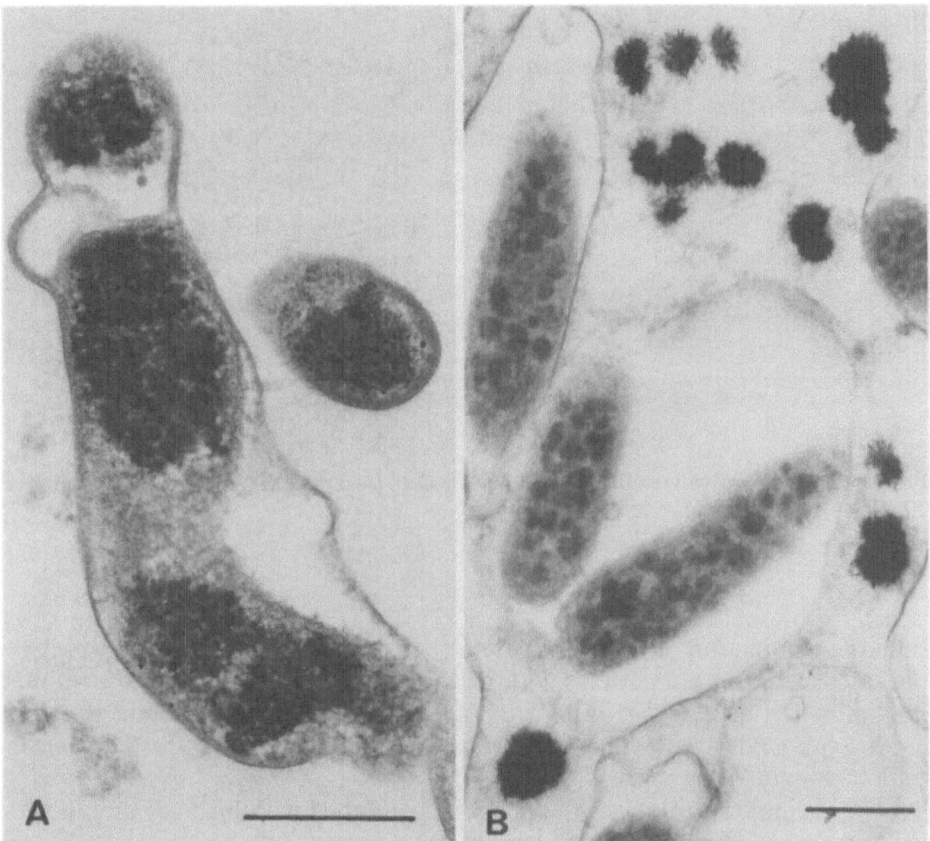

Fig. 3. A Structural degradation of *C. pylori* in vitro, produced by exposure of the culture to acidic conditions (pH 3) for 10 min. The cell wall separation and internal coagulation simulate the changes observed in vivo after CBS (De-Nol) administration. **B** Exposure of *C. pylori* culture to acidic conditions (pH 2) with addition of CBS (1000 mg/l) reproduced coarse deposition of bismuth complex around the degraded organisms (*bar* = 500 nm)

related to penetration of bismuth under the cell wall) the result would be to dislodge the organisms from their privileged site beneath the mucus. The gradient of increasing acidity across the mucus layer would then be sufficient to account for bacterial destruction as seen in vitro at or below pH 3.

Therapeutic Regimens to Eliminate *C. pylori*

Elimination of *C. pylori* from the gastric mucosa is better achieved by dual therapy with bismuth and a systemic antibiotic than a single therapy with either alone; in a double-blind placebo-controlled study CBS monotherapy re-

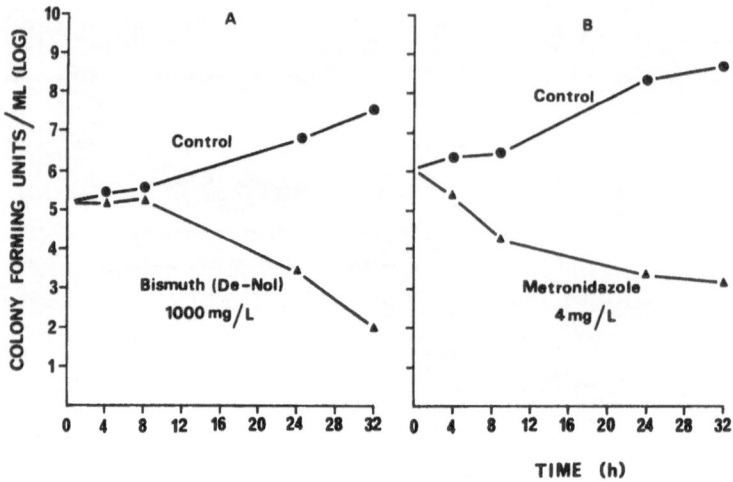

Fig. 4A,B. Quantitative viability curves for *C. pylori*, in control cultures and in the presence of CBS (**A**) and metronidazole (**B**)

sulted in elimination of *C. pylori* in 36% of patients, but dual therapy with CBS plus metronidazole (in patients with metronidazole-sensitive *C. pylori*) resulted in elimination of *C. pylori* in 85% of the patients [8]. At the present time bismuth compounds are the only agents known to be effective against *C. pylori* intraluminally in the stomach.

The systemic antibiotics which may be combined with bismuth offer a wide choice. Amoxycillin has a powerful action in vitro, but because beta-lactam antibiotics do not penetrate cells very well [9] this antibiotic is probably not the first choice to be given with a bismuth compound, as is borne out by the observation that only 47% of isolates were eliminated by this combination [8]. The first choice is probably metronidazole or tinidazole, although 20% of patients may have metronidazole-resistant *C. pylori* in their stomach [8]. Therefore a regimen of triple therapy to eliminate *C. pylori* is logical [2], which should include a bismuth compound such as CBS (De-Nol) probably for 4 weeks, together with metronidazole 400 mg thrice daily or tinidazole 1 g daily for the last 2 weeks, plus amoxycillin 500 mg every 6 h before meals for the last 2 weeks. Although monotherapy with ofloxacin has given rise to resistance [5], if a quinolone was given in place of amoxycillin this might yet be effective, because quinolones penetrate cells well. Alternatively in penicillin-hypersensitive patients tetracycline can be used as the third agent, but it must be remembered that chelation of tetracycline by bismuth would occur if these two drugs were given at the same time. Therefore it is our practice to give two tablets of CBS as the first thing in the morning and then again in the evening, with doxycycline 200 mg at lunchtime. Some patients may not take De-Nol in its most effective form because they do not wish to chew the tablets and stain their teeth and tongue. The tablets can be dissolved in water for a few hours before being swallowed or can be crushed to avoid blackening the tongue and teeth.

Implications of the Distribution of *C. pylori* in the Stomach

We now know that *C. pylori* occurs frequently in the fundus of the stomach as well as in the antrum. Organisms high in the stomach may not be so effectively exposed to oral antibacterials as those colonizing the antrum, thus fundus organisms may be the source of relapse after treatment. It is of interest to speculate whether lying down after ingestion of liquid bismuth would facilitate more effective exposure of *C. pylori* to the medication.

Conclusion

Appreciation of the sites of colonization of *C. pylori* and of the clinical experience that it is difficult to eliminate the organism in a high proportion of patients lead us to conclude that triple therapy with a bismuth compound, plus metronidazole or tinadazole, plus amoxycillin or a quinolone or tetracycline is required to achieve elimination of *C. pylori* in the highest percentage of patients. It is a good microbiological principle that if one antibacterial agent (such as amoxycillin) is to be given for a shorter period than a concurrent agent to which resistance rarely occurs (such as bismuth), then the second agent should be given in the latter part of the longer course.

Comparative in vivo and in vitro studies of *C. pylori*, following exposure to CBS, suggest that although this compound has bactericidal activity against the organism on prolonged exposure, this may not account for the rapid bacterial "knock-down" phenomenon observed in vivo. It is proposed that this may be due to an effect of bismuth causing microbial detachment from the mucosa, with resulting exposure of the organisms to lethal acidic conditions in the mucus layer and the gastric lumen.

References

1. Armstrong JA, Wee SH, Goodwin CS, Wilson DH (1987) Response of *Campylobacter pyloridis* to antibiotics, bismuth and an acid-reducing agent *in vitro*. An ultrastructural study. J Med Microbiol 24:343–350
2. Borody TJ, Carrick J, Hazell SL (1987) Symptoms improve after the eradication of gastric *Campylobacter pyloridis*. Med J of Aust 146:450–451
3. Chen XG, Correa P, Offerhaus J, Rodriguez E, Janney F, Hoffmann E, Fox J, Hunter F, Diavolitsis S (1986) Ultrastructure of the gastric mucosa harboring Campylobacter-like organisms. Amer J Clin Path 86:575–582
4. Czinn S, Carr H, Aronoff S (1986) Susceptibility of *Campylobacter pyloridis* to three macrolide antibiotics (erythromycin, rosithromycin [RU28965], CP62993) and rifampicin. Antimicrob Agents Chemother 30:328–329
5. Glupczynski Y, Labbe M, Burette A, Delmee M, Avesani V, Bruck C (1987) Treatment failure of ofloxacin in *Campylobacter pylori* infection. Lancet i:1096
6. Goodwin CS, Armstrong JA, Marshall BJ (1986) *Campylobacter pyloridis*, gastritis, and peptic ulceration. J Clin Pathol 39:353–365

7. Goodwin CS, Blake P, Blincow E (1986) The minimum inhibitory and bactericidal concentrations of antibiotic and anti-ulcer agents against *Campylobacter pyloridis*. J Antimicrob Chemother 17:309–314

8. Goodwin CS, Marshall BJ, Blincow ED, Wilson DH, Blackburn S, Phillips M (1987) Prevention of nitroimidazole resistance in *Campylobacter pylori* by co-administration of colloidal bismuth subcitrate: clinical and in vitro studies. J Clin Pathol 41:207–210

9. Jacobs RF, Wilson CB (1983) Intracellular penetration and antimicrobial activity of antibiotics. J Antimicrob Chem 12:C, 13–20

10. Lambert T, Megraud F, Gerbaud G, Courvalin P (1986) Susceptibility of *Campylobacter pyloridis* to 20 antimicrobial agents. Antimicrob Age and Chemother 30:510–511

11. Langenberg ML, Rauws EAJ, Schipper MEI, Widjojokosumo GN, Tytgat J, Rietra PJGM, Zanen HC (1985) The pathogenic role of *Campylobacter pyloridis* studied by attempts to eliminate these organisms. *Campylobacter III:* Proceedings of the third international workshop on *Campylobacter infections*. London: Public Health Laboratory Service 162–163

12. Marshall BJ, Goodwin CS (1987) Revised nomenclature for *Campylobacter pyloridis*. Internat J Systemat Bacteriol 37:68

13. Marshall BJ, Warren JR (1984) Unidentified curved bacilli in the stomach of patients with gastritis and peptic ulceration. Lancet i:1311–1315

14. Marshall BJ, Armstrong JA, Francis GJ, Nokes NT, Wee SH (1987) The antibacterial action of bismuth in relation to *Campylobacter pyloridis* colonisation and gastritis. Digestion 37: Supp. 2, 16–30

15. Marshall BJ, Royce H, Annear DI, Goodwin CS, Pearman JW, Warren JR and Armstrong JA (1984) Original isolation of *Campylobacter pyloridis* from human gastric mucosa. Microbios Letters 25:83–88

16. McNulty CAM, Dent J, Wise R (1985) Susceptibility of clinical isolates of *Campylobacter pyloridis* to eleven antimicrobial agents. Antimicrob Agents Chemother 28:837–838

17. McNulty CAM, Gearty JC, Grump B, Davis M, Donovan IA, Melikian V, Lister DM, Wise R (1986) *Campylobacter pyloridis* and associated gastritis: investigator blind, placebo controlled trial of bismuth salicylate and erythromycin ethylsuccinate. Brit Med J 293:645–649

18. Taylor DE, Hargreaves JA, Ng LK, Sherbaniuk RW, Jewell LD (1987) Isolation and characterization of *Campylobacter pyloridis* from gastric biopsies. J Clin Pathol 87:49–54

19. Tricottet V, Bruneval P, Vire O, Camilleri JP, Bloch F, Bonte N, Roge J (1986) Campylobacter-like organisms and surface epithelium abnormalities in active chronic gastritis in humans: an ultrastructural study. Ultrastruct Pathol 10:113–122

Discussion

Flemström: Regarding the lengths of "bacteria-free survival" as you showed in your second to the last slide: did this refer specifically to gastric ulcer or all types of ulcer?

Goodwin: Only to duodenal ulcer.

Ober: What were the numbers there? I ask this because at the AGA meeting in Chicago in May, a similar study was shown with bismuth subsalicylate without adding a second drug and with fewer relapses in the bismuth group.

Goodwin: There were about 27 or 29 in each group — very small numbers.

O'Moráin: I would like to ask some questions about drug therapy preparation. You mentioned the liquid and tablets. This may have something to do with the work which I will present tomorrow showing that the time of administration is critical. In our study when we gave one tablet q.i.d., we obtained almost the same results that you got with antibiotic and bismuth.

Goodwin: I showed you actually two treatments. As in Marshall's study, the double-blind trial, we were giving one tablet four times a day. But when I gave it with tetracycline, I realized that this is a bad idea, so I now give two in the morning and two in the evening.

Rösch: Was the ulcer relapse related to a recurrence of *Campylobacter pylori?*

Goodwin: Yes it was. Some patients can retain *Campylobacter* and stay ulcer-free. But this is a very complicated study, and I can not yet present the details. On the whole, if you get rid of *Campylobacter* and the patient stays free of this, he will not experience an ulcer relapse. But there is an overlap between the two groups. In other words, some patients can retain *Campylobacter* and are also healed; but this depends upon how long you follow them up. We have only followed-up for a year, and we are finding one or two relapses after a year. So if you follow-up for two years, you may find more.

Kraft: You spoke of metronidazole resistance. How did you measure resistance? Did you determine in vitro MICs or conclude that relapse after drug therapy was due to resistance development?

Goodwin: We measured in vitro by ordinary MIC testing.

Tytgat: I would like to return to the difference between the in vivo and the in vitro effects of bismuth. I do not think it is all that simple. For bismuth to enter the mucus gel it must probably remain in solution. With an acid pH in the stomach, colloidal bismuth will precipitate. Theoretically it should not, then, penetrate the mucus gel. In vivo one finds quite dramatic effects, as we have seen in Amsterdam. So I would like to ask you what the true differences are between the in vitro and in vivo effects. Was bismuth in solution in your in vitro situation? How did you provide bismuth in your in vitro test situation?

Goodwin: I think you make a very interesting theoretical comment that bismuth must be in solution to get to the mucusa, but, as in John Armstrong's picture, close to the macrovilli you could see bismuth around the organism. I do not know the actual pH of the gastric juice in that patient. But in vitro you can dissolve bismuth. This is quite complicated, but we obtain a powder from the makers of Denol which dissolves perfectly well. So in our in vitro work we use not a suspension but a solution.

Dammann: I would like to ask you about the development of the resistant strains under the combination therapy and the antibiotic therapy.

Goodwin: The only results were the metronidazole-resistant strains; we obtained two out of the 22 persons given both antibacterial drugs. Giving one drug alone we found a 70% resistance rate; this paper will be published shortly. If you have metronidazole-sensitive strains in vitro and plate them on metronidazole-containing agar, at least 10% of the strains show organisms that are metronidazole-resistant.

Brunner: Do you know, or does anyone else in the audience know whether and, if so, how much bismuth can enter the body via resorption. Does this have any influence on mitochondrial metabolism. Bacteria look very similar to mitochondria, and when bismuth enters michochondria, might it do damage?

Goodwin: I think much more work should be done on bismuth-organism interaction. Bismuth enters the blood stream in a small amount, and some governments are unwilling to licence this drug because of bismuth toxicity. Bismuth does enter to a certain extent the mucosa.

Axon: There is no doubt that bismuth is absorbed to some extent and accumulates to a small degree as well, because we have shown that patients who have been continued to excrete bismuth following cessation of therapy.

Marshall: There is one other possibility with the development of antibiotic resistance. In our trial we gave tinidazole with cimetidine, and in a recent study Glupczynsky reported giving ofloxacin with a H_2 antagonist — I think this was ranitidine. In both studies we see the development of antibiotic resistance. If you give an antibiotic in a stomach which contains acid, there will be no other bacteria in the lumen to pass on an antibiotic-resistant plasmid to *C. pylori.* However if you ablate the hydrochloric acid, the stomach flora will resemble that in the colon rather than that in the stomach. Therefore, if you are trying to treat *C. pylori* with a single antibiotic, I think we should consider that with single-agent therapy H$_2$ blockers may be contraindicated.

Axon: Are you saying that the number of *C. pylori* in the stomach increases when cimetidine is given?

Marshall: No, I believe that if you do not give cimetidine, the only organism in the stomach will be *C. pylori.* If you do give cimetidine, you have *C. pylori* floating in a sea of bowel flora, and there is the opportunity for another organism which has a resistant plasmid to pass this on to *C. pylori.* Dr. Goodwin has found that 20% of the isolates can be trained to be metronidazole-resistant in vitro, and yet we have 77% developing resistance when we give tinidazole alone with cimetidine. And in the case of ofloxacin resistance may occur in 100% of cases.

Goodwin: I think this is a very important observation. Anyone who has actually looked at cultures from the stomach can tell whether the patient is on cimetidine or not. In other words, if they are virgin persons who have just come up for biopsy, you obtain beautiful, clear plates in your culture. Your selective media will show only *C. pylori.* Whereas if you give cimetidine you sample a broth culture of every mouth organism. So I personally would never take cimetidine. It really would make my stomach, I would say, like the colon.

von Wulffen: I would like to comment on this *C. pylori* resistance. I have read the recent "Lancet" letter on quinolone resistance of *C. pylori,* and I would not think that the presence of other organisms in these cases were responsible for transferring this resistance. As far as I know, there has been no description yet of quinolone-resistance transfer between different species of bacteria via plasmids. So there are probably other mechanisms involved in the appearance of quinolone resistance that are still poorly understood.

Goodwin: There are many different ways of transferring DNA between bacteria, for example transformation by phage and by plasmids. And we will certainly see some papers published on restrictional endonucleases which show that the genome is incredibly variable. The organism is far more clever than we are.

In Search of Animal Models for *Campylobacter pylori* Induced Disease

M. WARRELMANN, S. EHLERS, and H. HAHN

Introduction

One of Koch's postulates indicating the pathogenicity of a given microorganism is that the microorganism be cultivable outside the host and that it elicits, in other animal species, symptoms similar to those elicited in the originally infected host. In addition, for microorganisms of pathogenetic relevance to humans it is important to establish an animal model as simple as possible in order to study mechanisms and assess the efficacy of therapeutic agents. Mice and rats are particularly well suited as experimental animals since there is available a considerable amount of information on genetics, immunology, and pathogenesis of their infections. For these reasons, we have tried to establish a rodent experimental model of *Campylobacter pylori* infection using various mouse strains and one rat strain.

Material and Methods

Campylobacter pylori (NCTC strain 11637) was cultured for 3 days in a brain-heart infusion broth supplemented with Skirrow supplement, amphotericin B, 10% fetal calf serum, and 5 µg/l haemin under continuous shaking in a microaerophilic atmosphere at 37°C. The concentration of microorganisms was determined by preparing appropriate dilutions of the bacterial suspension and plating 0.1 aliquots on Columbia chocolate agar.

Eighty C57-Bl/6 mice received 1×10^8 microorganisms each. The bacteria were injected i.v. into a lateral tail vein in a volume of 0.5 ml. Spleen, liver, kidneys, and heart from five animals each were removed aseptically after 6 h, 1, 3, and 12 days postinjection, respectively. The organs were homogenized in 5 ml thioglycollate broth. Appropriately diluted aliquots of 0.1 ml each were plated on Columbia chocolate agar, and the number of microorganisms was determined after 5 days of incubation at 37°C in a microaerophilic environment. In order to determine whether *Campylobacter pylori* was present in the gastric mucosa, the animals were left without food and water for 4–6 hours before stomachs were removed. Stomachs were removed as total organs and put into thioglycollate broth. Subsequently they were opened along the large curvature and rinsed with thioglycollate broth. The upper layer of the gastric mucosa was then carefully removed using scissors and forceps in order to expose the deeper layers and the mucosal membrane crypts. The latter were then imprinted on Columbia chocolate agar. The plates were incubated for 5 days in a microaerophilic atmosphere at 37° C. *Campylobacter* strain NCTC 11637 was used as reference strain.

Results

The results of the first experiment are presented in Fig. 1. After 6 h spleens contained about 10^5 microorganisms per organ; after 24 h the bacterial content had decreased below the detection level (< 50) (Fig. 1). After 6 h livers contained 1×10^7 microorganisms per organ. After 72 h only few *C. pylori* organisms could be demonstrated. After 12 days *C. pylori* could no longer be cultured. In kidneys there were 2.5×10^4 organisms per organ 6 h postinjection; later, the organs appeared culturally sterile. After 6 h postinfection there was only scant growth of *C. pylori* in hearts; later, *C. pylori* could no longer be cultured. Stomachs yielded no *C. pylori* organisms at any time.

In a second experiment, similar conditions were chosen as in the first one, except that the number of organisms administered was 5×10^8 per animal. Time points for plating the homogenized organs were more closely spaced here in or-

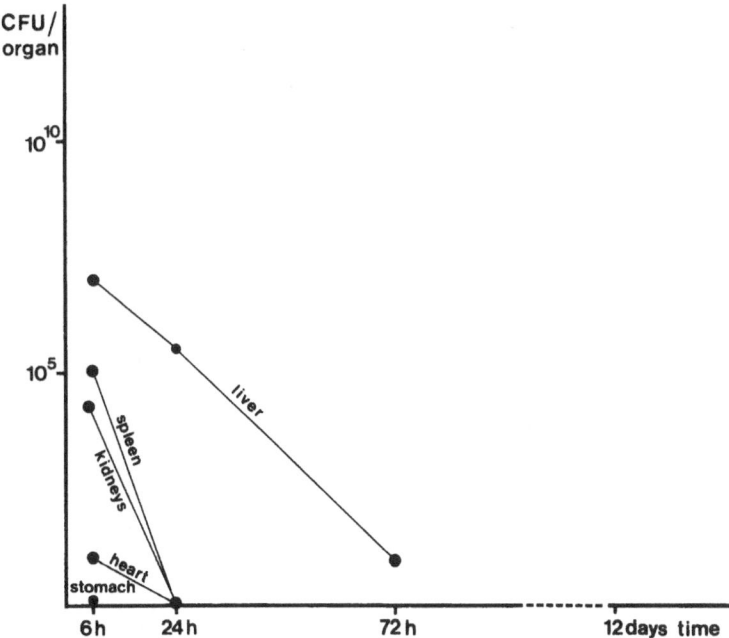

Fig. 1. Colony-forming units (CFU) of *Campylobacter pylori* (C.p.) in various organs at different points in time after i.v. application of 1×10^8 live C.p. per animal in the tail vein of C57-B1/6 mice. The data are the means of five observations each

der to document more exactly the kinetics of the decline of bacterial organ concentrations. Moreover, in order to lower the threshold for the demonstration of *C. pylori*, the organs were homogenized in 2 ml of thioglycollate broth instead of 5 ml, and the homogenates were plated in 0.5 ml aliquots. The results of this experiment were very similar to those obtained in the first, except that here the bacterial concentrations in the organs were slightly higher after 6 and 24 hours postinfection, due to the higher bacterial inoculum applied (Fig. 2).

In a third series of experiments, Lewis rats were injected with 1×10^8 bacteria per animal in a volume of 0.5 ml i.v. into the tail vein. Spleen, liver, kidneys, and stomach from three animals each were removed after 6 h, 24 h, 48 h, and 10 days. The organs were homogenized, and homogenates were plated according to the experimental protocol outlined above. After six hours there were 1×10^3 bacteria per organ in spleens and livers. Later, *C. pylori* could not be demonstrated in any organ (Fig. 3).

In summary, the results of the i.v. application of *C. pylori* in C57-Bl/6 mice and Lewis rats show that this leads to a transient colonization in various organs. Of the injected bacteria, 90% are removed by the liver. There follows a loglinear removal of bacteria (probably due to killing) without symptoms of disease appearing in the injected animals. There is no septicaemia demonstrable and, as judged by inspection, the infected mice appear to be healthy. There is no colonization of the gastric mucosa.

Since nothing is known about the possible transmission and mode of infection of *C. pylori* in humans, in a further series of experiments the behaviour of *C. pylori* in various mouse strains was investigated after oral application. A

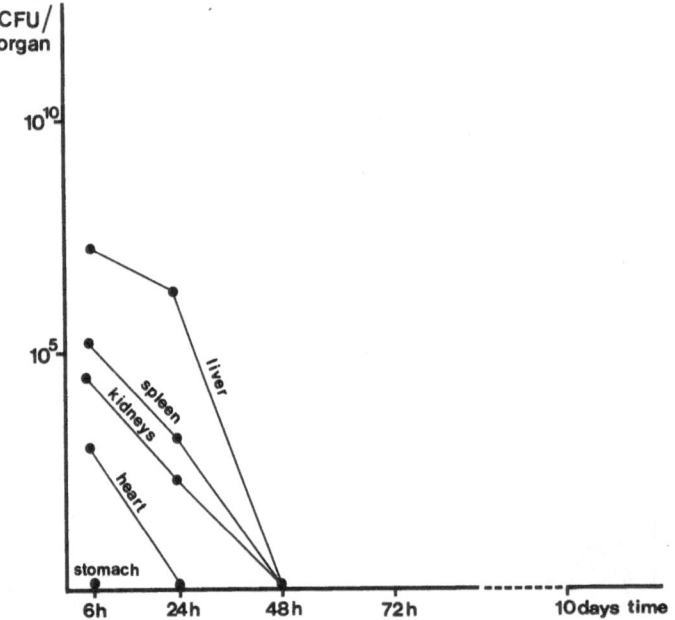

Fig. 2. Colony-forming units (CFU) of *Campylobacter pylori* (C.p.) in various organs at different times after i.v. application of 5×10^8 live C.p. per animal in the tail vein of C57-Bl/6 mice

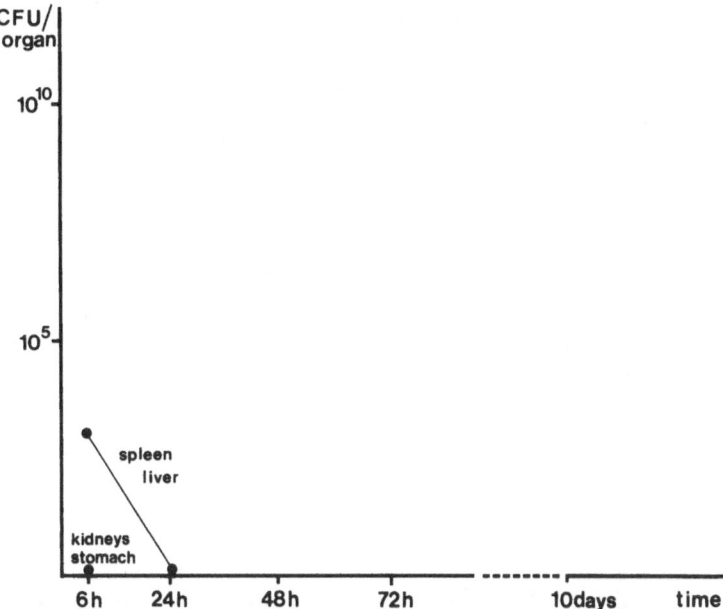

Fig. 3. Colony-forming units (CFU) of *Campylobacter pylori* (C.p.) in various organs at different times after i.v. application of 1×10^8 live C.p. per animal in the tail vein of Lewis rats

Table 1. Experimental protocol for the oral application of *Campylobacter pylori* (C.p.) in C57-Bl/6 mice

Group	Animals	Application
A	C57-Bl/6 mice	1×10^9 live C.p.
B	C57-Bl/6 mice	20 μmol/kg Omeprazol in PEG 400 i.v., −16 h and −4 h; 1×10^9 live C.p.
C	C57-Bl/6 mice	PEG 400 i.v.; −16 h and −4 h; 1×10^9 live C.p.

total of 1×10^9 microorganisms were applied orally using a 15-cm feeding cannula. The animals had been left without food and water for 24 h before the beginning of the experiment. Table 1 outlines the experimental protocol.

Omeprazol is a newly developed inhibitor of gastric acid secretion which specifically blocks the H^+-K^+-ATPase. Under the dose regimens used, gastric acid production in the stomachs of the animals was suppressed for at least 24 h. Thus it is to be concluded that the oral application of *C. pylori* occurred under complete achlorhydria. As in the first series of experiments, livers and spleens from five animals each were removed at 6 h, 1, 2, 3, and 10 days postinfection, homogenized and plated in appropriate dilutions. *C. pylori* (strain NCTC 11637) was used as a control. *C. pylori* could not be cultured at any time from any organ. The stomachs were prepared as described for the first series of experiments. Again, no *C. pylori* could be cultured.

Table 2. Experimental protocol for the oral application of *Campylobacter pylori* (C.p.) in various mice strains

Group	Animals	Application
A	Balb/c mice	1×10^9 live C.p.
B	DBA mice	1×10^9 live C.p.
C	athymic nude mice (nu/nu), Balb/c background	1×10^9 live C.p.
D	C57-Bl/6 mice	1×10^9 live C.p.
E	C57-Bl/6 mice	20 µmol/kg Omeprazol PEG 400 i.v.; − 16 h and −4 h; 1×10^9 live C.p.
F	C57-Bl/6	PEG 400 i.v.; − 16 h and −4 h; 1×10^9 live C.p.

In order to test different mouse strains for their response to orally applied *C. pylori*, in a second series of experiments the protocol as outlined in Table 2 was chosen. There was no *C. pylori* demonstrable in the liver, spleen, or stomach of any animal after 4 h, 1, 2, 3, 6, or 12 days.

Collectively, the experiments indicate that *C. pylori* after oral application of 1×10^9 microorganisms per animal could not be found in any of the mouse strains at any time in any of the investigated organs. Therefore, one must conclude that *C. pylori* does not colonize the gastric mucosa of the investigated animals, nor does it penetrate into the blood stream and cause bacteraemia.

Discussion

Under our experimental conditions *C. pylori* does not lead to disease symptoms, septicemia, nor colonization of gastric mucosa in mice strains or in Lewis rats. Neither rats nor mice appear particularly well suited as experimental animals for the establishment of an animal model for the study of *C. pylori*.

Technical difficulties in the preparation of stomachs which do not allow perfect working conditions may in part account for the negative findings. Also, due to the fact that stomachs could not be completely homogenized, we cannot exclude with certainty that *C. pylori* might have been present in some layer. Another question which we have not been able to answer concerns the behaviour of *C. pylori* after intravenous or oral application in the gastric mucosa after the latter has been damaged b stress lesions. Since nothing is known about the kinetics and conditions of *C. pylori* colonization of the gastric mucosa in patients, it appears possible that the microorganism can only gain a foothold in predamaged gastric mucosa. This would have to be investigated employing a stress model.

In view of the great interest in *C. pylori* infection and the importance of establishing an animal model it needs to be investigated whether the microorganisms could possibly be adapted to mice by frequent mouse passages. Appropriate experiments are currently in progress.

Summary

C. pylori (strain NCTC 11637) under the conditions chosen by us does not after oral and intravenous application elicit sepsis, disease symptoms, or colonization of the gastric mucosa in mice nor in rats.

After oral application the microorganism cannot be found even as early as 4 h after infection. After i.v. application there is a short bacteraemia with transient colonization of the liver and spleen. There is a loglinear bacterial killing without specific symptoms in the animals which could be related to damage caused by *C. pylori*. Further experiments are in progress to produce *C. pylori* strains which might be adapted to mice. In addition, we are working on a stress model and are examining other conditions for the colonization of gastric mucosa by *C. pylori*.

Discussion

Marshall: Did you look at the flora of these mice before you commenced the experiment for other *Campylobacter* or *Campylobacter*-like organisms, either by culture or by histology of the gastric mucosa? And secondly, were your mice allowed to eat their own feces in their cages during the experiment, or were they in special cages where the feces dropped through?

Warrelmann: We did not look at the stomachs before starting the experiments or used special cages in order to prevent the animals from eating their own feces.

Marshall: A point to remember with animal models for spiral bacteria colonizing the stomach is that many animals have their own gastric spiral bacteria; for instance, some mice have a spiral organism present. Also because they are coprophagous, it is possible that spiral bacteria which colonize the crypts of the colon, as shown by Adrian Lee in Sydney, could be passing through the stomach all the time, and the mice may therefore have a very high immunity to these types of bacteria. Perhaps the serological studies of these mice might be worthwhile.

Konturek: I think that you should study the colonization of *C. pylori* in a damaged gastric or duodenal mucosa, particularly using chronic types of damage, for example chronic gastric or duodenal ulcers. It is very simple to develop such ulcerations, and this would be a useful model to see whether bacteria can be colonized in the area of damage.

Warrelmann: No, we have not tried to establish a stress model.

Konturek: I am not talking about a stress ulcer model because this is acute mucosal damage, but rather about chronic damage induced by, for example, acetic-acid application to the gastric mucosa. You can develop chronic gastric or duodenal ulcers for several months or even years with the tendency to reulcerate after some time, and this might be a better model to see whether bacteria colonize in the ulcerated area.

Warrelmann: This obviously must be done.

An Animal Model of Gastritis Induced by *Campylobacter pylori*

W. G. KRAFT, D. R. MORGAN, R. D. LEUNK, and S. KRAKOWKA

Introduction

Following confirmation of the findings [1, 5, 10–12] first reported by Warren and Marshall [13] that gastritis and peptic ulcers are frequently associated with *Campylobacter pylori* colonization of gastric and duodenal mucosae, the major unresolved question concerns the role of the bacterium in these disease states. Unknown is whether *C. pylori* causes the inflammation and ulceration or simply secondarily colonizes the diseased tissue. Evidence is accumulating which suggests that the bacterium is a pathogen. We have previously reported that *C. pylori* produces a toxic factor that induces intracellular vacuolization in cultured mammalian cells. Similar intracellular vacuolization has been observed in tissues from patients suffering chronic gastritis [11]. Marshall [8] and Morris [9] have described their personal experiences on the development of gastritis following ingestion of the organism.

The want of an absolute therapy for gastrointestinal (GI) disease associated with *C. pylori* precludes further human challenges. Consequently, an alternative approach for further investigation into the nature of this organism has been a primary objective for our group. Preliminary work involving challenges of adult and neonatal mice, guinea pigs, and rabbits was unsuccessful. The gastrointestinal system of rodents and lagomorphs, however, is notably different from that of humans. The pig is a functional monogastric mammal with dietary habits and anatomical and physiological characteristics of the GI tract similar to humans [4].

The objective of the present study was to investigate the susceptibility of neonatal gnotobiotic piglets to oral challenge with a suspension of *C. pylori*. Results of the study are presented in this report.

Materials and Methods

Animals. In order to confirm susceptibility three separate litters with a total of 20 gnotobiotic domestic Yorkshire piglets were studied. The litters were derived from date-mated pregnant sows by cesarean section. Neonatal piglets were housed in partitioned germ-free isolation units. Challenged and control piglets were housed separately. All piglets received 100−150 ml of Similac plus iron *per os* three times daily.

Bacterial Inoculum. For the challenge inoculum bacteria were grown, as a shaking culture, in Brucella broth (Difco, Detroit, Michigan, USA) supplemented with 10% fetal bovine serum and 1% Isovitalex under a microaerobic environment for 48 h at 37 ° C. Cultures were centrifuged, resuspended in peptone water, and enumerated by a standard plate-count method before being used as the challenge inoculum.

Experimental Design. Piglets of less than 7 days of age were fasted for 12 h before receiving orally administered cimetidine (60 mg/kg) to effect temporary achlorhydria. Challenged piglets received orally approximately 10^9 colony-forming units (cfu) of *C. pylori* suspended in 2 ml of peptone water. Controls received either no treatment (litter 1) or 2 ml of peptone water (litters 2 and 3). At weekly intervals for up to 4 weeks following challenge, piglets were sacrificed, and tissue samples collected from the cardia, fundus, and pylorus of the stomach and the oropharynx, esophagus, duodenum, jejunum, ileum, spiral colon, terminal colon, and rectum. Fecal swabs were taken daily.

Bacteriological Examination. Samples of GI tract tissues and fecal swabs were inoculated onto GCHI agar plates supplemented with trimethoprim, vancomycin, amphotericin, and polymyxin B (Remel Media, Lenexa, Kansas, USA). Plates were incubated in GasPak jars (BBL, Cockeysville, Maryland, USA), and the desired microaerobic atmosphere was generated by CampyPak (BBL) envelopes. Incubation was at 37 ° C for 3−7 days. Isolates were classified as *C. pylori* on the basis of their typical appearance as Gram negative rods and of their positive reactions for oxidase, catalase, and urease.

Histopathological Examination. Tissue samples for histopathological examinations were taken from sites adjacent to those at which samples for bacteriological examinations were removed. After tissues were fixed, embedded, and sectioned, replicates were stained with hematoxylin and eosin (H&E), Warthin-Starry silver, and Alcian blue periodic acid-Schiff (PAS) stains.

Antibody Assay. At necropsy a terminal serum sample was collected from each piglet. Sera were tested for antibody to *C. pylori* using a standard ELISA procedure. Formalinized *C. pylori* cells (10^7 cfu/well) were used as the coating antigen. Alkaline phosphatase conjugated to goat anti-swine IgG was used as the probe for porcine antibody.

Results

Clinical Signs and Gross Visual Observations of Tissues

Except for mild, transient diarrhea noted for many of the piglets within the first 2 days after challenge and transient anorexia among a few piglets, clinical disease was not apparent. Infection did not result in grossly visible gastric epithelial erosions or ulcerations, although by 4 weeks after challenge prominent submucosal/mucosal lymphoid follicles (nodules) were observed. Accumulation of mucus within the gastric lumen of infected but not control piglets was especially prominent by 2 weeks after challenge. Other tissues, including the intestine, were unremarkable.

Tissue Distribution of *C. pylori*

For the procedure employed no viable bacteria were recovered from fecal swab samples at any time in the study. In contrast, by the time of the initial tissue examination following challenge *C. pylori* had established colonization of gastric and duodenal mucosae.

Composite results of both Warthin-Starry silver stain and bacterial culture of gastric and duodenal tissues are shown in Table 1. Notable is that colonization is persistent. Bacteria were recovered from at least one anatomical region of all challenged piglets for each examination interval over the 4 weeks of observation. No bacteria were found in tissues from control piglets at any examination.

Consistent with data from the study of gastric tissues removed from humans suffering chronic gastritis associated with *C. pylori*, the organism in challenged piglets colonizes all anatomical regions of the stomach and the duodenal bulb. As in the human disease the bacterium appears to establish discrete foci rather than being evenly distributed in the tissue.

As illustrated in the silver-stained tissue section (Fig. 1) the bacteria are limited to the mucus layer covering the epithelium. Organisms were ex-

Table 1. Distribution of *C. pylori* in gastric and duodenal tissues of piglets challenged orally

Weeks after challenge	Anatomical region[a]			
	Cardia	Fundus	Pylorus	Duodenal bulb
1	3/4	3/4	3/4	2/4
2	4/4	2/4	3/4	3/4
3	5/5	5/5	5/5	4/5
4	1/2	2/2	2/2	2/2
Control	0/5	0/5	0/5	0/5

[a] Number of piglets colonized/number of piglets sampled

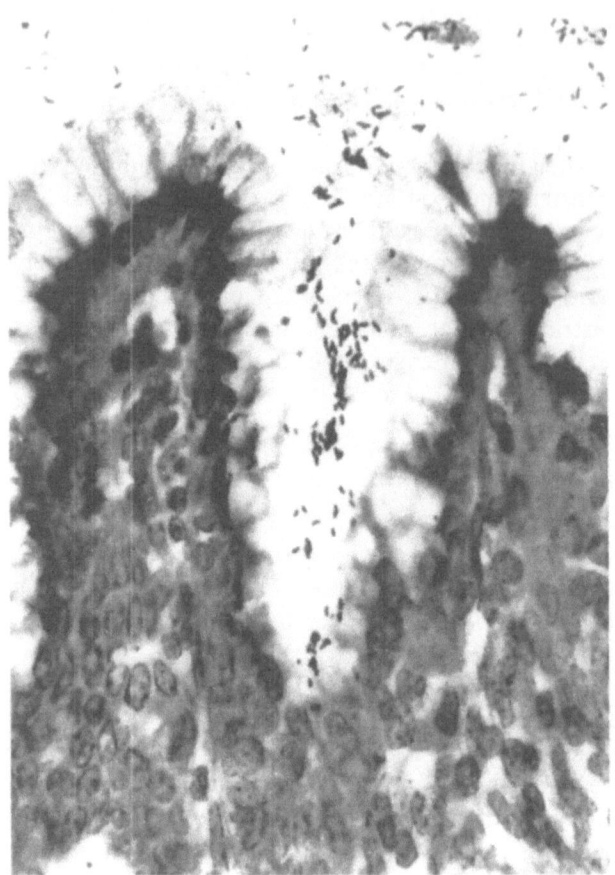

Fig. 1. *C. pylori* in the superficial mucus layer of gastric epithelium 1 week after challenge (Warthin-Starry silver stain)

traepithelial and appeared to be attached to the glycocalyx of the cells beneath the acellular mucus layer. Occasionally bacteria were noted in deeper portions of the mucosa. Here, also, the organism appeared to be extracellular and restricted to the lumens of dilated pits. No bacteria were seen in the submucosa and lamina propria.

Although *C. pylori* was detected in GI tract tissues outside the stomach, specifically in the esophagus and the duodenum, these tissues did not exhibit the histopathologic lesions characteristic of gastric epithelium colonized by *C. pylori*. Most likely, the bacteria found in tissues adjacent to the stomach reflect spillover from the stomach during gastric ligation and resection. Whereas *C. pylori* was detected in gastric tissue for all piglets at each examination interval, the presence of bacteria at other sites in the GI tract was not observed for every piglet or for every sample time.

The distribution data suggest a specificity of *C. pylori* for gastric tissue. This observation is consistent with reports that the organism in humans is associated only with gastric epithelial cells [2, 3, 7].

Microscopic Lesions

As shown in Table 2, histopathological lesions indicative of chronic active gastritis were observed in all three anatomical regions of the stomach and the duodenal bulb of piglets challenged with *C. pylori*. At the first examination (1 week after challenge), neutrophilic infiltrates, primarily limited to the nonglandular region (e.g., epithelial), were noted in the gastric cardiac region. Neutrophils formed intraepithelial aggregates and were present in the lamina propria. Mononuclear leukocytes were detected, mostly in the nonglandular regions. Cell aggregates were present in submucosal regions, occasionally obliterating crypt regions. Small lymphoid follicles were found in the cardia.

Severity and intensity of the lesions continued to increase with time. By the 2nd week after challenge the neutrophilic response had resolved and a significant increase in mononuclear cells was evident in both the submucosa and the lamina propria. Within the lamina propria discrete lymphofollicular aggregates were apparent.

Through the 3rd and 4th weeks the lesions intensified as mononuclear cell infiltration and proliferation into the lesions increased. Lymphoid follicles were prominent and occasionally coalesced to form sheets of cells spanning both the submucosa and the lamina propria.

Unchallenged piglets remained essentially unchanged through the 4 weeks of examination (Fig. 2). Infrequently, mononuclear cells were observed in the submucosa of the fundic and pyloric regions. Also within the submucosa rare lymphoid aggregates were seen. No neutrophils were ever observed in gastric tissues of control piglets.

At GI tract locations outside the stomach, microscopic lesions, in the form of lymphoreticular hyperplasia, were noted in tissues from challenged piglets. Such lesions, observed in all piglets and at each examination interval, were not consistent with the histopathology characteristic of chronic, active gastritis and were not associated with detectable bacteria. The significance of these immune-cell aggregates is uncertain.

In the human disease state marked mucus depletion is associated with *C. pylori* colonization of the gastric mucosa [2]. To determine whether the mucus layer is similarly eroded when the stomach of a piglet is colonized by the

Table 2. Microscopic lesions in gastric and duodenal tissues of piglets orally challenged with *C. pylori*

Weeks after challenge	Anatomical region[a]			
	Cardia	Fundus	Pylorus	Duodenal bulb
1	4/4	3/4	3/4	2/4
2	4/4	2/4	3/4	3/4
3	5/5	5/5	2/5	2/5
4	1/2	1/2	2/2	0/2
Control	1/5	2/5	1/5	0/5

[a] Number of piglets with tissue inflammation/number of piglets sampled

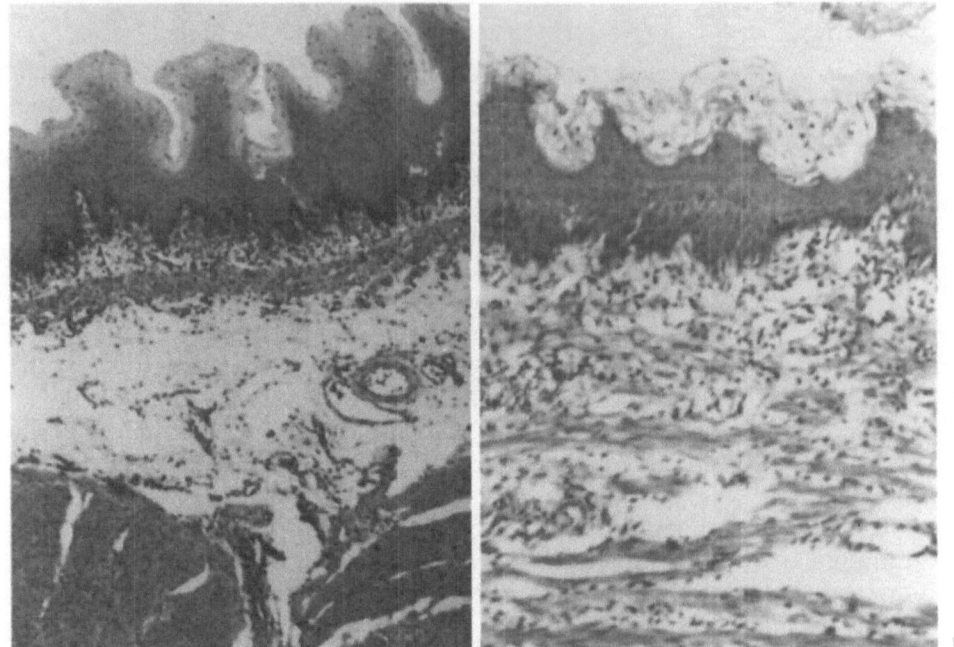

Fig. 2. a Cross-section from the gastric cardia of a control piglet demonstrating normal histology and **b** from an infected piglet 1 week after challenge demonstrating characteristic lymphoreticular infiltration and epithelial cell degeneration

bacterium, PAS-stained tissue sections were examined. Changes in the mucus layer were apparent by 2 weeks after challenge, primarily in the fundic and pyloric regions. Marked depletion of both the acid and neutral mucopolysaccharides were noted. Areas of depletion corresponded to those where microscopic lesions associated with *C. pylori* colonization were most prominent and where bacteria were detected. No changes in the covering layer occurred over time in control piglets.

Serology

Antibody specific to *C. pylori* was present in the serum of all piglets 2 weeks after bacterial challenge and at the final examination interval but not at 1 week after challenge. Control piglets did not produce antibody specific for the organism.

Discussion

The results of this study demonstrate that the neonatal gnotobiotic piglet is susceptible to infection by *C. pylori*. Under conditions that failed to induce bacterial colonization in several animal species, a persistent infection of the piglet stomach was established. Although competing bacteria which could limit the sites for colonization were eliminated by maintaining the piglets in germ-free isolators, *C. pylori* colonization following oral challenge was essentially restricted to the stomach. This tissue tropism corresponds to a similar site of colonization in humans.

In parallel with the development of bacterial colonization the gastric mucosa was first infiltrated by neutrophils which, after 2 weeks following challenge, dissipated and was replaced by an infiltration of mononuclear leukocytes. Early in the infection small aggregates of inflammatory cells became apparent. As the infection intensified these aggregates of immune cells increased in size and number. No ulcers, however, were observed through the 4 weeks of observation.

The histopathological and microbiological results in this report were recently confirmed by Lambert *et al.* [6]. Also working with neonatal gnotobiotic piglets, the Australian group demonstrated that when piglets were challenged only 3 h after derivation, infection was affected with a suspension of 10^6 cfu of *C. pylori.*

Antibody specific for *C. pylori* developed in response to the bacterium, further indicating that an infection developed from the challenge. First detected in sera collected 2 weeks after challenge, the antibody titer remained high through the remainder of the study period. Control piglets did not have antibody specific for the organism in their serum.

The model of gastritis was remarkably similar to the human disease state. Bacterial colonization and inflammation was dispersed over all anatomical regions of the piglet stomach and the duodenal bulb but not in other tissues of the GI tract, just as occurs in human gastritis associated with *C. pylori.* As in the natural disease mucus depletion was apparent in the model. The neonatal gnotobiotic piglet appears to be a useful host for further characterization of the pathogenicity of *C. pylori.*

References

1. Buck GF, Gourley WK, Lee WK, Subramanyam K, Latinus JM, DiNuzzo AR (1986) Relation of *Campylobacter pyloridis* to gastritis and peptic ulcer. J Infect Dis 153:664–669
2. Goodwin CS, Armstrong JA, Marshall BJ (1986) *Campylobacter pyloridis,* gastritis, and peptic ulceration. J Clin Pathol 39:353–365
3. Jones DM, Eldridge J, Fox AJ, Sethi P, Whorwell PJ (1986) Antibody to the gastric *Campylobacter*-like organism *(Campylobacter pyloridis)* – Clinical correlations and distribution in the normal population. J Med Microbiol 22:56–72
4. Jubb KVF, Kennedy PC, Palmer N (1985) Pathology of domestic animals, 3rd edn. Academic Press, New York, pp 24–49 (Vol 2)
5. Kasper G, Dickgieber N (1984) Isolation of *Campylobacter*-like bacteria from gastric epithelium. Infection 12:179–180
6. Lambert JR, Borromeo M, Turner H, Korman MG, Hansky J (1987) Colonization of gnotobiotic piglets with *Campylobacter pyloridis.* Gastroenterology 92:1489
7. Marshall BJ (1986) *Campylobacter pyloridis* and gastritis. J Infect Dis 153:650–657
8. Marshall BJ, Armstrong JA, McGechie DB, Glancy RJ (1985) Attempt to fulfil Koch's postulates for pyloric campylobacter. Med J Aust 142:439–444

9. Morris A, Nicholson G (1987) Ingestion of *Campylobacter pyloridis* causes gastritis and raised fasting gastric pH. Am J Gastroenterol 82:192 – 199
10. Rollason TP, Stone J, Rhodes JM (1984) Spiral organisms in endoscopic biopsies of the human stomach. J Clin Path 37:23 – 26
11. Tricottet V, Bruneval P, Vire O, Camilleri JP, Bloch F, Bonte N, Roge J (1986) *Campylobacter*-like organisms and surface epithelium abnormalities in active chronic gastritis in humans: An ultrastructural study. Ultra Pathol 10:113 – 122
12. Tytgat GNJ, Langenberg ML, Rauws E, Rietra PJGM (1985) *Campylobacter*-like organisms (CLO) in the human stomach. Gastroenterology 88:1620 – 1628
13. Warren JR, Marshall BJ (1983) Unidentified curved bacilli on the gastric epithelium in active chronic gastritis. Lancet I:1273 – 1275

Discussion

Langenberg: Did the neutrophilic infiltrate disappear completely after a few weeks, or did it merely decrease?

Kraft: Essentially, to our level of detection the neutrophilic response disappeared.

Goodwin: Did you do transmission electron microscopy to see adherence pedestals in the lesions?

Kraft: No, we have not done so to this time.

Goodwin: Did you notice in the duodenum what the tissue normally is in the piglet? In the human there are different types of histology of the duodenum; you may find what we call gastric metaplasia. Do you know the histology of the duodenum in infected piglets?

Kraft: No, we have not characterized the tissue of the piglet duodenum.

Mégraud: You mentioned that you have cultured rectal swabs. Were these positive?

Kraft: No, all rectal samples were negative. Essentially we recovered no organism outside the stomach or duodenal bulb.

Wyatt: Was the detection of *C. pylori* from the esophagus and the duodenum made on the basis of histology or on the basis of microbiological culture?

Kraft: Detection was made on the basis of microbiological culture. As I have stated in my paper, we expect that recovery from the esophagus or duodenum below the bulb is simply an artifact of tissue preparation.

Wyatt: You did not observe colonization on the duodenum?

Kraft: Not in the esophagus or remainder of the duodenum below the duodenal bulb.

Börsch: Prof. Goodwin raised a point which I think is very important and which we should make very clear. One of the most pressing questions of *Campylobacter* physiology and pathophysiology is its high association with duodenal ulcer disease. We know that *Campylobacter* does not live in normal duodenal mucosa, and you have shown that in your model *Campylobacter* did inhabit the duodenal bulb. You have also shown on your slides that it caused microscopic lesions. It is very important to look at the kind of duodenal mucosa which your piglets had — whether or not there was gastric metaplasia — because it is the only theoretical model to explain infestation in the human duodenum.

Kraft: The comments are well accepted.

O'Moráin: You mentioned that you rendered the gnotobiotic piglets achlorhydric. How did you do this? Was it essential?

Kraft: Yes, we did. The method was orally to administer cimetidine 3 h prior to challenge. The need for cimetidine administration is not certain. Basically, our protocol follows that for the human challenge studies.

Tytgat: Do you know whether other investigators have used the same model and failed?

Kraft: The results of our study have been confirmed recently by Lambert and coworkers. Their report was given at the AGA meeting in May. We have tried to use conventional piglets and were not successful.

Tytgat: Did the strain which you used come from one single subject or did you use a mixture of various strains?

Kraft: We used a mixture of strains which were human isolates.

von Wulffen: When you infected the gnotobiotic piglets, did you see any signs of general disease which could indicate acute inflammation, fever, high leukocyte count etc.?

Kraft: No we did not. There was a transient diarrhea and an apparent anorexia in many of the piglets, but otherwise the piglets did not indicate a clinical disease.

Tytgat: You mentioned that there was an accumulation of mucus in the stomachs of the infected pigs. Can you tell us a bit more about this, for example the volume? Was there increased mucus production or delayed gastric emptying in the pigs?

Kraft: I can say that mucus accumulation was substantial in the early days after challenge. Very solid plugs of some one-half inch in length were noted, but these seemed to be resolving in the later phases of infection when mucus depletion became evident. The production of mucus appeared to us to be a typical inflammatory response to the bacterium that would resolve with time.

Section 2

Pathophysiology of Gastritis and Peptic Ulcer Disease

Current Theories on Pathogenesis of Peptic Ulcer Disease

W. Roesch

While in the nineteenth century duodenal ulcer was extremely rare and gastric ulcer was essentially a disease of young women, epidemiology changed during the first half of this century, with male predominance and duodenal ulcers leading by about 4:1 (Langman, 1979). Recently there has been a constant decrease, at least in hospital admissions, for peptic ulcer disease, especially in duodenal ulcers, while the complication rates remain constant or even show a considerable increase in older patients, with hemorrhage and perforation, most probably due to consumption of nonsteroidal anti-inflammatory drugs (Wait et al., 1985).

The reasons why people develop ulcers are poorly understood. Whereas 50 years ago the poor were believed to be prone to gastric ulcers whilst the more affluent were thought to be more likely to develop duodenal ulcers, this apparently no longer holds true: mortality statistics and incidence studies suggest that both duodenal and gastric ulcer are now more frequent among the poorer in society. Although smokers are marginally more prone to ulcers than nonsmokers, there is a lack of coincidence in the trends of peptic ulcer mortality and cumulative cigarette consumption (Sonnenberg, 1986). As far as dietary habits are concerned students who drink coffee and cola-like drinks as well as those who smoke have been shown to be more likely to develop ulcers than those who do not (Paffenberger et al. 1974). The assertion that milk consumption protects against later ulcer whilst alcohol intake has no specific effect must be questioned in view of recent findings that a diet with high milk content has an adverse effect on the healing rate of duodenal ulcers (Kumar et al. 1986). Scandinavian authors have suggested that a diet low in fiber makes people more prone to develop ulcers whereas a high-fiber diet is more protective, but the data of a 6-month ulcer prevention study are not very convincing. There is some evidence that dietary salt may be a risk factor in gastric ulcer disease (Sonnenberg 1985), but individual consequences remain doubtful. There is good evidence to suggest that habitual aspirin intake will predispose one to gastric ulceration, although the risk is small. Nonsteroidal antirheumatic agents are probably ulcerogenic whereas small doses of corticosteroids do not cause ulcers (Conn and Blitzer 1976). In terms of erosions and microbleeding aspirin is significantly more toxic than other NSAIDs; the mechanism of impaired adaptation to continued ingestion is still poorly understood.

Concerning pathogenesis of peptic ulcer many facts are known on impaired function in the context of imbalance of aggressive and protective factors, but natural history and relapse rates are difficult to explain with current theories. Most probably, peptic ulceration is not a single disease; especially gastric ulcers seem to be a heterogenous condition: the common single gastric ulcer on the lesser curve is associated with normal or decreased acid secretion and moderately increased gastrin production, while prepyloric ulcers are characterized by increased acid and gastrin levels and by increased active pepsin. Pyloric and prepyloric ulcers have a lower peak pentagastrin-stimulated acid output (<20 mmol/l) than duodenal ulcers and may be caused by a primary pyloroantral motor disturbance.

There is no doubt that the 1910 maxim of Schwarz – "no acid no ulcer" – is still relevant and forms the basis for all successful therapeutic efforts against parietal cell function. With the currently known four receptors at the parietal cell (histamine, acetylcholine, gastrin and prostaglandin E_2) the intracellular pathway with ATP as energy source and the Ca^{2+} dependence of acid secretion as well as the proton pump exchanging K^+ and H^+, we are offered many ways to interfere with acid secretion (Fig. 1). There is a close correlation between acid suppression and healing of duodenal ulcer, especially in cases involving nocturnal acid suppression, whereas the situation for gastric ulcer is not as clear-cut (Hunt et al. 1986).

However, acid and pepsin are only one facet of peptic ulcer disease although in duodenal ulcers parietal cell mass, gastrin sensitivity, postprandial gastrin release, peak acid output and enhanced gastric emptying speak in favor of an acid overload to the duodenal mucosa. Recently Isenberg et al. (1986) have shown an impaired proximal duodenal mucosal bicarbonate secretion

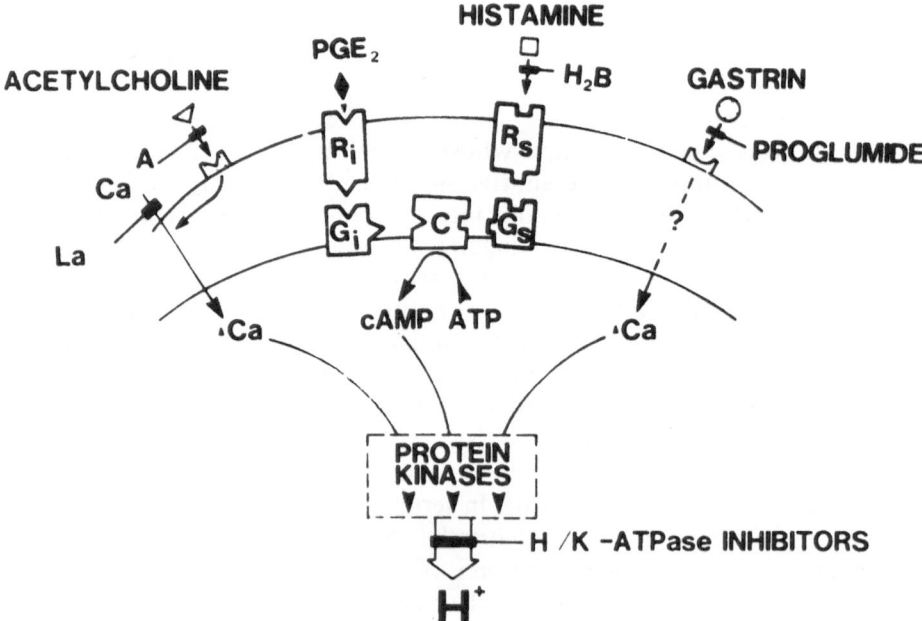

Fig. 1. Model for the regulation of parietal cell function (according to Soll 1986) with gastrin, histamine, acetylcholine and PGE_2 receptors at the surface

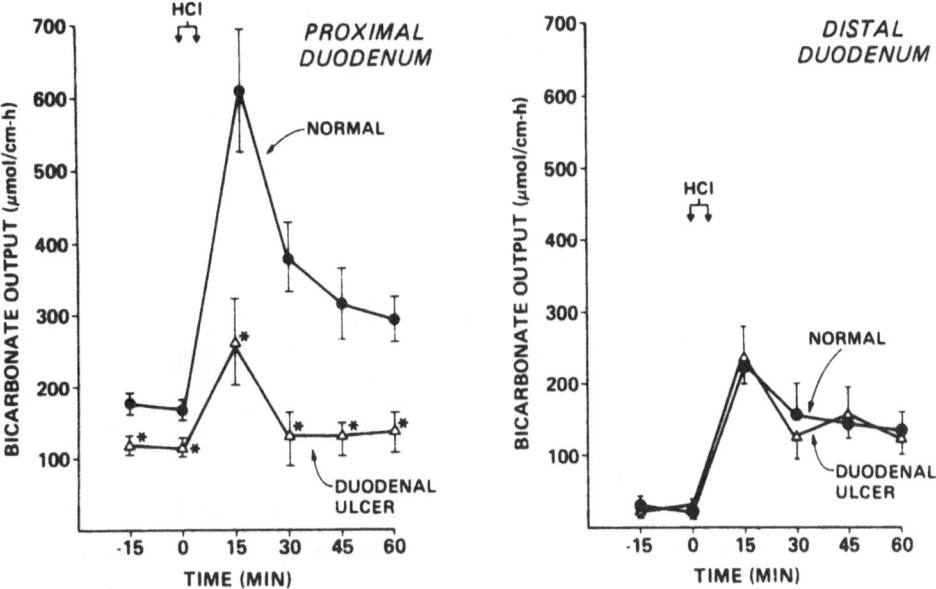

Fig. 2. Impaired bicarbonate output in the proximal and distal duodenum in duodenal ulcer patients (according to Isenberg et al. 1987)

(Fig. 2) in which in response to a physiologic amount of hydrochloric acid peak bicarbonate output was only 41% of the normal response. An unstirred layer of adherent mucus acts as a permeability barrier to luminal pepsin: in patients with peptic ulcer disease the structure is deficient because of decreased polymerization of the component glycoproteins. This impairment is associated with increased amounts of pepsin 1, which digests the mucus layer more aggressively than does the major pepsin, pepsin 3 (Allen et al. 1986) (Fig. 3).

It has been suggested that a deficiency in locally synthetized prostaglandins underlies gastric and duodenal ulcer disease, mediating mucosal lesions induced by nonsteroidal antiinflammatory drugs. There is good evidence that prostanoids protect deeper mucosal cells from necrotic damage by local irritants, enhance the process of epithelial restitution, stimulate bicarbonate secretion, and increase mucosal blood flow. However, therapy combining antisecretory with cytoprotective properties does not offer superiority to conventional treatment. During cigarette smoking prostaglandin synthesis within the gastric mucosa decreases (Cohen et al. 1986). At the same time bile reflux increases (Müller-Lissner 1986), and pancreatic bicarbonate output decreases. There is also some evidence that acid output and pepsinogen I concentration are increased in smokers (Parente et al. 1985; Whitfield and Hobsley 1985). All these phaenomena may interfere with ulcer healing and relapse.

The role of infectious agents, such as herpes simplex virus and *Campylobacter pylori*, and of chemical irritants, such as nitrites, is speculative (Wormsley 1983). Although there is substantial evidence that antimicrobial therapy using tripotassium dicitratobismuthate or gyrase inhibitors heal re-

LUMEN

SOLUBLE MUCUS - LUBRICANT   HCL   PEPSIN   DEGRADED MUCUS

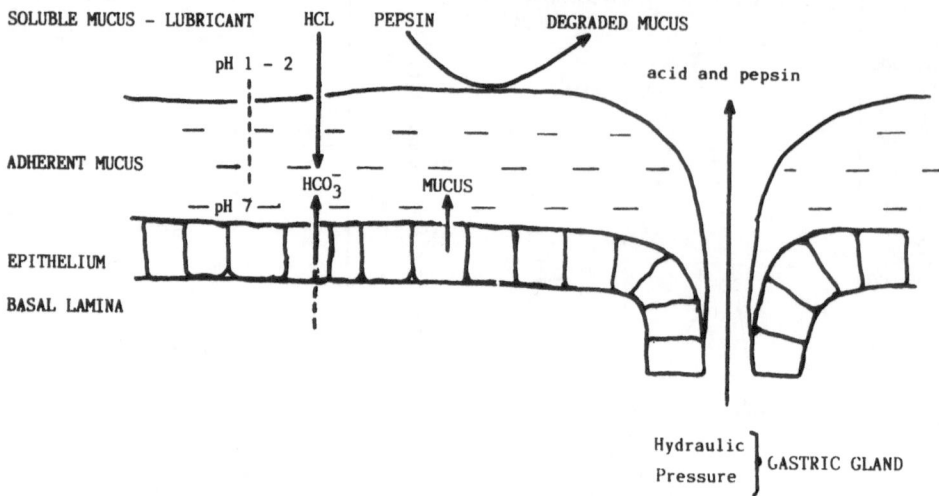

Fig. 3. The mucus-bicarbonate barrier protecting against endogenous aggressors, acid and pepsin (according to Allen 1986)

fractory ulcers (McLean et al. 1985; Ottenjann and Bayerdörffer, 1987), controlled tests are urgently needed to confirm or falsify the hypothesis that peptic ulcer is an infectious disorder.

One interesting aspect of recent clinical trials is the fact that up to 40% of peptic ulcers and under H_2-blocker treatment even up to 80% are asymptomatic (Jorde et al. 1986). Follow-up studies performed by Wormsley indicate that these asymptomatic ulcers may persist for years, however about 70% eventually become symptomatic, but when treated medically, these heal within 4−8 weeks. The other aspect which is of clinical relevance is the maintenance of ulcer healing. Relapse rates may be influenced by the choice of drug, with conflicting data in favour of noninhibitory drugs (McLean et al. 1985). For instance, bismuth subcitrate, which kills *Campylobacter*-like organisms, has a reported relapse rate between 43% and 62% versus a relapse rate of 80% with H_2-blocker treated patients. Smokers and patients with high gastric secretory capacities have a greater tendency to relapse during maintenance treatment (Battaglia et al. 1985; Ippoliti 1985). Furthermore, patients whose duodenal ulcers heal slowly and those with prepyloric ulcers tend to relapse earlier (Wormsley 1986) and may need a higher maintenance dose, i.e., cimetidine 400 mg twice daily. If ulcers remain in remission during the first 12 months of maintenance, treatment remission usually persists as long as treatment is continued; apparently the natural history of these ulcers is changed as long as maintenance treatment lasts. Although we do not yet have data that maintenance treatment reduces ulcer mortality (most complications occur without warning in elderly patients taking nonsteroidal antiinflammatory drugs) break-through ulcers are clinically benign.

Peptic ulcer disease remains an unknown entity as far as pathogenesis is concerned. An argument against the currently practiced favouring of the

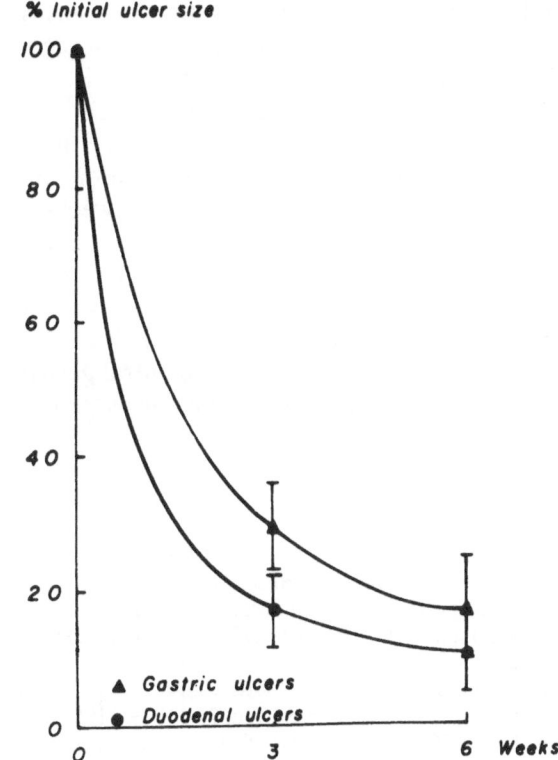

% Initial ulcer size

▲ Gastric ulcers
● Duodenal ulcers

Fig. 4. Healing-time course of incompletely healed gastric and duodenal ulcers as a function of time (According to Scheurer et al. 1977)

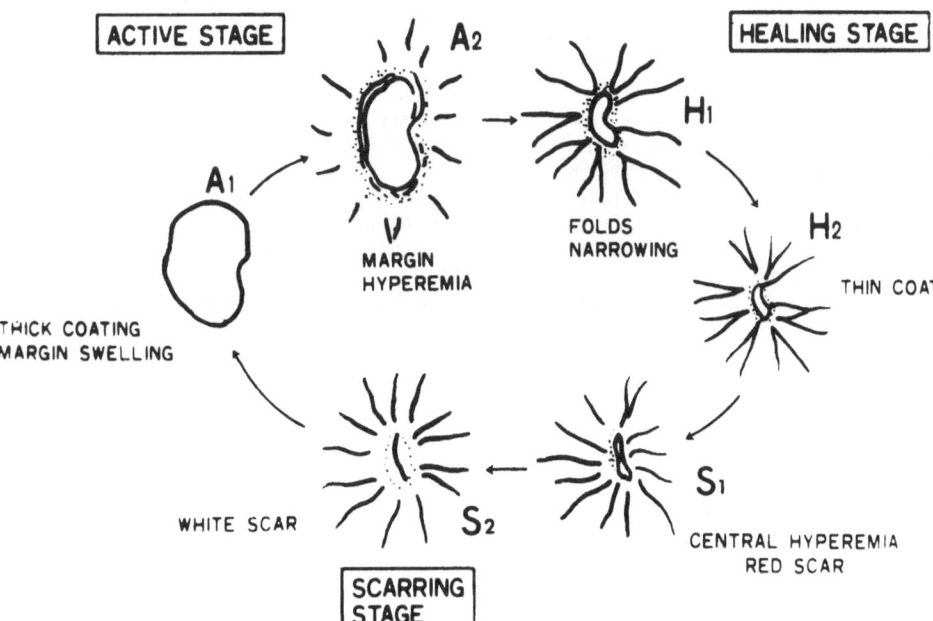

Fig. 5. Life cycle of benign ulcer

Schwarz dictum is the observation that gastric and duodenal ulcers exhibit the same healing kinetics when treated with placebo (Scheurer et al. 1977) (Fig. 4). Morphogenesis of the healing process is, according to Japanese authors, relatively uniform: the benign cycle of ulcer healing shows characteristic features with concentric or linear diminution of the ulcer crater, converging folds, and finally a red scar due to capillarization underneath a thin atrophic mucosa (Fig. 5). It usually takes another 4–6 weeks before a white scar develops which remains visible for 1 or 2 years unless recurrence occurs usually at the same site. However, in some patients ulcer shows a tendency to change localization depending upon the extent of gastritis, wandering from the duodenum towards the cardia within several years (Rösch et al. 1975). We may therefore consider the therapeutic interference with antral gastritis which is closely related to *Campylobacter pylori* infection, to be one way to prevent ulcer relapses.

References

1. Allen A, Hutton DA, Leonard AJ, Pearson JP, Sellers LA (1986) The role of mucus in the protection of the gastroduodenal mucosa. Scand J Gastroenterol 21 (suppl 125) 71–77
2. Battaglia G, Farini R, DiMario F, Vianello F, Piccoli A, Plebani M, Naccarato R (1985) Is maximal acid output useful in identifying relapsing duodenal ulcer patients? J Clin Gastroenterol 7:375–378
3. Cohen MM, McCready DR, Clark L (1985) Cigarette smoking reduces human gastric luminal prostaglandin E_2. Gut 26:1192–1196
4. Conn HO, Blitzer BL (1976) Non-association of adrenocorticosteroid therapy and peptic ulcer. New Engl J Med 294:473–479
5. Hunt RH, Howden CW, Jones DB, Burget DW, Kerr GD (1986) The correlation between acid suppression and peptic ulcer healing. Scand J Gastroenterol 21 (suppl 125), 22–29
6. Isenberg JI, Selling JA, Hogan DL, Koss MA (1987) Impaired proximal duodenal mucosal bicarbonate secretion in patients with duodenal ulcer. New Engl J Med 316:374–379
7. Ippoliti AF (1985) Prognostic factors in ulcer disease: are they real, are they relevant? J Clin Gastroenterol 7:445–446
8. Jorde R, Bostad L, Burhol PG (1986) Asymptomatic gastric ulcer: A follow-up study in patients with previous gastric ulcer disease. Lancet I, 119–121
9. Kumar N, Kumar A, Broor SL, Vij JC, Anand BS (1986) Effect of milk on patients with duodenal ulcers. Br med J 293:666
10. Langman MJS (1979) The epidemiology of chronic digestive disease. London, Arnold
11. McLean AJ, Harrison PM, Joannides-Demos L, Byrne AJ, McCarthy P, Dudley FJ (1985) The choice of ulcer healing agent influences duodenal ulcer relapse rate and long-term clinical outcome. Aust NZ J Med 15:367–374
12. Müller-Lissner SA (1986) Bile reflux is increased in cigarette smokers. Gastroenterology 90:1205–1209
13. Ottenjann R, Bayerdörffer E (1987) Campylobacter pyloridis. Opportunist oder Pathogen im oberen Magen-Darm-Trakt. Dt Ärztebl 84:1045–1046
14. Paffenberger RS, Wing AL, Hyde RT (1974) Chronic disease in former college students. Amer J Epidemiol 100:307–315
15. Parente F, Lazzaroni M, Sangaletti O, Baroni S, Bianchi-Porro G (1985) Cigarette smoking, gastric acid secretion, and serum pepsinogen I concentrations in duodenal ulcer patients. Gut 26:1327–1332
16. Rösch W, Kinzler E, Demling L (1973) Das Ulcusrezidiv-Langzeitbeobachtungen. In: Demling L, Moser K, Rösch W (eds) Das peptische Ulkus. Pathophysiologie, Diagnose, Therapie. Schattauer, Stuttgart-New York
17. Scheurer U, Witzel L, Halter F, Keller HM, Huber R, Galeazzi R (1977) Gastric and duodenal ulcer healing under placebo treatment. Gastroenterology, 72:838–841

18. Schwarz K (1910) Über penetrierende Magen- und Jejunalgeschwüre. Bruns Beitr Klin Chir 67:96−128
19. Soll AH (1986) Mechanisms of action of antisecretory drugs. Scand J Gastroenterol (suppl 125) 21:1−6
20. Sonnenberg A (1986) Smoking and mortality from peptic ulcer in the United Kingdom. Gut 27:1369−1372
21. Sonnenberg A (1986) Dietary salt is a risk factor in gastric ulcer disease. Gastroenterology 90:1642
22. Wait R, Katschinski B, Logan R, Ashley J, Langman M (1986) Rising frequency of ulcer perforation in elderly people in the United Kingdom. Lancet I:489−491
23. Whitfield PF, Hobsley M (1985) Maximal gastric secretion in smokers and nonsmokers with duodenal ulcer. Brit J Surg 72:955−957
24. Wormsley KG (1983) Duodenal ulcer: does pathophysiology equal aetiology? Gut 24:775−780
25. Wormsley KG (1986) Ulcer disease: medical treatment. Current Opinion in Gastroenterology 2:855−868

Discussion

Classen: What do you think about the role of physical activity in the pathophysiology of duodenal ulcer? And secondly, is alcohol protective or aggressive?

Rösch: The second question is easier to answer than the first. Alcohol up to 20 g per day seems to speed healing. That constant alcohol consumption is protective, I would doubt, for this may be deleterious to further life; but small amounts of alcohol apparently do speed healing. Therefore we should not ask our patients to abstain from alcohol. Physical activity is difficult to quantify, and if you consider joggers losing small amounts of blood apparently because the abdominal perfusion is markedly decreased, one could speculate that this may also interfere with mucosal perfusion of the gastric mucosa. This might not be a good idea for a patient who is prone to develop gastric or duodenal ulcers. But there is considerable speculation as to this and I doubt whether one can quantify or recommend a certain amount of physical activity to an ulcer patient simply to prevent ulcer relapse.

Classen: You misunderstand me. Is hard physical labour, such as brick laying, a factor?

Rösch: It is very difficult to answer your question, but if you look back a little in ulcer history, you will find that ulcer incidence has always been especially high among heavy laborers. So one could argue that the decrease in ulcer incidence is due to a decrease in physical activity. But you seem to mean the opposite!

Konturek: I think that Professor Classen meant the physical activity of the stomach and duodenum rather than that of the whole body. Could you comment on this? Gastrointestinal motility, particularly gastric emptying is, of course, an important factor in the pathogenesis of peptic ulcer. Could you comment on what the role might be of changes in emptying of the stomach, of the motility of the duodenum, in the formation and therapy of peptic ulcer?

Rösch: I mentioned that the maladie antral of Liebermann-Meffert may be one reason why some people develop recurrent prepyloric or pyloric ulcers, and that motility interferes with ulcer development. In duodenal ulcers we find in many patients enhancement of gastric emptying and in gastric ulcer patients we find delayed gastric emptying, at least during the time of active ulceration. There are very few trials in which metoclopramide or domperidone was tried as an ulcer drug; these have yielded very conflicting data, some studies showing no effect, some showing enhancement of ulcer healing, but all these studies are impaired by a very small number of participants, only 10 or 20.

Ober: Professor Rösch, is it a wisdom based on the large number of theories as to the reason for peptic ulcer disease which have not held true? What would you require – as you shy away from embracing *Campylobacter pylori* as a cause for peptic ulcer disease – to accept *C. pylori* as a cause for peptic disease? If you look at the epidemiological data, at the fact that *C. pylori* produces toxins, at the antibodies that can be found in gastric juice as well as in blood, at the fact that strange drugs – strange for peptic ulcer disease (namely chemotherapeutic agents) – can cure the disease, at the self-experiments that have been done, and at those gnotobiotic piglets, the question really arises, what would a clinician want to be presented with in order to accept *C. pylori* as a cause of this disease.

Rösch: I purposely avoided *Campylobacter* because I had hope that by the end of this symposium we would be able to answer this question, although I now fear that we may not. What is very difficult to explain by this infection theory are the epidemiological changes which I have shown you – that about 70 or 80 or 100 years ago gastric ulcer was 20 times more common than duodenal ulcer, compared to nowadays. There must be a reason for this. Why do some people develop a gastric or duodenal ulcer only once in life, which, when treated, disappears. Why do many ulcers remain asymptomatic for 5 or 10 years and, upon finally becoming symptomatic and receiving treatment, heal within 4 weeks. So there are many questions to be answered. The infection theory comes up every 20 – 25 years. The last time it was herpes simplex virus that was the infectious agent as postulated by Danish authors, and now it is *Campylobacter,* and maybe in 10 years it will be another bug or another virus. So I think one really must prove that this agent causes the lesion, that the lesion disappears concomitant with the agent, and that recurrence is closely correlated with the recurrence of the infectious agent. I think that there are many problems involved here and many answers still to be given. It is a nice hypothesis, but no more.

Tytgat: You did not think that you would get that question, did you? Come now, *Campylobacter* proponents; where are you? Barry Marshall?

Marshall: Perhaps I have been presented with this problem longer than most people. I have come to the conclusion that the current theories of ulcer production are to gastroenterologists as Judaism is to Jews. I have Jewish friends whom I can tell how nice it is to eat bacon, and whom I can show an analysis of bacon, but they will still not eat the bacon. As with a religious belief, I do not think we will convert many gastroenterologists into thinking that ulcer disease is an infection. I think we must wait until they retire from practice and are replaced by new gastroenterologists.

Tytgat: Professor Rösch, does it surprise you that the bicarbonate secretory capacity proximally in the duodenum is abnormal in duodenal ulcer? That the mucosa is abnormal there has been very well shown by South African clinicians. Does this surprise you?

Rösch: It surprises me that it was attempted for a long time to prove this, and that nobody succeeded. It is an old postulate that the mucosa in the duodenal bulb is especially susceptible to H ions, and that the bicarbonate output might be impaired. One initially postulated that the pancreatic bicarbonate output was decreased, which is the case, as Konturek has shown, during cigarette smoking. These new findings are, in my opinion, somewhat surprising in showing that the decrease amounts to 60% in the duodenal bulb, where the ulcer is located. And we might interfere here with prostaglandins, for instance, and increase and normalize the bicarbonate output. Whether this causes healing or not, is entirely another matter.

Tytgat: What is then the most damaging effect of cigarette smoking?

Rösch: This is very speculative. It is multifactorial. There is some impairment of the mucosal bloodflow, there is impairment of the prostaglandin synthesis, there is apparently impairment in the volume, but not in the H ion output. What the decisive factor is, I cannot tell you.

Börsch: Because this is a *Campylobacter* meeting we should discuss the very old German gastroenterological notion that ulcer disease is gastritis-associated ulcer disease. We learned from Konjetzny many years ago that in patients with peptic ulcer we can almost invariably find antral gastritis. We should not go as far as to state that *Campylobacter* is the cause, the sufficient cause, for ulcers, but we should speculate as to whether, in addition to acidity, we should introduce *C. pylori* as one more factor into the pathophysiology of ulcer disease. I would like you to comment on this.

Rösch: It is true that especially gastric ulcer is closely associated with gastritis. But when the gastric ulcer is situated very close to the cardia, one finds severe chronic atrophic gastritis and almost no acidity in the stomach. This is another fact on which we can speculate as to whether the definite healing of ulcer disease is due to chronic atrophic gastritis developing in the stomach. And as soon as there is chronic atrophic gastritis, the *Campylobacter* disappears; but you still have ulcer disease. It takes a little longer for the ulcer to disappear. And we have many patients who began at the age of 30 with duodenal ulcer and by the age of 60 had developed a gastric ulcer situated very close to the cardia.

The Mucus Bicarbonate Barrier and Its Role in Gastroduodenal Mucosal Protection *

G. Flemström, L. Knutson, and E. Kivilaakso

The Gastroduodenal Mucus-Bicarbonate Surface Layer

Almost a hundred years ago Pavlov suggested that "alkaline mucus" lining the gastric mucosa neutralized luminal acid (Pavlov 1898). Much later, Hollander postulated that gastric secretion of an alkaline (non-parietal) fluid took place, and that this was produced at a constant rate (see Hollander 1963). He also provided experimental evidence for the occurrence of bicarbonate in the secretion from gastric fundic pouches in dogs after inhibition of the acid secretion by vagotomy and antrectomy. During the last 10 years it has been demonstrated that gastric antral and fundic mucosa in several species, including man, secretes bicarbonate to the lumen by processes which depend on tissue metabolism, and that the secretion can be stimulated and inhibited by a variety of means. Furthermore, the surface epithelium in the duodenum possesses a similarly metabolism-dependent ability to secrete bicarbonate. The rates of secretion are higher in the duodenum than in the stomach and higher in proximal than in more distal segments of the duodenum. In addition, the duodenum shows distinct differences from the stomach with respect both to the processes of the transport of bicarbonate and to the control of the secretion (Flemström and Turnberg 1984; Flemström 1987).

The mucus gel adherent to the epithelial surface, together with the gastric and duodenal secretions of bicarbonate, is most probably important in the mucosal protection against luminal acid and pepsin. The use of pH-sensitive microelectrodes inserted into the gel has shown that the pH within the gel is near neutral in spite of high acidities in the luminal bulk solution (cf. Fig. 1). In addition, there is a close correlation between the alkalinity of the surface gel and the rate of metabolic-dependent bicarbonate secretion. In human, rabbit, and frog gastric mucosa in vitro and human and rat stomach in vivo, the pH at the epithelial surface is near neutral when that in the luminal solution is $2.0 - 3.0$ (Bahari et al. 1982; Takeuchi et al. 1983; Quigley and Turnberg 1987). It should be noted that there is a leakage of bicarbonate across damaged mucosa and also that this passive diffusion increases pH at the surface to values considerably higher than that in the luminal bulk solution (Kiviluoto et al.

* This work was supported by the Swedish Medical Research Council (grant 04X-3515), the Tore Nilsson Foundation and the Medical Research Council of the Academy of Finland.

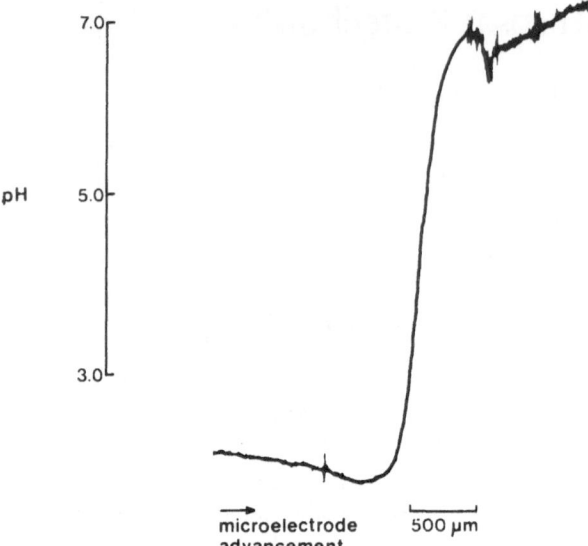

Fig. 1. Recording of pH at the surface of duodenum in situ (~25 mm distal to the pylorus) in an anesthetized rat. A pH-sensitive antimony microelectrode was advanced vertically from the luminal bulk solution (pH 2.0) across the surface layer into the mucosa at a constant speed. A surface pH gradient is demonstrated with neutral pH in the immediate vicinity of the luminal surface in spite of that in the lumen being as low as pH 2.0

1987). An unstirred layer supporting a pH gradient on top of damaged mucosa is probably made of a fibrin-based gel containing mucus and necrotic cells (Allen et al. 1986).

In the rat duodenum in vivo, the surface pH is neutral when the pH in the lumen is 2.0 and a surface pH gradient is maintained even at a luminal pH of 1.2 (Flemström and Kivilaakso 1983; Kivilaakso and Flemström 1984). Positioning of electrodes in proximal duodenum by endoscopy have recently enabled the identification of a similar pH gradient at the duodenal surface in humans (Quigley and Turnberg 1987). The pH in the duodenum seldom falls below 2.0, and the bicarbonate secretion by the surface epithelium may be its main defence mechanism against acid. In the stomach high luminal acidities (pH 1.0−2.0) predominate over the alkalinity of the surface gradient, with consequent acidification of the epithelial surface. It seems probable therefore that additional mechanisms for defence such as the restitution of the mucosa are more important in the stomach than in duodenum. It should also be noted that only the surface epithelium is covered with mucus in the stomach and that other mechanisms seem necessary for protecting the (chief and parietal) cells lining the gastric crypts. It has been reported that the apical membrane of gastric chief cells possesses remarkable inherent ability to resist luminal acid (Sanders et al. 1985).

The composition and structure of gastric and duodenal mucus have recently been reviewed in detail by Allen and Carrol (1985). The mucus forms a continuous thin layer of water-insoluble, visco-elastic gel adherent to the surface of the epithelium. The actual thickness of the gel reflects the balance between the secretion of mucus at the epithelial surface and the continuous degradation of the gel by pepsin at the lumen-facing surface. The mucus gel at the gastric surface is impermeable to pepsin, and the surface alkalinity should inactivate pepsin. The thickness of the surface gradient recorded with pH-sensitive microelectrodes in the stomach of the rabbit, rat, frog, and man ($350-1000 \, \mu m$) and in the duodenum of the rat ($\sim 700 \, \mu m$) is greater than the measured thickness of the gradient in the mucus gel ($50-500 \, \mu m$). This discrepancy may be partly due to inclusion of an unstirred layer of water outside the gel in the pH gradient (Allen et al. 1983).

Physiological Control of Mucosal Bicarbonate Secretion

The demonstration of an alkaline surface layer in the stomach and duodenum and of its dependence on mucosal alkaline secretion has made the study of the mechanisms for regulating this secretion particularly relevant. Three ways in which mucosal protection against the acid could be enhanced are:

1) simultaneous neural stimulation of gastroduodenal bicarbonate and gastric acid secretion,
2) local mucosal linkage between the process of parietal cell H^+ secretion and that of secretion of HCO_3^- by the surface epithelial cells,
3) stimulation of the gastric and duodenal bicarbonate secretion by the presence of acid in the lumen.

Recent studies have provided evidence that all three mechanisms do operate.

Neural Control

Sham-feeding is a stimulant of gastric secretion of bicarbonate (as well as of acid) in humans, an effect which is inhibited by anticholinergic drugs such as atropine and benzilonium bromide (Feldman 1985; Forssell et al. 1985). Similar stimulation of both gastric and duodenal mucosal bicarbonate secretion by sham-feeding has been demonstrated in dogs (Konturek and Thor 1986). Further evidence for the occurrence of central neural control of gastric and duodenal bicarbonate secretion are the facts that intrahypothalamic injection of corticotropine releasing factor (CRF) causes a 20-fold increase in the gastric bicarbonate content in the rat (Gunion et al. 1985), and that intracerebroventricular (but not intravenous) infusion of thyrotropin releasing factor (TRH) increases duodenal mucosal bicarbonate secretion in this species (G. Flemström, unpublished). Electrical stimulation of the vagal nerves increases both the gastric and the duodenal secretion of bicarbonate (and gastric secretion of acid) in cats and rats (Fändriks 1986; Jönsson et al. 1986; Nylander et al. 1987). Intravenous administration of pirenzepine which is classified as an M_1-selective muscarinic antagonist increases duodenal mucosal bicarbonate secretion in rats (Säfsten and Flemström 1986). Vagotomy eliminates this stimulation, suggesting that it is exerted centrally and mediated by the vagal nerves. The combined results suggest that gastroduodenal protective mechanisms are under central nervous influence (Fig. 2).

MUCOSAL PROTECTION — CNS CONTROL

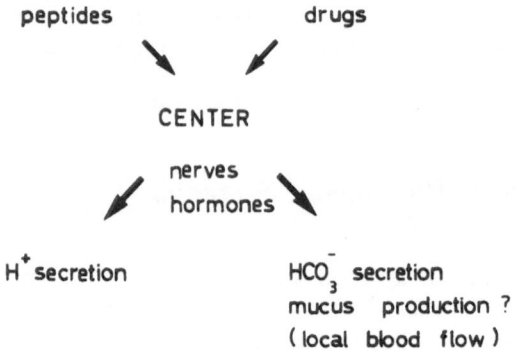

Fig. 2. Gastric and duodenal mucosal bicarbonate secretions (as previously known for gastric acid secretion) are under central nervous influence. There may therefore be a balance at the central nervous level between the control of protective bicarbonate secretion and that of acid secretion

Evidence indicating that duodenal mucosal bicarbonate secretion is also under sympathetic influence has been published recently. Adrenergic alpha$_1$-agonists stimulate the secretion in rats whereas alpha$_2$-agonists have an opposite effect (Nylander and Flemström 1986). Moderate hemorrhage, which is associated with increased sympathetic activity, also inhibits the secretion (Jönsson and Fändriks 1987). It should also be noted that ligating the adrenals increases the rise in mucosal bicarbonate secretion in response to (electrical) vagal stimulation (Jönsson et al. 1986). Catecholamines released from the adrenal medulla thus probably moderate the vagally mediated stimulation.

Role of the Acid Secretory Process

The process of acid secretion by the parietal cells is very probably important in mucosal protection. Thus, it has been demonstrated that stimulation of acid secretion (by histamine) increases the ability of the gastric mucosa to resist instilled intraluminal acid while inhibition of the secretion (by histamine H$_2$ antagonists) decreases this ability. Parenteral infusion of bicarbonate but not of other buffer species exerts a similar protective effect (Kivilaakso 1981). Furthermore, recent studies (Gannon et al. 1984) have indicated the presence of fenestrated capillaries in the rat and in human gastric mucosa. These may facilitate vascular transport of bicarbonate, released interstitially by the parietal cells during H+ secretion, to the surface epithelium for utilization in the bicarbonate secretory process.

Stimulation by Luminal Acid

The presence of acid in the lumen is a stimulant of mucosal secretion of bicarbonate in both the stomach and duodenum. This has been demonstrated in these organs in a variety of species, including humans (Heylings et al. 1984;

Isenberg et al. 1986; Flemström 1987). Mucosal endogenous production of prostaglandins, as well as humoral factors and neural mechanisms, are involved in mediating this rise in mucosal bicarbonate secretion in response to acid in the duodenum. The response to a luminal pH of 2.0 but not that to a pH of 5.0 in the rat duodenum is sensitive to inhibition of mucosal cyclooxygenase activity by aspirin (Flemström and Kivilaakso 1983), suggesting that prostaglandin production is mainly important in mediating the response at high luminal acidities.

Intake of a meat meal increases the surface epithelial bicarbonate secretion both in the stomach and in the duodenum in the conscious dog (Konturek et al. 1983). This may reflect neural stimulation of the bicarbonate secretion by the process of feeding per se, as well as local mucosal or humoral stimulation by the presence of food and/or acid in the gastroduodenal lumen.

Some Exogenous Stimulants and Inhibitors

Gastric bicarbonate secretion has been studied in amphibian mucosa in vitro, in mammals in vivo and in humans. Secretion is stimulated by dibutyryl cyclic GMP, cholinergic agents, prostaglandins, and some gastrointestinal hormones. Atropine does not affect basal (unstimulated) secretion but inhibits the response to cholinergic stimulation. Potent stimulants of gastric acid secretion such as gastrin and histamine have no effect on gastric bicarbonate secretion, indicating that the mechanisms for stimulation are different (see Flemström and Turnberg 1984; Flemström 1987).

The bicarbonate secretion by duodenal surface epithelium, devoid of Brunner's glands, has been studied in a variety of species, including humans. Prostaglandin E_2 and synthetic analogues of this prostaglandin, as well as the precursor arachidonic acid, stimulate secretion. In contrast to findings in the stomach, bicarbonate secretion by duodenal mucosa is stimulated by cyclic AMP while cyclic GMP has no effect. Vasoactive intestinal peptide (VIP) causes an up to fourfold increase in secretion in the rat and cat (Isenberg et al. 1984; Flemström et al. 1985). Stimulation of mucosal bicarbonate secretion by VIP has recently also been demonstrated in the human duodenum (Thomas et al. 1986). Very small amounts (20 ng/kg) of the endogenous opioid peptides beta-endorphin, methionine enkephalin, and leucine enkephalin increase bicarbonate secretion by the duodenal surface epithelium in man by acting on μ-opiate receptors (Flemström et al. 1986).

Future Prospects

Administration of E-type prostaglandins enhances the secretion of bicarbonate and mucus by gastric and duodenal mucosa, and the endogenous mucosal production of prostaglandins is important in the physiological control of these protective secretions. Vagal neural stimulation and administration of some peptides, including endorphins acting at μ-receptors and vasoactive intestinal polypeptide increase the bicarbonate secretion. Administration of adrenergic alpha$_2$-agonist or eliciting a sympathetic neural reflex inhibits the secretion by the duodenal mucosa in animals. Furthermore, impaired duodenal mucosal bicarbonate secretion and impaired ability of this mucosa to maintain a surface pH gradient have been reported in patients with chronic duodenal ulcer disease (Isenberg et al. 1987; Quigley and Turnberg 1987). The bicarbonate secretion by intact mucosa and bicarbonate leakage across damaged mucosa maintains a pH in the mucus gel adherent to the gastric surface which is considerably higher than that in the luminal bulk solution. This may facilitate the growth of acid-sensitive bacteria on this surface. It would seem very worthwhile to further study the local mucosal, neural, and humoral controls of gastroduodenal secretion of bicarbonate and mucus, their possible interactions, and their role in mucosal protection.

Summary

Bicarbonate secretion by the surface epithelium in the stomach and duodenum maintains a near neutral pH in the mucus gel adherent to the surface, in spite of acidities as high as pH $2.0-3.0$ in the gastric lumen, and pH $1.5-2.0$ in the duodenal lumen. This strongly suggests that the alkaline secretion together with the mucus gel provides a first line of protection in the stomach and that the secretion may be the main mechanism of defence in the duodenum. It is increased by physiological stimuli such as sham-feeding or the presence of acid in the lumen. Mucosal endogenous production of prostaglandins as well as humoral and neural mechanisms also influence the secretion. The fact that the pH in the surface mucus gel is higher than that in the gastric lumen, may facilitate growth of acid-sensitive bacteria on this surface.

References

1. Allen A, Carrol NJH (1985) Adherent and soluble mucus in the stomach and duodenum. Dig Dis Sci 30 [Suppl]: 6S – 13S
2. Allen A, Hutton D, McQueen S, Garner A (1983) Dimensions of gastroduodenal surface pH gradient exceed those of adherent mucus gel layers. Gastroenterology 85: 463 – 466
3. Allen A, Hutton A, Leonard JP, Pearson JP, Sellers LA (1986) The role of mucus in the protection of the gastroduodenal mucosa. Scand J Gastroenterol 21 [Suppl 125]: 71 – 77
4. Bahari HMM, Ross IN, Turnberg LA (1982) Demonstration of a pH gradient across the mucus layer on the surface of human gastric mucosa in vitro. Gut 23: 513 – 516
5. Fändriks L (1986) Vagal and splanchnic neural influences on gastric and duodenal bicarbonate secretions. Acta Physiol Scand 128 [Suppl 555]: 1 – 39
6. Feldman M (1985) Gastric H^+ and HCO_3^- secretion in response to sham feeding in humans. Am J Physiol 248: G 188 – G 191
7. Flemström G (1987) Gastric and duodenal mucosal bicarbonate secretion. In: Johnson LR et al. (eds) Physiology of the gastrointestinal tract, 2nd edn. Raven, New York, pp 1011 – 1029
8. Flemström G, Kivilaakso E (1983) Demonstration of a pH gradient at the luminal surface of rat duodenum in vivo and its dependence on mucosal alkaline secretion. Gastroenterology 84: 787 – 794
9. Flemström G, Turnberg LA (1984) Gastroduodenal defence mechanisms. Clin Gastroenterol 13: 327 – 354

10. Flemström G, Jedstedt G, Nylander O (1985) Effects of some opiates and vasoactive intestinal peptide (VIP) on duodenal surface epithelial bicarbonate secretion in the rat. Scand J Gastroenterol 20 [Suppl 110]:49−53
11. Flemström G, Jedstedt G, Nylander O (1986) β-endorphin and enkephalins stimulate duodenal mucosal alkaline secretion in the rat in vivo. Gastroenterology 90:368−372
12. Forssell H, Stenquist B, Olbe L (1985) Vagal stimulation of human gastric bicarbonate secretion. Gastroenterology 89:581−586
13. Gannon B, Browning J, O'Brien P, Rogers P (1984) Mucosal microvascular architecture of the fundus and body of human stomach. Gastroenterology 86:866−875
14. Gunion MW, Taché Y, Kauffman GL (1985) Intrahypothalamic corticotropin-releasing factor (CRF) increases gastric bicarbonate content. Gastroenterology 88:1407 (abstr)
15. Heylings JR, Garner A, Flemström G (1984) Regulation of gastroduodenal HCO_3^- transport by luminal acid in the frog in vitro. Am J Physiol 246:G 235−G 242
16. Hollander F (1963) The electrolyte pattern of gastric mucinous secretions: its implication for cystic fibrosis. Ann NY Acad Sci 106:757−766
17. Isenberg JI, Wallin B, Johansson C, Smedfors B, Mutt V, Takemoto K, Emås S (1984) Secretin, VIP, and PHI stimulate rat proximal duodenal surface epithelial bicarbonate secretion in vivo. Regul Pept 8:315−320
18. Isenberg JI, Hogan DL, Koss MA, Selling JA (1986) Human duodenal mucosal bicarbonate secretion. Evidence for basal secretion and stimulation by hydrochloric acid and a synthetic prostaglandin E_1. Gastroenterology 91:370−378
19. Isenberg JI, Selling JA, Hogan DL, Koss MA (1987) Impaired duodenal mucosal bicarbonate secretion in duodenal ulcer patients. N Eng J Med 316:374−379
20. Jönsson C, Fändriks L (1987) Bleeding inhibits vagally-induced duodenal HCO_3^- secretion via activation of the splanchnic nerves in anaesthetized rats. Acta Physiol Scand 130:259−264
21. Jönsson C, Nylander O, Flemström G, Fändrik L (1986) Vagal stimulation of duodenal HCO_3^- secretion in anesthetized rats. Acta Physiol Scand 128:65−70
22. Kivilaakso E (1981) High plasma HCO_3^- protects gastric mucosa against acute ulceration in the rat. Gastroenterology 81:921−927
23. Kivilaakso E, Flemström G (1984) Surface pH gradient in gastroduodenal mucosa. Scand J Gastroenterol 19 [Suppl 105]:50−52
24. Kiviluoto T, Voipio J, Kivilaakso E (1987). Is "H^+ back diffusion" following disruption of the gastric mucosal barrier in fact alkali (HCO_3^-) secretion? Gastroenterology 92:1470 (abstr)
25. Konturek SJ, Thor P (1986) Relation between duodenal alkaline secretion and motility in fasted and sham-fed dogs. Am J Physiol 251:G 591−G 596
26. Konturek SJ, Tasler J, Bilski J, Kania J (1983) Prostaglandins and alkaline secretion from oxyntic, antral, and duodenal mucosa of the dog. Am J Physiol 245:G 539−G 546
27. Nylander O, Flemström G (1986) Effects of alpha-adrenoceptor agonists and antagonists on duodenal surface epithelial HCO_3^- secretion in the rat in vivo. Acta Physiol Scand 126:433−441
28. Nylander O, Flemström G, Delbro D, Fändriks L (1987) Vagal influence on gastroduodenal HCO_3^- secretion in the cat in vivo. Am J Physiol 252:G 522−G 528
29. Pavlov JP (1898) Die Arbeit der Verdauungsdrüsen. Bergmann, Wiesbaden, pp 30−56
30. Quigley EMM, Turnberg LA (1987) pH of the microclimate lining human gastric and duodenal mucosa in vivo. Studies in control subjects and in duodenal ulcer patients. Gastroenterology 92:1876−1884
31. Säfsten B, Flemström G (1986) Stimulatory effect of pirenzepine on mucosal bicarbonate secretion in rat duodenum in vivo. Acta Physiol Scand 127:267−268
32. Sanders MJ, Ayalon A, Roll M, Soll AH (1985) The apical surface of canine chief cells resists H^+ back-diffusion. Nature 313:52−54
33. Takeuchi K, Magee D, Critchlow J, Matthews J, Silen W (1983) Studies of the pH gradient and thickness of frog gastric mucus gel. Gastroenterology 84:331−340
34. Thomas FJ, Hogan DL, Krejs GJ, Algazi M, Koss MA, Sackman JW, Isenberg JI (1986) The effect of secretin and VIP on duodenal bicarbonate secretion in humans. Gastroenterology 90:1663 (abstr)

Discussion

Konturek: There have been several reports recently that vasoactive intestinal peptide (VIP) is important, particularly in the duodenum for the stimulation of alkaline secretion also in response to duodenal acid application. Would you comment on the role of VIP in the mechanism of alkaline secretion?

Flemström: VIP is a very potent stimulant of duodenal mucosal bicarbonate secretion in animals and in man. I know of one recent abstract (Isenberg, AGA), where an antagonist of VIP was tried in the rat. It clearly decreased the rise in bicarbonate response to acid. But there is also a decrease in this response with aspirin and indomethacin. Further, such a decrease is easily demonstrable with atropine or hexamethonium.

Konturek: We have been looking at alkaline secretion in dogs and also in humans and what puzzled us was that this alkaline secretion in the stomach and duodenum was not stable but under fasting conditions it *always* fluctuated. This fluctuation was very closely associated with the changes in the motor activity of the stomach and the duodenum, the so-called migrating motor complex (MMC). We found that motilin which triggers the generation of premature MMC is also effective in the stimulation of alkaline secretion. You have been working mostly on in vitro preparations, so you probably never observed such alkaline fluctuations. But you also used intact cats and you may have observed such alkaline fluctuations. Could you comment on that?

Flemström: No, we did not. However, we have not worked with conscious animals. Your findings are further evidence for the role of the neural system in control of gastroduodenal bicarbonate secretion.

von Wulffen: Have you looked at the functional quality of different samples of mucus, different in respect to the biochemical composition of the mucus, whether they have high molecular or low molecular polymers? In view of the possible bacterial etiology one might conceive that products of a bacterium would deteriorate the mucus in some way, maybe break it down.

Flemström: We have never measured the composition of mucus but I can refer to the British work from Newcastle already referred to by Professor Rösch. A. Allen et al. have reported in *Gastroenterology* that the fraction of solubilized mucus is greater in the gel in gastric ulcer patients. This may indicate that this mucus has lower protective ability. Whether that is a cause or the consequence of the disease, is not known.

Gregor: There is a certain shortage of time but being in a meeting on *C. pylori*, I would like to ask you whether you could speculate on the interrelationship between *C. pylori* and the mucosal bicarbonate barrier.

Flemström: Nobody has tested that. I should like to know what the toxins of this bacterium are and what they do. The mere presence of a bacterium cannot be harmful. Could somebody answer this question?

Goodwin: Yes, there are plenty of toxins; there is lipid A, which is quite unusual with 3 hydroxyoctadecanoic acid, and almost certainly diffuses across the adherence pedestal. It may affect the mucus production; also you have cytotoxin and intracellular cytoplasmic vacuolization which has been described by Dr. Kraft, and there are many other toxins which may not have been discovered.

Flemström: Does this mean that you can buy them and test them?

Goodwin: Not yet, they will be available in the years to come. Nobody has produced them yet, but you could analyse lipid A as Inger Mattsby-Baltzer is doing in Göteborg.

Flemström: I feel a bit uneasy about studying ion transport in infected animals. The infection per se may affect so many systems and they may be difficult to anesthetize. What you would need would be an equally "toxic" bacterium without the gastric effects.

Marshall: There was a paper presented at the AGA in Chicago which studied the structure of mucus after incubation with *C. pylori* in vitro. *C. pylori* digested the protein substructure of the mucus and this resulted in a similar abnormality to that seen in the mucus of gastric ulcer patients when run through gel. There appears to be an alteration in the mucus induced by the organism.

Flemström: From which lab?

Marshall: I cannot remember the name.

Flemström: Mucus is difficult.

Semiquantitative Histopathology of Active Chronic Gastritis in *Campylobacter pylori* Infection and Its Relationship to Peptic Ulcer Disease and Gastric Carcinoma

H. J. Houthoff, E. A. J. Rauws, W. Langenberg, and G. N. J. Tytgat

Introduction

What is the precise relation between the presence of *Campylobacter pylori* in the mucus gel on the surface of the gastric mucosa and the simultaneous occurrence of various disease entities such as active chronic gastritis, peptic ulcer disease of the stomach or duodenum, or gastric carcinoma? Among the many publications following the renewed interest in bacteria in the stomach, several focussed on their relation to active chronic gastritis [1–4] and benign peptic ulcer disease [5, 6]. It barely needs further clarification that a relation with these disease entities exists; a relation with gastric carcinoma has so far not been documented.

What still remains to be elucidated is the type of relation between *C. pylori* and the various disease entities, especially, whether *C. pylori* infection is a consequence rather than a causal factor of the pathologic alterations, what are the source and natural history of a primo infection, and (in case of a causal relation) whether the bacterium is a necessary and sufficient etiologic factor or forms only one of the conditions in a multifactorial pathogenesis.

In this paper the contribution of semiquantitative histopathology in carefully selected patient groups is reviewed, as part of the answer to some of the questions raised. Most of the results are from previous studies of the authors [7–10], and for detailed information the reader is referred to these publications.

Methods and Patient Series

Endoscopic biopsies and surgically removed specimens from the stomach and duodenum, processed for routine histopathology, provide suitable material for scoring the presence and amount of *C. pylori* in the mucus gel and for semiquantitative grading of the type, intensity, and distribution of the inflammatory infiltrate and the mucosal damage.

C. pylori can be visualized with special staining techniques, such as Whartin-Starry silver staining (Fig. 1a), or with monoclonal or monospecific polyclonal antibodies in an immunohistologic procedure (Fig. 1b). However, in a preliminary double blind study (Houthoff et al., unpublished observations)

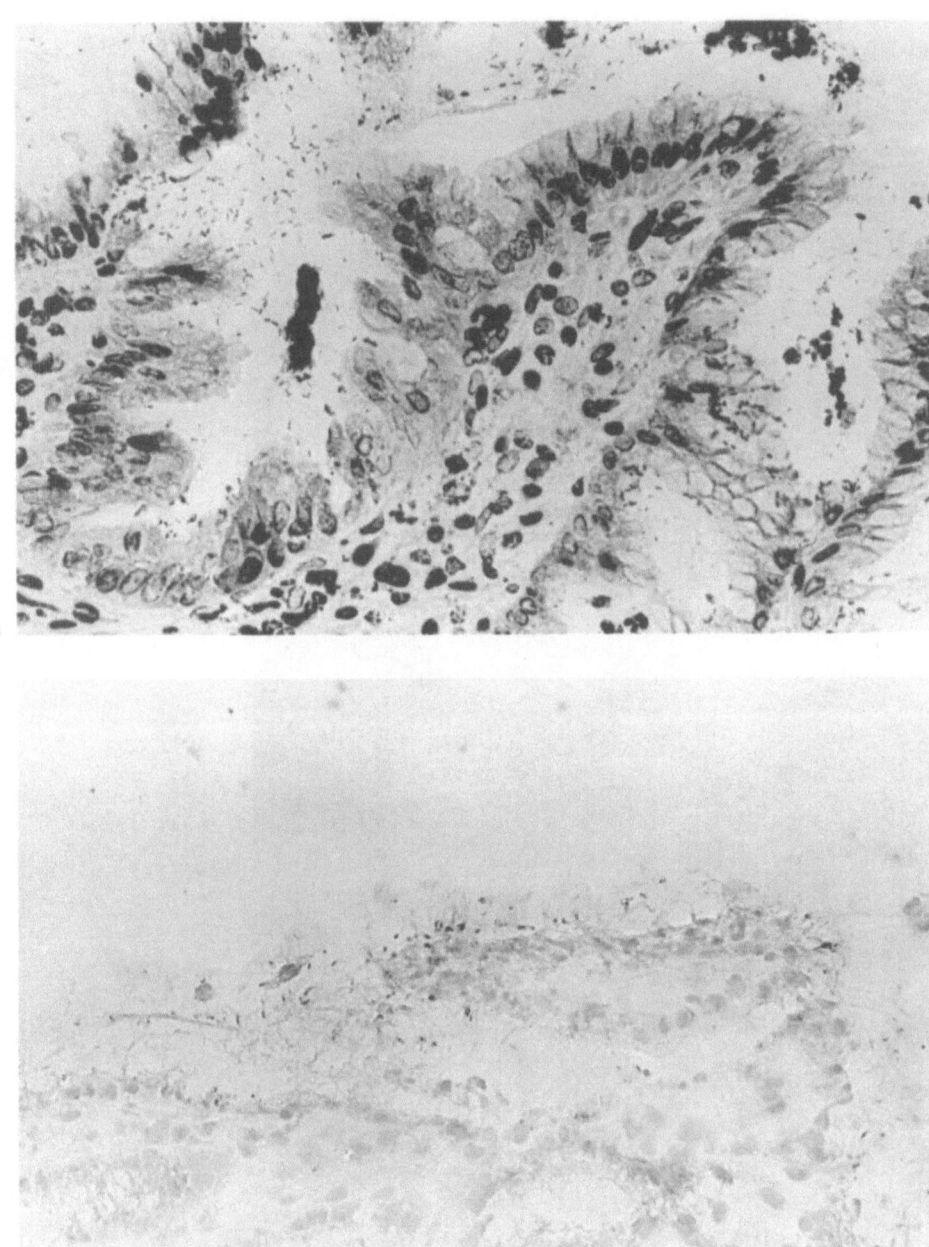

Fig. 1 a, b. Special staining techniques for the demonstration of *C. pylori*. Note the selective staining of the curved rods in the mucus gel. **a** Whartin-Starry silver staining, × 350. **b** Immunohistology using a polyclonal monospecific antibody in a direct immunoperoxidase technique, × 350

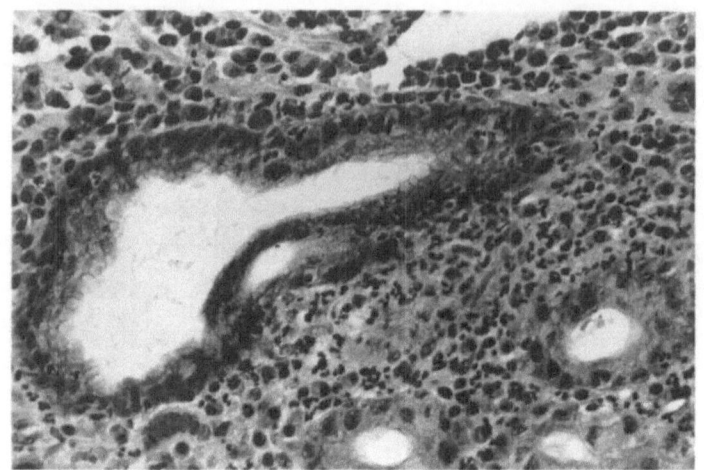

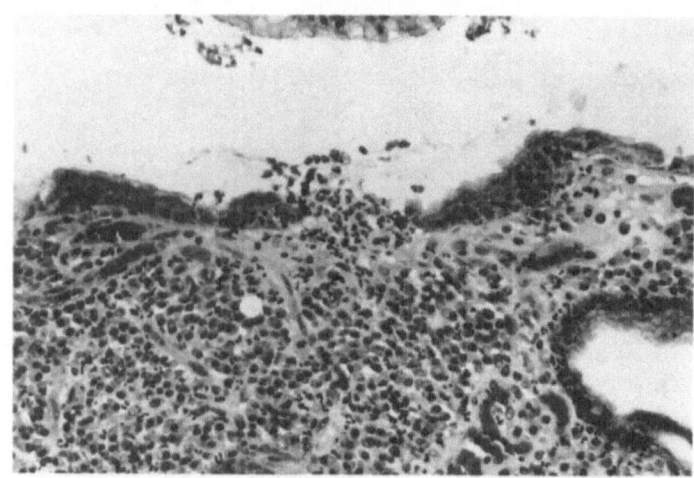

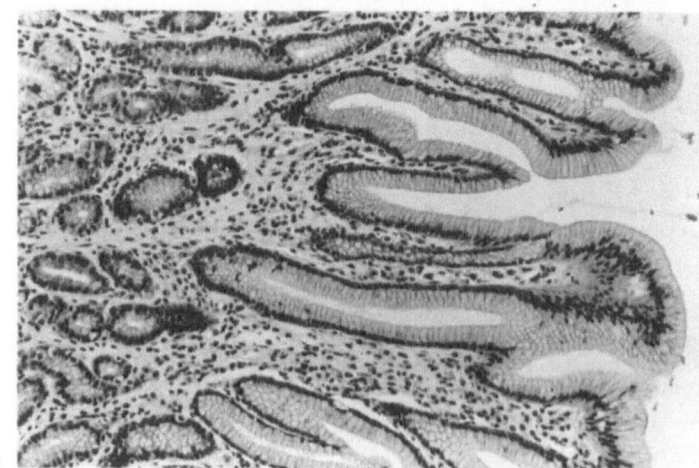

comparing H&E stained tissue sections (Fig. 2a) with *C. pylori* culture ($n = 337$), *C. pylori* was scored histologically in 95% of the culture positive biopsies. False positive histological scores were absent, provided that dubious cases (in which the characteristic curved morphology of *C. pylori* could not be detected unequivocally) were scored as negative. False negative histological scores amounted to 5% and coincided mainly with a restricted growth density in bacterial cultures. Special staining techniques or immunohistologic methods did not improve these results, made the interpretation sometimes easier at the expense of a more time-consuming method, and thus proved to be only of limited value.

To compare the histopathologic changes in the specimens with each other and with the presence or absence of *C. pylori*, an "inflammation score" can be useful. From the 12 histopathologic parameters that were used initially to document the inflammation and mucosal damage semiquantitatively, the following four parameters were selected for scoring the grade of active chronic gastritis.

		Score
Lamina propria:	total inflammatory infiltrate	0−2
	neutrophils (Fig. 2)	0−3
Epithelium:	neutrophils (Fig. 2a)	0−3
	superficial erosions (Fig. 2b)	0−2
Total (= Gastritis score)		0−10

The material consisted of

1) random antral biopsies,
2) duodenal biopsies from the margin of a peptic ulcer,
3) gastrectomy specimens for gastric carcinoma.

The random antral biopsies were taken in the course of a longitudinal follow-up study of 337 patients with peptic ulcer or nonulcer dyspepsia, referred for nonemergency endoscopy, without a history of gastric surgery or malignancy, without medication during the last month for anti-inflammatory drugs (including steroids) or antibiotics, and following informed consent. The study included 34 normal controls. According to initial endoscopic results the patients were allotted to one of the groups of gastric ulcer, duodenal ulcer or nonulcer dyspepsia, randomized for therapy and reevaluated endoscopically 1 day and 1, 3, 6, and 12 months after therapy with yearly controls thereafter. At each endos-

◄────────────────────────────────────

Fig. 2a – c. H&E stained paraffin sections for the combined demonstration of *C. pylori* in the mucus gel and the active chronic gastritis in the mucosa. **a** Junctional area between deep foveolar epithelium and antral glands. Note the presence of *C. pylori* in the lumen, the neutrophils in the foveolar epithelium, and the dense inflammatory infiltrate with many neutrophils in the lamina propria. Gastritis score 8. × 350. **b** Same biopsy, superficial foveolar epithelium with microerosion. Gastritis score 8. × 350. **c** Same patient, biopsy 1 month following successful treatment with amoxicillin. Note the essentially normal antral morphology. Gastritis score 1. × 140

copy, four random antral biopsies were taken for *C. pylori* culture and routine histology. The duodenal biopsies were taken from 20 patients with a benign peptic ulcer of the duodenum. The gastrectomy specimens were of 33 patients with gastric carcinoma and included multiple antral tissue samples.

Active Chronic Gastritis

Of the normal controls, 7 had both a positive *C. pylori* culture and a positive gastritis score; the remaining 27 were negative for both. These findings illustrate several points. In the first place, around 20% of the normal adult population has a *C. pylori* infection with active chronic gastritis, corresponding to literature data [7]. Secondly, an active chronic gastritis can remain silent, lacking the symptoms of dyspepsia; so far, a direct relation between the presence or severity of active chronic gastritis and the presence or severity of dyspepsia symptoms has not been documented. In the third place, a highly significant relation between the presence of active chronic gastritis and the presence of *C. pylori* exists.

Of the 240 patients with nonulcer dyspepsia, 164 of 166 with a positive gastritis score had also a *C. pylori* positive culture in the initial antral biopsies, while 69 of 74 with a negative gastritis score did not. Here too, a highly significant relation between active chronic gastritis and *C. pylori* infection exists. Furthermore, apart from a group with *C. pylori* infection and gastritis, the series of patients with nonulcer dyspepsia appears to include other groups (e.g., motility disturbances) that were not cleared by the entrance criteria of the study.

Benign Peptic Ulcer Disease

Of the 27 patients with gastric ulcer, 26 were positive for both the *C. pylori* culture and the gastritis score in the initial random antral biopsies. The remaining patient had neither gastritis nor a positive *C. pylori* culture, and after requestioning appeared not to have fullfilled the entrance criteria of the study. All 36 of the patients with duodenal ulcer were positive in the antral biopsies for both the *C. pylori* culture and the gastritis score. Apart from the highly significant relation between *C. pylori* infection and the gastritis score in the antral biopsies, several other conclusions can be drawn from these results. In the first place, peptic gastric and duodenal ulcer always coincide with antral *C. pylori* infection and chronic active gastritis. In the second place, given the entrance criteria of the study group, the 100% score for *C. pylori* infection and active chronic gastritis means that if an ulcer patient has not had a stomach operation or medication, he or she always has a *C. pylori* infection; thus, there is no rest group of unknown disease promoting factors and a *C. pylori* infection therefore appears to be a necessary condition for the occurrence of a benign peptic ulcer of either the stomach or the duodenum in this patient population. These findings and conclusions are not completely paralleled by the results of several other groups [2, 5, 6], a discrepancy that presumably can be explained by mutual differences in the entrance criteria for the respective patient groups, and therefore by differences in the populations studied.

In the duodenal biopsies from patients with an active ($n = 15$) or healing ($n = 5$) benign peptic ulcer of the duodenum, in 6 of 20 cases (30%) *C. pylori* was found exclusively in areas with antral metaplasia or with mucosal epithelium lacking differentiation characteristics. In all of these 20 patients, positive *C. pylori* culture and gastritis scores were found in the random antral biopsies, taken simultaneously. The interpretation of these findings is not equivocal, as the series is too small and the sampling from the duodenum too incomplete to warrant definite conclusions. However, the results suggest that an antral *C. pylori* infection with chronic active gastritis forms a necessary condition for the occurrence of benign duodenal ulcer, whereas gastric metaplasia with a *C. pylori* infection in the duodenum does not.

Gastric Carcinoma

Surgical resection specimens for gastric carcinoma ($n = 33$; Fig. 3) offer a wealth of tissue sampling possibilities. Light to severe dysplasia, a feature infrequently encountered in the patient groups with active chronic gastritis and/or benign peptic ulcer disease, were here regularly found in nearly every case. In the 20 specimens with a carcinoma of the antral region, *C. pylori* was found in only 3 of 8 cases with an active chronic gastritis. In the 13 specimens with a carcinoma of the cardial region, 6 cases had an active chronic gastritis but *C. pylori* was never found. In general, it appeared that prominent features of the antral mucosa included intestinal metaplasia, foveolar hyperplasia and dense lymphoplasmacellular infiltrates ("chronic gastritis"), while superficial erosions and a chronic active gastritis with neurophils were an inconsistent and less prominent finding. The presence of *C. pylori* in 3 of 33 (9%) gastric resection specimens remains well within the limits of the 20% *C. pylori* infection in the normal adult population (see before). Therefore, the results indicate that there is no relation between a *C. pylori* infection of the stomach and the occurrence of gastric carcinoma.

Follow-up and Treatment Studies

The patients with nonulcer dyspepsia and benign peptic ulcer disease from the study groups were randomly allotted to one of various treatment regimens of which only colloidal bismuth subcitrate (DeNol), amoxicillin, and a combination of these had an effect in the eradication of *C. pylori*. The results are shown in Table 1, where the other treatment regimens are taken together with the placebo group. As shown in the table, the therapeutic effect did not last in a

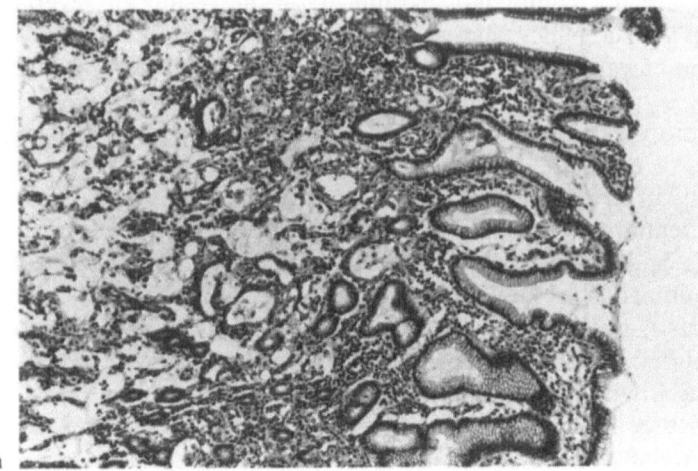

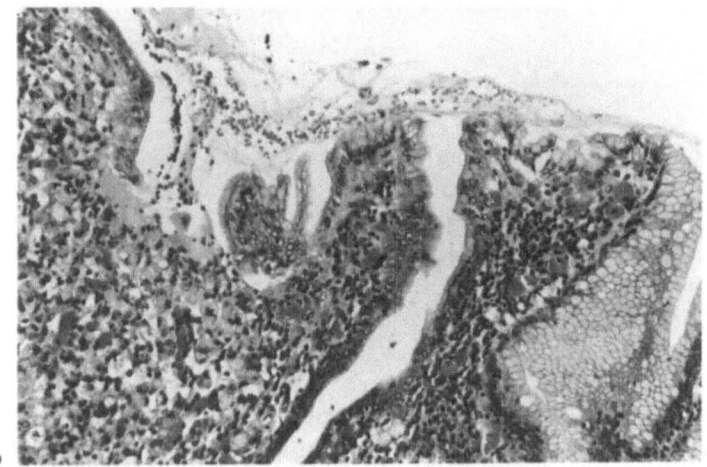

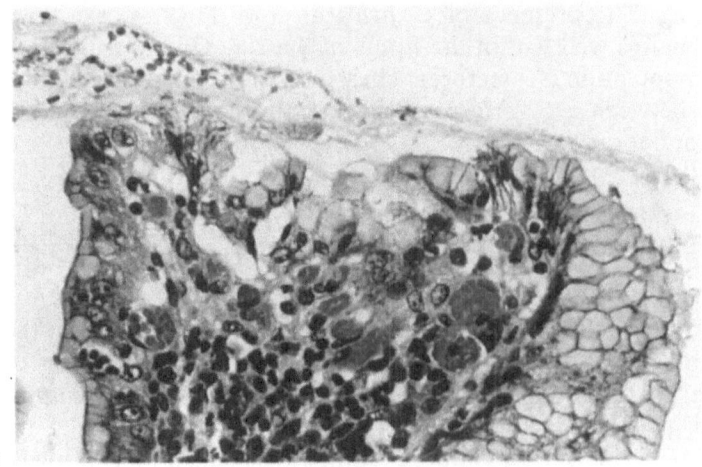

Table 1. *C. pylori* culture results of antral biopsies following various therapeutic regimens. Follow-up period of 1 year

Treatment	Total (n)	Patients with negative culture after		
		1 day (n)	1 month (n)	1 year (n)
CBS	67	30	12	7
amoxicillin	22	15	5	5
CBS + amoxicillin	20	18	8	7
other/placebo	124	0	0	0

CBS, colloidal bismuth subcitrate

majority of patients with an initially negative *C. pylori* culture. This underlines the necessity of long-term follow-up in the evaluation of initial therapeutic success in the eradication of *C. pylori;* the period of follow-up in this study was at least 2–3 years.

A comparison of the gastritis scores following a treatment course between the *C. pylori* culture positive and negative patients during a follow-up period of 12 months revealed highly significant differences in the mean absolute gastritis scores. The mean gastritis scores before treatment varied from 5 to 6, following successful treatment the mean score decreased below 1 within a month, whereas in the patient groups where treatment was not or only temporarily successful the mean score stabilized again between 5 and 6 within 3 months. Also, in looking at the successive biopsies and culture results of individual patients (Fig. 2), a near 100% correlation between the disappearance and reappearance of *C. pylori* and that of gastritis was found. These results in follow-up of both individual patients and patient groups taken together imply that there is a direct correlation between *C. pylori* in the mucus gel and chronic active inflammation in the gastric mucosa. In contrast to colloidal bismuth subcitrate, amoxicillin is known to have only bacteriotoxic effect and notably lacks a cytoprotective effect. This means that the disappearance of gastritis in the patients treated only with amoxicillin is causally related to eradication of *C. pylori*.

In 250 *C. pylori* positive nonulcer dyspepsia patients of the study group, the occurrence rate of benign peptic ulceration (0.008%) and gastric carcinoma (0.004%) remained negligible during a 3-year follow-up period.

Fig. 3a–c. Gastric adenocarcinoma. **a** Intramucosal carcinoma with an intact superficial foveolar epithelium. The inflammatory infiltrate can be designated as chronic gastritis, but signs of an active chronic gastritis and of *C. pylori* are lacking. H&E, × 90. **b** Intramucosal carcinoma with tumor erosion of the superficial foveolar epithelium. H&E, × 140. **c** Detail of **a**, showing the presence of *C. pylori* in the transitional area between the carcinoma and the adjacent foveolar epithelium: an exceptional finding. H&E, × 350

Concluding Remarks

A direct relation exists between *C. pylori* and active chronic antral gastritis, as evidenced by the follow-up in the treatment studies. In individual patients, *C. pylori* and the gastritis vanish or reappear simultaneously with a near 100% correlation. *C. pylori* causes active chronic gastritis, as evidenced by

a) the disappearance of gastritis during amoxicillin treatment (a bacteriotoxic drug lacking cytoprotective properties),
b) the reappearance of the gastritis during *C. pylori* recrudescence.

Strong but still circumstantial evidence is presented that *C. pylori* is a disease promoting factor but not a direct cause for the occurrence of benign peptic ulceration, based upon

a) the fact that *C. pylori* was always found when the strict entrance criteria for the study group were fullfilled,
b) the low occurrence rate of ulcer development in the follow-up of nonulcer patients with *C. pylori*.

This holds for both gastric and duodenal benign ulcer disease; in the latter a relation with a *C. pylori* induced antral gastritis seems stronger than with local factors, such as gastric metaplasia with or without *C. pylori*.

The results suggest that there is no relation between gastric carcinoma and *C. pylori* as evidenced by an occurrence rate of *C. pylori* in carcinoma patients not surpassing that of normal controls.

In the terminology of clinical epidemiology [11], patients become susceptible to disease by risk factors, the occurrence of the disease is dependent upon etiologic factors and the susceptibility of the patient. In this terminology, the results can be summarized as follows.

Disease	CP as etiologic factor	CP as risk factor
Chronic active gastritis	+	+
Gastric peptic ulcer	−	+
Duodenal peptic ulcer	−	+
Gastric carcinoma	−	− (?)

References

1. Warren JR, Marshall BJ (1983) Unidentified curved bacilli on gastric epithelium in active chronic gastritis. Lancet i:1273−1275
2. Marshall BJ, Warren JR (1984) Unidentified curved bacilli in the stomach of patients with gastritis and peptic ulceration. Lancet i:1311−1315
3. Rollason TP, Stone J, Rhodes JM (1984) Spinal organisms in endoscopic biopsies of the human stomach. J Clin Pathol 37:23−26

4. Jones DM, Lessells AM, Eldridge J (1984) Camylobacter like organisms on the gastric mucosa: culture, histological, and serological studies. J Clin Pathol 37:1002–1006
5. Price AB, Levi J, Dolby JM et al. (1985) Campylobacter pyloridis in peptic ulcer disease: microbiology, pathology, and scanning electron microscopy. Gut 26:1183–1188
6. Buck GE, Gourley WK, Lee WK et al. (1986) Relation of Campylobacter pyloridis to gastritis and peptic ulcer. J Inf Dis 153:664–669
7. Langenberg ML, Tytgat GNJ, Schipper MEI, Rietra PJGM, Zanen HC (1984) Campylobacter-like organisms in the stomach of patients and healthy individuals. Lancet 1:1348
8. Langenberg ML, Rauws EAJ, Schipper MEI et al. (1985) The pathogenic role of Campylobacter pyloridis studied by attempts to eliminate these organisms. In: Pearson AD, Skirrow MB, Lior N, Rowe B (eds) Campylobacter III. Proceedings of the third international workshop on Campylobacter infections. Public Health Laboratory Service, London, pp 162–163
9. Rauws EAJ, Langenberg ML, Houthoff HJ, Zanen HC, Tytgat GNJ (1987) Campylobacter pyloridis-associated chronic active antral gastritis. Gastroenterology (to be published)
10. Langenberg ML, Rauws EAJ, Houthoff HJ et al. (1987) A study of the natural history of C. pyloridis-associated gastritis. To be published
11. Fletcher RH, Fletcher SW, Wagner EH (1982) Clinical epidemiology – the essentials. Williams and Wilkins, Baltimore

Discussion

Classen: The low frequency of 30% CLO in the bulbar mucosa of duodenal ulcer patients in your study could be due to technical reasons. I think all these biopsies were taken endoscopically. There may soon be some improvement available in targetting endoscopic biopsies in magnification endoscopy. We can then much better detect gastric metaplasia or heterotopia in the duodenal bulb. In this context I recall a presentation given by a Danish colleague at the European Gastroenterology Conference in 1972 in Paris. He had performed systemic examinations of the duodenal bulb in duodenal ulcer patients and found a high frequency, about 50%, of gastric mucosal heterotopia. You should study resection specimens from previous years again.

Houthoff: In general I agree with your remarks, however, we do not often get resection specimen of duodenal ulcers. An alternative to your suggestion would be a follow-up study with duodenal biopsies both for CLO culture and histopathology. During my presentation I pointed out that our results did not provide definite conclusions but only circumstantial evidence on this point. I also pointed out that from the circumstantial evidence the frequency of ulcer development in CLO-positive patients was an important factor, as the patients may have the bacterium and the gastritis for a long time and never develop an ulcer. The incidence of ulcer in a large-scale study of CLO-positive patients should confirm the circumstantial evidence presented.

Hahn: I wonder about the relationship between the inflammatory cells and the bacteria. Was there any evidence of phagocytosis in those inflammatory foci?

Houthoff: The CLO do not invade intact mucosal lining and to my knowledge have never been observed in macrophages. Only phagocytosis of cellular debris in areas of superficial erosion has been observed.

Tytgat: With the electron microscope one can see bacteria within permeating neutrophils or within neutrophils in the lumen.

Houthoff: I think what you are asking for is a study with several monoclonals to the epitopes of soluble and insoluble bacterial macromolecules, or with DNA in situ hybridisation to detect bacterial DNA as a remnant of phagocytosed material of bacterial debris. But in general CLO do not invade the stomach wall and the diffusion of soluble bacterial antigens could very well explain the host's immune response.

Hahn: To my simple understanding, it is the rule that when you find bacteria in the tissue and an inflammatory reaction around it, there is phagocytosis involved. You see this in the microscope; you do not need the electron-microscope nor monoclonal antibodies. But here it seems to me that phagocytosis is obviously not very much present.

Houthoff: I cannot fully agree with you. Phagocytosis of necrotic cell debris does occur. As with many bacterial strains in other parts of the gut, CLO may remain confined to the surface and not invade the tissue.

Tytgat: I have a related question. Have you, or has anyone else in the audience, found a relationship between the density of bacterial load and the number of polymorphs in the mucosa?

Houthoff: I think that there is no direct relation between them. We have many cases with many bacteria and many granulocytes. In the biopsy the places with many granulocytes are not necessarily the places with many bacteria.

Tytgat: That was exactly my point. Do you want to comment upon that?

Marshall: A statement has been made by Robin Warren, that in some cases the bacteria are not where the polymorphs are found. In other words, it seems that the polymorphs, once they start appearing in large numbers and invading the gland necks, are consuming the bacteria. And I find it very easy to see polymorphs with bacteria within them in Gram's-stained mucus smears.

Rösch: Among the drugs you excluded was cortisone. What happens if you give cortisone to patients with *Campylobacter pylori* – since you change the mucus quality?

Houthoff: I think that your question should be answered by the gastroenterologists who will discuss this topic tomorrow. As a pathologist, I think it is beyond my scope to try to give an answer.

Börsch: I want to return briefly to the question of the activity of gastritis. You have devised your own score for gastritis, and this makes it difficult to compare your data with those of others. The usual way to measure gastritis is either the method of Whitehead or the method of Hafter and Siebenmann. Whitehead defines the activity of gastritis merely by the presence or absence of polymorphs. If you reevaluate your data according to this definition, would you find *Campylobacter* invariably associated with this form of active gastritis defined by polymorph cellular infiltration? There is considerable debate on this question.

Houthoff: If we eliminate the density of the inflammatory infiltrate and the superficial erosions, the scores for the granulocytes in the lamina propria and in the epithelial layer would have added up to much the same result. In fact, we also could have used a score for granulocytes ranging from 0 to 10 in a quantitative or semiquantitative study.

Wyatt: I would like to make some further comments on the question of activity. Firstly, I think that when you consider the activity of the gastritis to be specifically neutrophils within the epithelium, we have certainly seen that *Campylobacter* is much more prevalent in biopsies showing active than inactive gastritis; the percentages are about 95% of the active cases compared to about 60% of inactive. We have devised a scoring system for the population density of colonizing *C. pylori* on the biopsies and found that the density of population is higher among the active than among the inactive cases. There has also been some work from Steer in Southampton; he has seen cimetidine sections in which he counted the numbers of polymorphs, counted the numbers of bacteria, and has shown that there is a correlation between the two. So I think they certainly are associated. If I could just follow this up with a question about clearance and about improvements of histology in your patients after the clearance. Did the histology in those patients who later suffered a relapse with their gastritis return to normal to the same extent as in those patients who remained clear of the organism?

Houthoff: Initially, yes.

Wyatt: They both became completely normal?

Houthoff: No, but there were no differences between both groups. In fact, in the biopsies 1 day following treatment the gastritis scores had decreased significantly, but in most cases did not yet equal 0 or 1.

Ó'Moráin: You told us that you followed up 250 *Campylobacter*-positive patients for a period of 2 or 3 years, and that none of these developed a peptic ulcer while only one developed a gastric cancer. Did these patients receive any treatment to make them negative? And secondly, did you follow-up any patients who were negative but who became positive in this time and, if so, did they develop ulcers or gastritis?

Houthoff: I think your questions should be answered by Tytgat or Rauws as gastroenterologists, preferably following their presentations on the same topic.

Marshall: I want to comment on the classification of histology. I think we should not carry the millstone of previous classifications around our necks when we look at *Campylobacter pylori*. In previous literature on gastritis many of the benchmark papers did not include pictures of the histology and did not include clinical data about the patients. When you begin looking at these papers, it is not possible to work out exactly what type of gastritis was present.

One of the confusing things in the literature is that people call intestinal meta-plasia chronic atrophic gastritis. If you take a biopsy which contains only in-testinal metaplasia, there is often no inflammation within it, and you cannot de-duce from such a specimen what the rest of the gastric mucosa is like. I think it is better to ignore the previous papers and say that we have a classification or a method which is based on the terminology of Whitehead in which each aspect of the mucosa is described separately; that is, neutrophils, mononuclear cells, metaplasia, atrophy and epithelial cell damage. If we talk about each of these individually for the present, then in a few years we may be able to reconstitute them back into a coherent terminology for gastritis. At the moment, once we start getting away from the individual description of each component and start using terms like "atrophic gastritis" or "superficial gastritis" we will not know what anyone else is talking about. The classification used by Dr. Houthoff was an excellent one, and it is very easy to compare with Dr. McNulty's paper, with Whitehead's papers, and also with my own.

Section 3

Epidemiology of
Campylobacter pylori Infection

Incidence of *Campylobacter pylori* in Patients with Gastritis and Peptic Ulcer Disease in Various Countries

B. J. RATHBONE, J. I. WYATT, and R. V. HEATLEY

The organism that we now know as *Campylobacter pylori* was first isolated in 1982 by Marshall et al. [1] in Australia. The organism had, however, been intermittently noted on gastric epithelium by a variety of investigators in several countries since the turn of the century.

Human gastric spiral organisms were first reported in association with ulcerating carcinomas in the German literature [2, 3]. Doenges [4] in the USA in a histological study of 242 autopsy stomachs found spiral organisms present in 43% of cases. Autolysis made detailed histological assessment impossible. To avoid this Freedberg and Barron [5] studied gastric resection specimens using haematoxylin and silver stain. They reported that 37.1% of their 35 cases were colonised. Interestingly, in 13 duodenal-ulcer patients with associated chronic gastritis only two were found to be positive. In an attempt to confirm the presence of gastric spiral organisms Palmer [6] in the USA studied 1180 suction biopsies by haematoxylin and eosin stains and found no evidence of spiral organisms. In 1975 Steer and Colin-Jones [7, 8] in the UK described bacteria on the luminal surface of epithelial cells of gastric ulcer patients, and in 1979 Fung et al. [9] in Australia noted bacteria in association with chronic gastritis.

Although thus intermittently identified, the strong association of spiral organisms with gastric mucosal inflammation and peptic ulceration was not fully appreciated until Warren [10] and Marshall's [11] letters in the *Lancet* in 1983. Independently of one another Steer [12] and Rollason et al. [13] submitted papers in 1983 regarding spiral organisms and chronic gastritis. Following Marshall's report on the isolation of these organisms there has been an avalanche of literature on *C. pylori* from all over the world, describing the prevalence of *C. pylori* in various diseases and various groups of patients.

C. pylori and the Normal Gastroduodenal Epithelium

The prevalence of *C. pylori* in normal and gastritic mucosa is shown in Table 1. The figures presented are generally based on relatively small numbers of patients with the prevalence of *C. pylori* in stomachs with entirely normal gastric histology varying between 0% and 40%. In our own studies we always perform a biopsy on gastric antrum and body and judge colonisation by examination of sections stained by a modified Giemsa technique [26]. We have yet to find a

Table 1. Prevalence of *C. pylori* colonisation with normal gastric histology and chronic gastritis in various countries (figures in parentheses refer to population size where known)

Country	Normal histology		Chronic gastritis	Reference
Australia	0% (21)		96% (54)	14
Holland	7% (15)		89% (35)	15
UK	11% (119)		71% (86)	16
Yugoslavia	0% (8)		52% (62)	17
Spain	10% (10)		91% (33)	18
USA	11% (37)		63% (96)	19
Canada	0% (26)		60% (10)	20, 21
Japan	–	65%[a]	–	22
Hongkong	40%		78%	23
Italy	31%		43%	24
Peru	–		100% (103)	25

[a] Overall prevalence in endoscopy patients, not taking into account histology

colonised stomach which is histologically normal in both antrum and body. *C. pylori* are commonly present on morphologically normal body-type mucosa but always in association with antral gastritis [27]. Differences between figures for various groups are most likely due either to sampling errors, especially when only a single gastric biopsy is used, to differences in the interpretation of the histology, or to differences in techniques for diagnosing *C. pylori* colonisation.

C. pylori fail to colonise intestinal metaplasia in the stomach despite the adjacent gastric-type often being colonised. Normal duodenal epithelium has never been reported to be colonised [28].

C. pylori and Chronic Gastritis

The association of *C. pylori* with chronic gastritis is confirmed in all groups (Table 1), however the percentage varies considerably (43% – 100%), both between groups in the same country and between countries. The association of *C. pylori* with gastritis was reported originally to be strongest with active gastritis [14] (activity, referring here to polymorphe invading the epithelium); however, as can be seen in Table 1, some researchers dispute this. The differences between groups are most likely due to sampling errors or interpretation errors, but it is also possible that in different countries investigators are studying different gastritis populations.

Chronic gastritis can be divided into autoimmune and non-autoimmune gastritis [29]. The former, associated with pernicious anaemia, gives a histological picture similar to that of the latter but shows a different pattern of involvement, the body being more affected than the antrum (type A gastritis); in the more usual (type B) gastritis the antrum is affected more than the body [30]. O'Connor et al. [31] have demonstrated histologically that *C. pylori* is poorly associated with autoimmune gastritis. Among patients with this type of gastritis, however, there may be a tendency to underestimate colonisation due to the high prevalence of intestinal metaplasia on which *C. pylori* is never found [32].

We have examined this group in more detail and have found that serologically less than 50% of autoimmune gastritis patients have *C. pylori* IgG antibodies in the range expected with colonisation. Among our non-ulcer dyspepsia patients those with type A gastritis (typical of autoimmune gastritis) had a highly significant reduction in *C. pylori* colonisation compared to those with type B gastritis (12 of 25 *C. pylori* negative in type-A gastritis versus 5 of 112 *C. pylori* negative in type B gastritis, $p < 0.0001$). Another, more recently described type of histological gastritis is reflux gastritis which also appears to be poorly associated with colonisation [33]. Clearly chronic gastritis is not a single disease, and this may contribute to some of the differences we see across nations.

C. pylori and Duodenitis

There is a strong association between *C. pylori* colonisation of the duodenum and histological duodenitis [28], which may occur with or without duodenal ulceration. In the latter group of cases *C. pylori* colonisation of the duodenum in addition to the antrum occurs in 55% – 73% of cases [12, 28, 34]. *C. pylori* does not normally colonise small-intestinal epithelium, but the presence of islands of metaplastic gastric epithelium (a feature of duodenitis) appears to allow colonisation in patients who have *C. pylori* associated chronic gastritis. There is evidence linking gastric metaplasia in the duodenum to acid production by the stomach [35, 36], which provides a hypothesis accounting for the association of *C. pylori* gastritis, high acidity, duodenitis and duodenal ulceration.

C. pylori and Peptic Ulceration

Much attention has focussed on the association between *C. pylori* and peptic ulceration. The relationship between antral gastritis and ulceration, particularly duodenal ulceration, has been documented previously [37, 38]. Table 2 summarises some of the cross-national data concerning gastric *C. pylori* colonisation and peptic ulceration. In general the association between gastric ulcers and *C. pylori* is less pronounced than that between duodenal ulcers and *C. pylori.* Care must be taken, however, in directly comparing data from one country to another, for both gastric and duodenal ulcers appear multifactorial in origin, and their prevalence varies considerably around the world.

Most populations in which *C. pylori* has been studied have been Western in style, and little is consequently known about this in the Third World. We have recently had the opportunity to study a group of symptomatic patients from Kumasi, Ghana (J. de Caestecker, J. Wyatt, B. Rathbone, R. Heatley, unpub-

Table 2. Prevalence of *C. pylori* in gastric and duodenal ulceration in various countries (figures in parentheses refer to population size where known)

Country	Gastric ulcer		Duodenal ulcer	Reference
Australia	68% (40)		90% (70)	14
Holland	67% (3)		100% (9)	15
UK	57% (21)		78% (32)	16
Yugoslavia	83% (6)		71% (28)	17
Spain	–	86% (28)[a]	–	18
USA	54% (28)		60% (25)	19
Canada	43% (42)		27% (26)	20, 21
Japan	–	100%[a]	–	22
Hongkong	–	80%[a]	–	23
Italy	79% (14)		71% (28)	24

[a] Published figures do not differentiate between gastric and duodenal ulcers.

lished work). Duodenal ulcers are common in the Ghanese population, but benign gastric ulcers appear to be quite a rarity. In a total of 39 patients undergoing endoscopy we found 38 were *C. pylori* positive, with 23 having duodenal ulcers or duodenitis, but none with benign gastric ulceration. Although this group of patients is relatively small the prevalence of *C. pylori* colonisation here is one of the highest reported. Thus if one assumes *C. pylori* colonisation to be implicated in benign gastric ulcer disease, different factors seem to be operating in the Ghanese population than in Western populations, such as that in the UK, where the prevalence of gastric ulcers is approximately one-half that of duodenal ulcers.

A recent UK study of *C. pylori* positive and negative gastric ulcers revealed a significantly higher prevalence of histological reflux gastritis amongst the *C. pylori* negative group, suggesting two different agents of mucosal damage (*C. pylori* colonisation and gastroduodenal reflux), each predisposing to gastric ulceration [39].

The role of non-steroidal anti-inflammatory drugs in ulcer disease has recently been much debated, and it has certainly been reported that ingestion of these drugs may account for a proportion of the *C. pylori* negative gastric ulcers which have been seen [40]. Clearly the prescribing of these drugs is likely to vary widely between countries and hence may contribute to prevalence differences.

C. pylori and the Normal Healthy Population

Unlike patients with symptoms, the normal healthy population is a difficult group to study, particularly with regard to gastric inflammation and colonisation with bacteria. Large prevalence studies carried out in Finland and Estonia in the 1960s and 1970s demonstrated that histological antral gastritis is a common phenomenon in the general population, with an overall prevalence of 68%

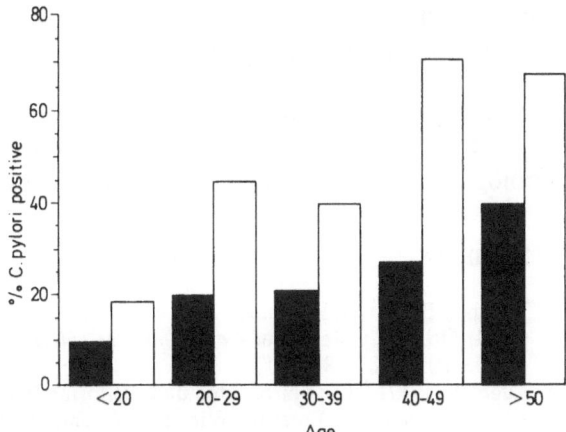

Fig. 1. Age-related prevalence of *C. pylori* colonisation among Leeds blood donors (*shaded bars*) and non-ulcer dyspepsia patients (*unshaded bars*)

of cases in an Estonian rural population [41, 42]. When age was taken into account, a steady increase in prevalence was found with increasing age [43]. More recently Kreuning et al. [44] in Holland showed that 18 of 50 asymptomatic volunteers had evidence of chronic gastritis. Atrophic gastritis appeared age-related, with the majority of such cases in patients over 40 years old.

The prevalence of *C. pylori* in the healthy population is clearly important, yet very few studies have examined this. The demonstration of specific systemic antibody responses in association with *C. pylori* colonisation has provided a suitable marker for studying *C. pylori* associated chronic gastritis in large populations without the need for endoscopy and biopsy. A number of investigators in Australia and the UK [45–47] have demonstrated by serology a steady increase in the prevalence of *C. pylori* with age, thus supporting the histological data. In our own studies we have compared prevalence in healthy blood donors to a population of patients with non-ulcer dyspepsia (Fig. 1). In both groups the prevalence of *C. pylori* colonisation increased with age, but in the non-ulcer group the actual prevalence for each age group was approximately twice that among the blood donors. Such data suggest a relationship between *C. pylori* associated gastroduodenitis and dyspeptic symptoms, but clearly more work is required to confirm this.

Conclusions

All studies to date from over 15 countries confirm the association between *C. pylori* and chronic gastritis, gastric and duodenal ulceration. Individual prevalence rates vary, and care must be taken in interpreting such differences. The type of population studied and the methods of diagnosing *C. pylori* colonisation or mucosal inflammation may contribute to apparent differences. It must also be remembered that the gastroduodenal mucosa, like other parts of the gastrointestinal tract is limited in the means by which it can respond to various injuries, and conditions such as peptic ulceration are multifactorial in origin. Thus the importance of various factors in different populations may vary considerably.

Careful study in future on well defined populations in various countries may help to answer many important questions about peptic ulcer disease, the aetiology of dyspeptic symptoms and the role of *C. pylori*.

References

1. Marshall BJ, Royce H, Annear DI, Goodwin CS, Pearman JW, Warren JR, Armstrong JA (1984) Original isolation of *Campylobacter pyloridis* from human gastric mucosa. Microbios Letters 25:83–88
2. Luger A (1917) Über Spirochäten und fusiforme Bazillen im Darm, mit einem Beitrag zur Frage der Lamblien-Enteritis. Wien klin Wochnschr 52:1643–1647
3. Krienitz W (1906) Über das Auftreten von Mageninhalt bei Carcinoma ventriculi. Dtsch Med Wochenschr 22:872
4. Doenges JL (1939) Spirochaetes in the gastric glands of Macacus rhesus and of man without related disease. Arch Path 27:469–477
5. Freedburg AS, Barron LE (1940) The presence of spirochaetes in human gastric mucosa. Am J Dig Dis 7:443–445
6. Palmer ED (1954) Investigation of the gastric mucosa spirochetes of the human. Gastroenterol 27:218–220
7. Steer HW, Colin-Jones DG (1975) Mucosal changes in gastric ulceration and their response to carbenoxolone sodium. Gut 16:590–597
8. Steer HW (1975) Ultrastructure of cell migration through the gastric epithelium and its relationship to bacteria. J Clin Pathol 28:639–646
9. Fung WP, Papadimitriou JM, Matz LR (1979) Endoscopic, histological and ultrastructural correlations in chronic gastritis. Am J Gastroenterol 71:269–279
10. Warren JR (1983) Unidentified curved bacilli on gastric epithelium in active chronic gastritis. Lancet i:1273
11. Marshall B (1983) Unidentified curved bacilli on gastric epithelium in active chronic gastritis. Lancet i:1273–1275
12. Steer HW (1984) Surface morphology of the gastroduodenal mucosa in duodenal ulceration. Gut 25:1203–1210
13. Rollason TP, Stone J, Rhodes JM (1984) Spiral organisms in endoscopic biopsies of the human stomach. J Clin Pathol 37:23–26
14. Marshall BJ, Warren JR (1984) Unidentified curved bacilli in the stomach of patients with gastritis and peptic ulceration. Lancet i:1311–1315
15. Langenberg M-L, Tytgat GNJ, Schipper MEI, Rietra PJGM, Zanen HC (1984) Campylobacter-like organisms in the stomach of patients and healthy individuals. Lancet i:1348
16. Pearson AD, Bamforth J, Booth L, Holdstock G, Ireland A, Walker C, Hawtin P, Millward-Sadler H (1984) Polyacrylamide gel electrophoresis of spiral bacteria from the gastric antrum. Lancet i:1349–1350
17. Kalenic S, Faliseva V, Scukanec-Spoljar M, Vodopija I (1985) *Campylobacter pyloridis* in the gastric mucosa of patients with gastritis and peptic ulcer. In: Pearson AD, Skirrow MB, Lior H (eds) Campylobacter III, Proceedings of the Third International Workshop on Campylobacter Infections, Public Health Laboratory Service, London, p 193
18. Lopez-Brea M, Jimenez ML, Blanco M, Pajares JM (1985) Isolation of *Campylobacter pyloridis* from patients with and without gastroduodenal pathology. In: Pearson AD, Skirrow MB, Lior H (eds) Campylobacter III. Proceedings of the Third International Workshop on Campylobacter Infections, Public Health Laboratory Service, London, pp 193–194
19. Pettross CW, Cohen H, Appleman MD, Valenzuela JE, Chandrasama P (1986) *Campylobacter pyloridis:* relationship to peptic disease, gastric inflammation and other conditions. Gastroenterol 90:1585

20. Bohnen J, Krajden S, Kempston J, Anderson J, Karmali M (1985) *Campylobacter pyloridis* in Toronto. In: Pearson AD, Skirrow MB, Lior H (eds) Campylobacter III, Proceedings of the Third International Workshop on Campylobacter Infections, Public Health Laboratory Service, London, p 175–177
21. Drumm B, O'Brien A, Cutz E, Sherman P (1986) *Campylobacter pyloridis* are associated with primary antral gastritis in the paediatric population. Gastroenterol 90:1399
22. Ishii E, Inoue H, Tsuyuguchi T, Shimoyama T, Tanaka T, Wada M, Kishi T, Masui M, Tamura T, Yanagase Y, Shoji K (1985) *Campylobacter pyloridis* in cases of stomach diseases in Japan. In: Pearson AD, Skirrow MB, Lior H (eds) Campylobacter III, Proceedings of the Third International Workshop on Campylobacter Infections. Public Health Laboratory Service, London, p 179–180
23. Hui WM, Lam SK, Ho J, Chan PY, Lui I, Lai CL, Lok A, Ng MMT (1986) Campylobacter-like organisms do not affect the healing of gastric ulcers. Gastroenterol 90:1468
24. Marcheggiano A, Iannoni C, Agnello M, Paoluzi P, Pallone F (1986) Campylobacter-like organisms gastritis and peptic ulcer. Gastroenterol 90:1533
25. Barreda C, Gilman RH, Leon-Barua R, Koch J, Quevedo N, Ramirez-Ramos A, Recavarren S, Rodriguez C, Spira WM, Stephensen C (1985) Differential colonisation of the stomach by *Campylobacter pyloridis* studied by a novel sheathed brush. In: Pearson AD, Skirrow MB, Lior H (eds) Campylobacter III. Proceedings of the Third International Workshop on Campylobacter Infections, Public Health Laboratory Service, London, p 192
26. Gray SF, Wyatt JI, Rathbone BJ (1986) Simplified techniques for identifying *Campylobacter pyloridis*. J Clin Pathol 39:1279–1280
27. Wyatt JI, Rathbone BJ, Heatley RV (1986) Local immune response to gastric campylobacter in non-ulcer dyspepsia. J Clin Pathol 39:863–870
28. Johnston BJ, Reed PI, Hali M (1986) Campylobacter like organisms in duodenal and antral endoscopic biopsies: relationship to inflammation. Gut 27:1132–1137
29. Rathbone BJ, Heatley RV (1986) Gastritis. In: Losowsky MS, Heatley RV (eds) Gut Defences in Clinical Practice. Churchill Churchill Livingstone, London
30. Strickland RG, Mackay IR (1973) A reappraisal of the nature and significance of chronic atrophic gastritis. Am J Dig Dis 18:426–440
31. O'Connor HJ, Axon ATR, Dixon MF (1984) Campylobacter-like organisms unusual in type A (pernicious anaemia) gastritis. Lancet ii:1091
32. Meyrick Thomas J (1984) Campylobacter-like organisms in gastritis. Lancet ii:1217
33. Dixon M, O'Connor HJ, Axon ATR, King RFGJ, Johnston D (1986) Campylobacter-like organisms and reflux gastritis. J Clin Pathol 39:531–534
34. Wyatt JI, Rathbone BJ, Dixon MF, Heatley RV (1987) *Campylobacter pyloridis* and acid-induced gastric metaplasia in the pathogenesis of duodenitis. J Clin Pathol, in press
35. James AH (1964) Gastric epithelium in the duodenum. Gut 5:285–294
36. Patrick WJA, Denham D, Forrest APM (1974) Mucous change in the human duodenum: A light and electron microscopic study and correlation with disease and gastric acid secretion. Gut 15:767–776
37. Schrager J, Spink R, Mitra S (1967) The antrum in patients with duodenal and gastric ulcers. Gut 8:497–508
38. Earlam RJ, Amerigo J, Kakavoulis T, Pollock DJ (1985) Histological appearances of oesophagus, antrum and duodenum and their correlation with symptoms in patients with a duodenal ulcer. Gut 26:95–100
39. O'Connor HJ, Dixon MF, Wyatt JI, Axon ATR (1986) Campylobacter-positive and campylobacter-negative gastric ulcers – have they a different aetiology? Gut 27:1282A
40. Marshall BJ, McGechie DB, Rogers PA, Glancy RJ (1985) Pyloric campylobacter infection and gastroduodenal disease. Med J Aust 142:439–444
41. Villako K, Tamm A, Savisaar E, Ruttas M (1976) Prevalence of antral and fundic gastritis in a randomly selected group of an Estonian rural population. Scand J Gastroenterol 11:817–822
42. Siurala M, Isokoski M, Varis K, Kekki M (1968) Prevalence of gastritis in a rural population. Scand J Gastroenterol 3:211–223
43. Siurala M, Salmi HJ (1971) Long term follow-up of subjects with superficial gastritis or a normal gastric mucosa. Scand J Gastroenterol 6:459–463

44. Kreuning J, Bosman FT, Kuiper G, van de Wal AM, Lindeman J (1978) Gastric and duo-denal mucosa in healthy individuals. J Clin Pathol 31:69 – 77
45. Eldridge J, Jones DM, Sethi P (1985) The occurrence of antibody to *Campylobacter pyloridis* in various groups of individuals. In: Pearson AD, Skirrow MB, Lior H (eds) Campylobacter III, Proceedings of the Third International Workshop on Campylobacter Infections, Public Health Laboratory Service, London, p 183 – 184
46. Hawtin PR, Pearson AD, McBride H, Gibson J, Booth L (1985) Specific IgG and IgA responses to *Camylobacter pyloridis* in man. In: Pearson AD, Skirrow MB, Lior H (eds) Campylobacter III, Proceedings of the Third International Workshop on Campylobacter Infections, Public Health Laboratory Service, London, p 186 – 187
47. Marshall BJ, Whisson M, Francis G, McGechie D (1985) Correlation between symptoms of dyspepsia and *Campylobacter pyloridis* serology in Western Australian blood donors. In: Pearson AD, Skirrow MB, Lior H (eds) Campylobacter III. Proceedings of the Third International Workshop on Campylobacter Infections, Public Health Laboratory Service, London, p 188 – 189

Discussion

Marshall: I would like to ask whether are you suggesting, that there are other causes of type B gastritis besides *C. pylori?* And if so, what percentage? This is a totally new concept to me.

Rathbone: One cannot assume that a histological picture is necessarily caused by one factor, and with gastritis we have explained why we find *C. pylori* negative cases.

Marshall: So what percentage of type B chronic gastritis is not caused by *C. pylori?*

Rathbone: In our study it has been less than 5%.

Pearson: You quote incidence and prevalence figures for populations; do you have any information on the actual population denominator or on further studies to which you have compared detection rates of antibody to *C. pylori?*

Rathbone: Yes, we have done this, but I do not have the data here.

Marshall: Dr. Pearson, just clarify this for me: When we refer to the number of patients in a group of endoscopy patients who have *C. pylori*, should we call this is a "prevalence rate" or the "prevalence of the incidence?" What is the correct term here?

Pearson: Neither. This is a frequency as I understand it. An incidence rate is the number of new cases in a defined population; a prevalence rate is the total number of cases, e.g. the new and old cases in a defined population. Adherence to the correct meaning of the definition is required in order to compare incidence and prevalence rates in different populations. You have compared age-related data on *C. pylori* antibody from various countries. The age distribution of your sample and the age structures in the different countries need to be taken into account before saying the frequencies of *C. pylori* antibody are similar. I do not believe that the data you presented are strictly comparable. This age adjustment may be especially important if you compare the population of Peru with the population of England or Australia.

Börsch: In one of your first slides you showed a frequency of *Campylobacter pylori* in normal mucosa in Hong Kong at 40%. Was this a mistake, or could you comment on this extremely high frequency?

Rathbone: This is a problem in the interpretation of what is normal and what is gastritis. The Hong Kong data refer to endoscopic gastritis rather that to histological gastritis.

Marshall: I would suggest that, if the pathologist rarely sees biopsies from endoscopically normal patients, his concept of normality is uncertain, and his threshold for gastritis is likely to be raised. If the clinician is only taking a biopsy from patients with an endoscopic lesion, there will be very few normal biopsies reaching the pathologist.

Rathbone: Yes, I think that I must point out that clinicians often take undue notice of endoscopic appearance and talk about endoscopic gastritis. There is very little relation between endoscopic appearance and histological gastritis.

Börsch: I want to return to the important question of whether *Campylobacter pylori* is the only cause of chronic antral type B gastritis or not. In our experience using CLO tests and histologic examination, *C. pylori* is associated in only 70% − 80% of cases. About 20% − 30% of chronic antral type B gastritis is negative. I think a very strong further candidate for causing such chronic antral type B gastritis is duodenal-gastric reflux. There is a need to differentiate between the fasting state, which Professor Axon and his group investigated, and the postprandial state, which is quite different. The postprandial state is characterized by cellular infiltration just as is that kind of gastritis which we see in *C. pylori* infestation. There was an important paper in the *Scandinavian Journal of Gastroenterology* in 1987 by Niemelä and Lehtola from Finland, who pointed out this fact. So I suggest that the postprandial duodenal-gastric reflux is a serious candidate for causing an identical picture of histology.

Rathbone: I would like to point out that the histological lesion that Dr. Dixon talks about is, in fact, very rare among our dyspeptic patients and certainly accounts for very few of the *C. pylori* negative gastritis cases among our non-ulcer patients.

Axon: May I comment, that reflux gastritis is not common compared to *C. pylori* gastritis, but patients who have had operations such as gastrojejunostomy, which allow gastric reflux, do have it frequently. In this group the histological appearances are different from those of the gastritis found with *C. pylori* and can be termed "reflux gastritis." Patients with gastric ulcer have histological gastritis, those who are *C. pylori* negative have the appearances of reflux gastritis, so although in the general population reflux gastritis is uncommon, it is relatively frequent in those with gastric ulcer. Dr. Dixon's work suggests that there are two types of gastric ulcer, those possibly secondary to *C. pylori* gastritis and those maybe occurring secondary to reflux gastritis.

Tytgat: Do you know whether anyone has looked at gastric tissue obtained a long time ago or at blood samples taken long ago to find out whether the same frequencies of *C. pylori* infection were present? In other words do we know whether *C. pylori* infection is a recent disease or a very old one? Could the *C. pylori* infection perhaps be an iatrogenically transmitted disease?

Rathbone: Answering your last question first, we have not actually looked at this. But it is an interesting point. Concerning old material, I think people have looked back at specimens taken at the turn of the century. One problem is that most are resection specimens, and unless they are put into formalin quickly *C. pylori* is difficult to see. Serologically I do not know if anyone has gone back to old serum. It would be interesting, but I do not know if anyone has serum that is 40 or 50 years old.

Molecular Epidemiology and Natural History of *Campylobacter pylori* Colonization

W. LANGENBERG

Not long after the first attempts to cure *C. pylori*-associated gastritis by antibacterial treatment, it became clear that it was necessary to develop a method for typing *Campylobacter pylori* isolates. It is still the case that bacteria soon reappear in many patients with negative cultures immediately after cessation of therapy [1, 2]. It must be assessed whether this is due to reinfection or to relapse. In addition, a method for typing *C. pylori* is needed to identify the source(s) of human infection, to study the routes of transmission, etc.

As the development of a serotyping scheme is time consuming and the preliminary results of biotyping and SDS-PAGE analysis of the proteins of *C. pylori* looked unpromising, restriction endonuclease DNA analysis was used for precise identification of *C. pylori* isolates [3]. Isolates recovered from different patients produced clearly different DNA patterns after digestion with *Hin*dIII as well as after digestion with *Eco*R1. In addition, the patterns seemed stable, both in vivo (during prolonged colonization of the gastric mucosa) and in vitro (during repeated subculturing in the laboratory).

Using restriction endonuclease DNA analysis, posttreatment recurrence of *C. pylori* infection was attributed to recrudescence of surviving bacteria rather than to reinfection [3]. This technique was also used to study the natural history of *C. pylori*-associated gastritis (Fig. 1). Untreated, *C. pylori* infected patients were reexamined regularly or irregularly for 1−2 years. The infection persisted in all with the same strain. During the same study, no *C. pylori* infections were observed in noninfected patients who were also followed up for 1−2 years.

Although on one occasion a few colonies of *C. pylori* were grown from the gastric biopsies of one of these patients, DNA analysis indicated that the biopsy specimens were contaminated by *C. pylori* of the patient immediately before, who was examined with the same (though cleaned and ethanol-treated) endoscope.

It was found that the DNA patterns of *C. pylori* isolates recovered subsequently from the same patient showed differences of more than one band in about a third of both the treated and the untreated patients. These differences were minor as compared to the clearly different patterns produced by isolates from different patients and were usually only apparent in the *Hin*dIII but not in the *Eco*R1 digests (Fig. 1). It is therefore probable that these subsequent isolates represent variants of the same strain rather than different strains. Further studies of this phenomenon are needed to establish its cause and its importance for restriction endonuclease DNA analysis as a method for precise identification of *C. pylori* isolates.

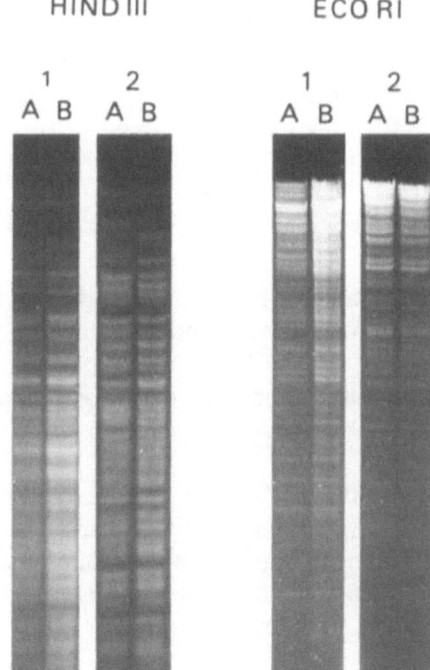

Fig. 1. Restriction enzyme analysis of whole cell bacterial DNA. DNA preparations digested with *Hin*dIII and with *Eco*R1 of the initial (*a lanes*) and the most recent (*b lanes*) *C. pylori* isolates from two untreated patients (*1* and *2*). Note the clearly different patterns produced by isolates from different patients, and the slight differences between the *Hin*dIII digests of the isolates of patient 2, which are not present in the *Eco*R1 digests

References

1. Jones DM, Eldrigde J, Whorwell PJ, et al. (1985) The effects of various anti-ulcer regimens and antibiotics on the presence of *Campylobacter pyloridis* and its antibody. In: Pearson AD, Skirrow MB, Lior H, Rowe B (eds) Campylobacter III: proceedings of the third international workshop on campylobacter infections. Public Health Laboratory Service, London, p 161
2. Langenberg ML, Rauws EAJ, Schipper MEI, et al. (1985) The pathogenic role of *Campylobacter pyloridis* studied by attempts to eliminate these organisms. In: Pearson AD, Skirrow MB, Lior H, Rowe B (eds) Campylobacter III: proceedings of the third international workshop on campylobacter infections. Public Health Laboratory Service PHLS, London, pp 162—163
3. Langenberg W, Rauws EAJ, Widjojokusumo A, et al.(1986) Identification of *Campylobacter pyloridis* isolates by restriction endonuclease DNA analysis. J Clin Microbiol 24:414—417

Discussion

Marshall: Dr. Pearson, what do you think about the terminology in the conclusion on prevalence and incidence?

Pearson: You may give us the population base data, but I suspect, you are actually talking about an isolation rate from a group of patients that you studied.

Langenberg: Yes, this is true. We studied a group of healthy volunteers and found infection in 24%. These figures have been confirmed by serological examinations in many other groups of asymptomatic subjects. So, although it is a frequency, I do think that *C. pylori* associated gastritis is present in many people, in many countries.

Goodwin: I think your work with the restriction endonuclease has been very valuable. In Perth we have isolates from the same patient over a period of 1 or 2 years, and the two original isolates were similar in terms of endonuclease, but the second two of four were quite different from the first two. We have also found in Perth that the second isolate from patients has been different in about 50% of cases. I think it remains to be seen whether you are right that if you have a similar profile on *E. coli,* that they are the same; I am not sure that it is necessarily true, because if the *Hin*dIII profiles show major differences, it does suggest that the isolates are different; but I would entirely agree with you that they are variants probably of the same original isolate of course. In microbiology we know that in the colon, for instance, with *E. coli* serotypes you can find two, three or more types occurring in the same patient. I think this is a very important observation, because *C. pylori* is an extremely widespread pathogen throughout the world; everywhere you look for it you find it. And one of the attributes of successful pathogens is the ability to undergo genomic variations and this could well be an example of it by endonuclease study.

Tytgat: You suggested that the patient who did not develop persistent infection had a previous CP exposure, in view of his immune profile. Might this be the reason why he cleared the organism spontaneously? Question also to Dr. Marshall: At the time you ingested the organism, did you have antibodies in your blood prior to ingestion? And then my second question, related to that is, why do people who have antibodies in their serum not clear the organism?

Marshall: My serum was examined by Jacob Caldor and by Professor Goodwin and after many months working with the organism, I did have a rise in titer into the equivocal range, but I never developed positive serology. We did culture numerous biopsies from the 14-day examination, but unfortunately, the organism had disappeared. The other question you asked was, why infected patients cannot clear the organism. Professor Goodwin mentioned yesterday, this organism is located in very unusual sites throughout the gastric mucosa. Firstly, we do not know enough about the immunity of gastric mucosa and gastric mucus. The stomach is a sterile organ and before *C. pylori* colonized man there was no reason to have immune response in the gastric mucosa, because there were no viable organisms there. Secondly, there is the occasional colonization of the parietal cells by *C. pylori*. The parietal cell canaliculus must be a very acidic environment. *C. pylori* organisms here may not be exposed to antibodies. Thirdly because of its toxins and inhibition of phagocytosis, even the fact that CP is coated with this Ig does not help the phagocytic cells and the bacterium is not properly cleared.

Pearson: Could we go back to the question of persistence versus reinfection, I am not totally convinced by going down the line of a single interpretation of your very nice Brenda pictures. If the majority of the strains are very similar, and if there is a common source, then surely, one could have reinfection rather than, as in your interpretation, persistence of the existing infection.

Langenberg: It could be that there is in the environment of the patient a remaining source and that the patient can perhaps be reinfected from that source with the same strain. But I do not think that the strains that are present in a wider environment are very similar as far as their Brenda patterns are concerned.

Marshall: I agree, because the pattern is the same. This does not necessarily mean that the patient has a persistent infection, because the patient could have a family member with exactly the same organism. In our data from Perth reinfection was relatively rare, probably not more than 10% per annum. This figure is based on a negative biopsy taken at least 3 months after treatment. If the biopsy was clear 3 months after treatment, that patient could be relied upon to remain negative with occasional exceptions.

Campylobacter pylori in Children

S. Cadranel, Y. Glupczinsky, M. Labbe, and C. de Prez

Chronic abdominal pain, a very common complaint in children, includes a wide variety of etiologies, such as constipation, food allergy, and the so-called psychosomatic diseases, which have been thoroughly studied in the classic work by Appley [1]. However most children complain of pain located in the periumbilical region. During the past decade, with the advent of small, flexible, fiberoptic endoscopes, upper gastrointestinal (GI) investigation has become available and is now widely used in children complaining from epigastric pain, resulting in a more frequent recognition of peptic ulcer disease and gastritis in children [2].

Despite the apparently increased incidence of childhood peptic disease its cause remains obscure. Few studies on chronic gastritis in children with biopsy material obtained blindly have been published [3−5]; and a granular aspect of the gastric antral mucosa was reported from Spain [6]. Since the report by Marshall and Warren [7] of the presence of *Campylobacter*-like organisms on the gastric mucosa of adults with chronic active gastritis and ulcers of the stomach and duodenum, great interest has been aroused concerning the possible etiological role of these microorganisms. Until now, only three papers [8−10] have been published concerning the presence of *Campylobacter pylori* (CP) in the gastric mucosa of 6, 8 and 5 children, respectively. The aim of the present study is to evaluate the presence and significance of CP colonization in children undergoing upper GI endoscopy and mucosal biopsy.

Material and Methods

From September 1986 to May 1987 a total of 385 mucosal biopsies could be obtained for histological and bacteriological studies from 137 endoscopic procedures in 114 infants, children and adolescents undergoing examination for a variety of indications such as recurrent vomiting, chronic abdominal pain, haematemesis, post-operative revision after Nissen's anti-reflux fundoplication and follow-up examinations for gastroduodenal ulcers and oesophageal caustic injuries. The age range of the children was 2 months to 16 years; the mean was 6.7 years. Seven young adults (18−21 years old) who had been followed for many years as children were also included in this series. There were 59 females and 55 males. The ethnic origins were as follows: 59 Belgians, 35 North Africans, 6 Italians, 4 Spaniards, 4 African Bantus, 2 Greeks, 2 Turks and 2 Yugoslavians.

Endoscopies were carried out with Olympus 7.9 mm GIF-XP or 8.7 Olympus GIF-P10. When possible, four biopsies were taken at each site, two for CP culture and two for histology. The specimens were transported in semi-solid agar transport medium and processed within 2 h of collection for direct examination (Gram's staining) and incubated on two chocolate agar plates for 5 days at 37 °C in microaerophilic atmosphere (5% O_2, 10% CO_2). Histologic specimens were stained with haematoxylin-eosin and examined, without knowledge of patient data, for chronic gastritis (mild, moderate, severe) and chronic active gastritis (mild, moderate, severe) according to Whitehead's criteria. Finding of CP either by direct examination, culture or histology was considered positive.

Results

The clinical features of children with and without *C. pylori* are given in Table 1. CP was found positive in 47 out of 137 endoscopic examinations (35%) and in 36 out of 114 children (31.6%). The youngest children were aged 3 and 4 years

Table 1. Clinical features in children with and without *C. pylori* (CP) in gastric biopsy samples

Clinical features	CP−	CP+	Total
Chronic epigastric pain	7	19	26
Duodenal ulcer	0	2	2
Gastric ulcer	1	0	1
Stress ulcer in neonates	2	0	2
GD ulcer follow-up	3	3	6
Total	13	24	37
Gastro-oesophageal reflux	27	0	27
Hiatal hernia (+/− Nissen)	2	7	9
Caustic oesophageal injuries:			
(<2 months)	2	0	2
(>1 year)	0	5	5
Total	31	12	43
Cow's milk intolerance	5	1	6
Malabsorption	2	0	2
Coeliac disease	6	3	9
BID (Crohn, UHRC)	3	0	3
Liver cirrhosis	2	2	4
Others	9	1	10
Total	27	7	34

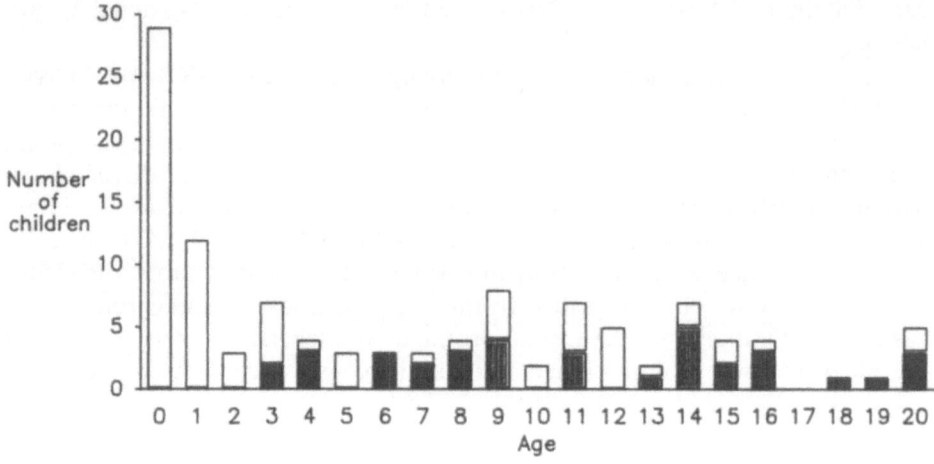

Fig. 1. Distribution of patients according to age ($n = 114$). *Shaded bars, C. pylori* negative ($n = 78$); *unshaded bars, C. pylori* positive ($n = 36$)

Table 2. Prevalence of *C. pylori* (CP) in gastric biopsy samples in relation to the ethnic origin of the children

Ethnic origin	CP−	CP+	Total
Belgians	49	10	59
Moroccans	16	19	35
Italians	5	1	6
Zairians	2	2	4
Spaniards	4	0	4
Turks	0	2	2
Greeks	2	0	2
Yugoslavians	1	1	2
Total	78	36	114

(Fig. 1). The ethnic origin of the children with and without CP is given in Table 2. The high incidence of CP in North African children corresponds to the distribution among the adult population in our hospital.

Direct examination was positive, together with positive culture, in seven cases and associated with a negative culture in one case. On one occasion CP was found by histology while it appeared negative on direct examination and in culture. In 27 cases direct examination was negative while culture gave a positive result for CP. Chronic epigastric pain characterized 19 of the 24 children with suspicion of peptic disease. CP was also present in seven of the nine children with hiatal hernia and all five children with caustic oesphagitis of more than 1 year of evolution. CP was present in the gastric mucosa of three of the nine children with untreated coeliac disease.

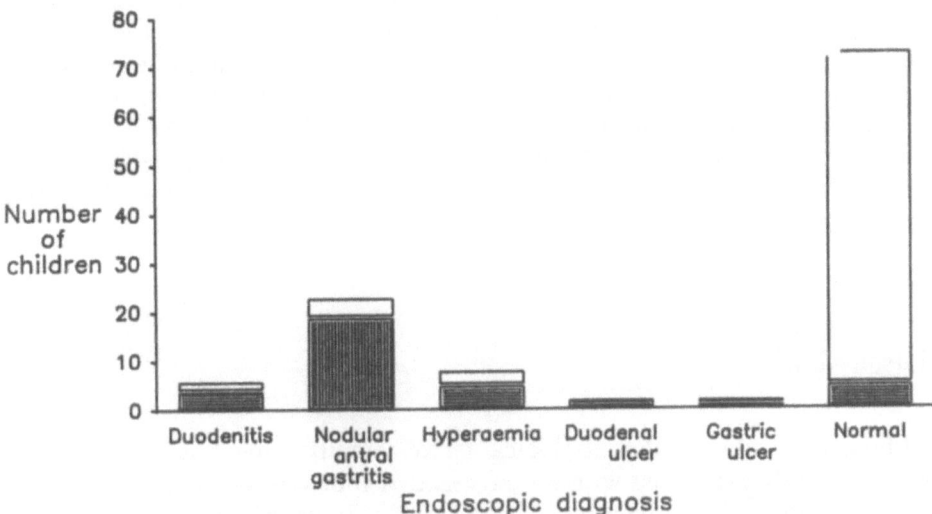

Fig. 2. Antral biopsies (*n* = 114) by endoscopic diagnosis and *C. pylori* finding. *Solid bars, C. pylori* negative (*n* = 78); *striped bars, C. pylori* positive (*n* = 36)

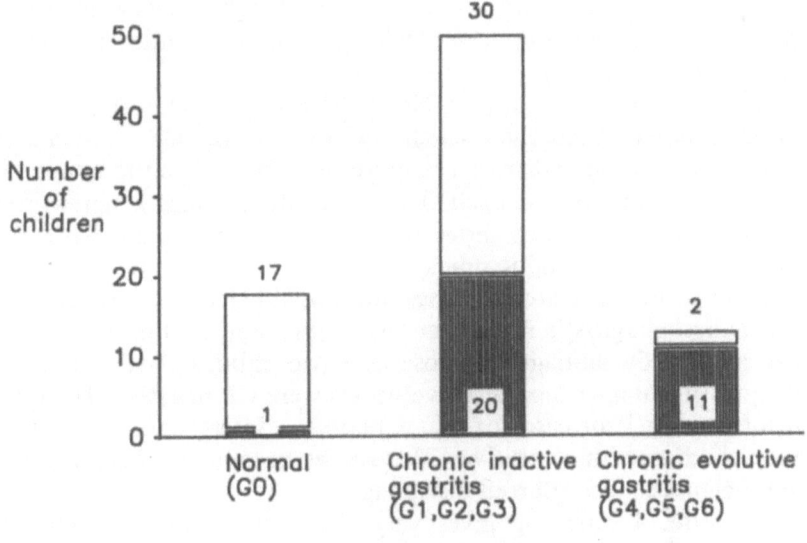

Fig. 3. Antral biopsies (*n* = 81) by histologic diagnosis and *C. pylori* finding. *Solid bars, C. pylori* negative (*n* = 49); *striped bars, C. pylori* positive (*n* = 32)

Endoscopic features in children with and without *C. pylori* in gastric biopsy samples are given in Fig. 2. CP was found positive only in five cases with normal mucosa while the occurrence of a micronodular pattern, sometimes associated with erosions at the level of the antrum, was very frequent. Positive CP was found in only one out of 18 cases with a histologically normal mucosa

(Fig. 3), but found positive in 20 out of 50 cases with chronic gastritis (40%) – 32% in mild, 56% in moderate and 66% in severe chronic gastritis – and in 11 out of 13 cases with chronic active gastritis (84%) – 83% in mild and 86% in moderate active chronic gastritis, but no case of severe chronic gastritis.

The site of biopsy is also interesting since, out of 385 biopsies examined, CP was found positive in 94 (24%) with the following distribution: jejunum 0/14; duodenum 2/38 (5%); duodenal bulb 13/103 (12%); antrum 47/119 (39%); fundus 29/62 (46%) and cardia 3/40 (7.5%).

Discussion

Although the role of CP as etiological factor remains a hypothesis, its presence seems strongly associated with the presence of mucosal lesions in children, reproducing the classical features of gastritis already described in adults but perhaps with a less severe course. It is interesting to note the very high incidence of endoscopically recognizable lesions, especially the so-called micronodular antral pattern. Indeed, when this pattern was present, CP was found in 19 cases, while the same pattern was associated with negative CP in only four. This finding might be of some importance when dealing with children complaining from chronic epigastric pain.

The high incidence among North Africans in our series has already been noted in the adult patients as well, and some of the CP+ associated with such indications as coeliac disease are more probably related to ethnic origin of patients than to the disease itself. The age of the patients is noteworthy since the youngest children in our series were aged 3 and presented the characteristic micronodular antral endoscopical pattern.

Among the associated diseases, the coincidence of CP in five children with caustic oesophagitis is important and might indicate that CP is ready to colonize an already damaged mucosa; the two children with fresh caustic oesophagitis (less than 1 month of evolution) were CP negative. The relatively high incidence of CP in cases of hiatal hernia is interesting, especially in that all three children with a positive CP from the oesophagus belonged to this group and each presented a Barrett oesophagus.

The site of sampling gives very clear-cut results: the antral and fundic biopsies are more often positive than any other site of sampling and should be explored with priority over any other site.

Conclusion

This preliminary series of 36 CP colonizations of the upper GI tract in children draws attention to the relatively high incidence of CP in paediatrics. Unlike in adult patients, gastric and duodenal ulcers are rare while chronic gastritis is frequent. Of course, further studies are necessary, aimed at proper treatment and follow-up as are also careful epidemiological studies on the families of these children.

References

1. Appley J (1975) The children with abdominal pains. Blackwell Scientific Publications, Oxford
2. Christie DL, Ament ME (1976) Gastric acid hypersecretion in children with duodenal ulcer. Pediatr Res 10:353
3. Apostolov BG (1973) Chronic gastritis in children and their treatment. Pediatriia 23:15
4. Sokolova MI (1973) Functional and morphological state of the duodenum in children with chronic gastritis. Pediatriia 52:20
5. Lebedev VP (1973) Chronic diffuse gastritis in young patients. Vrach. Delo 5:103
6. Beltran S, Varea V, Vilar P, Cusi V, Vila J, Farré C (1978) Gastritis cronica infantil. An Esp Pediat 11:383
7. Marshall B, Warren JR (1984) Unidentified curved bacilli in the stomach of patients with gastritis and peptic ulceration. Lancet i:1311
8. Hill R, Pearman J, Worthy P, Caruso V, Goodwin S, Blincow E (1986) Campylobacter pyloridis and gastritis in children. Lancet i:387
9. Cadranel S, Goossens H, De Boeck M, Malengreau A, Rodesch P, Butzler JP (1986) Campylobacter pyloridis in children. Lancet i:735
10. Czinn SJ, Everly BD, Jacobs GH, Kaplan B, Rothstein FC (1986) Campylobacter-like organisms in association with symptomatic gastritis in children. J Pediat 109:80

Discussion

Classen: May I ask a question concerning the incidence and prevalence of peptic ulcers in children? Are the figures precisely known and can they be compared to those in adults?

Cadranel: No, I do not think they are known. This, of course, was a very special population that was referred to us. So I cannot say, unless we have at our disposal something less invasive than gastroscopy to evaluate this problem, because we cannot perform endoscopy on every child. It is almost impossible until we get some easier way of evaluation.

Ó'Moráin: Have you treated any children with chronic abdominal pain who are CP-positive, and, if so, how have they done?

Cadranel: I have, but not all of them, because we knew the results of Tytgat and colleagues. So we were reluctant to use bismuth salts in children and did so only with those who were over the age of 12. These did well. But I cannot say just now how many of them became CP-negative and how many remained CP-positive. But generally I would say that most of them remained positive.

Classen: Can you draw any therapeutic conclusions concerning treatment in children?

Cadranel: No, of course not. I am here just for the purpose of discovering how to treat them; I hope to draw from the audience suggestions as to how children as young as 3 years of age could be treated, for instance, without too much harm to their further growth.

Börsch: Did micronodular antral gastritis resolve in those few patients that you have treated?

Cadranel: Of the two slides I showed you, the first was micronodular gastritis without too many erosions; the second endoscopy slide had heavy erosions. And I would say that these showed some improvement. But none of them really disappeared. Histologically it was improved but it was not a complete cure. But maybe I did not treat them long enough.

Classen: Micronodular gastritis seems rather infrequent in adults.

Cadranel: This is correct.

Ottenjann: What is the histological feature of this so-called micronodular gastritis? Is there lymphatic hyperplasia or the like?

Cadranel: No, I do not think there is any difference. Our histologist has tried to ascertain a difference between our series and the adult series (she is the pathologist for both clinics), and she sees no difference whatever. She also sees no difference between the histological pattern of heavy and light colonization. So there seems to be no relationship between the number of colonies we can culture and the infiltration or the histological pattern.

Ottenjann: Can you tell something about the diameter of the nodules?

Cadranel: Yes, I would say they are about 1 mm.

Classen: Do they look like lymphoid follicles?

Cadranel: Yes, this is how we published it earlier, as lymphoid follicles.

Pearson: Have you compared the biochemical properties, the protein profiles or the results of Brenda on any of your strains with isolates from adult patients?

Cadranel: This work is in progress. I cannot tell you anything about it now, but this is one of our aims at present. And besides, we can do it because it is the same clinic, and most of our children have parents with epigastric pain or have been referred to an adult gastroenterologist for ulcers or dyspepsia. What we are trying to do now is to collect family data for serological determination and, when possible, for strains and CP culture in their biopsies.

Goodwin: Just to answer this last query for you. The restriction endonuclease pattern of children's isolates is no different from that of adult isolates. If you place them together, you cannot see a difference.

Cadranel: Yes, that is right.

Riecken: You pointed out that you found *Campylobacter pylori* in 3 out of 9 patients with coeliac disease. Did you mean to imply by mentioning this especially that this finding has some bearing on the malabsorption syndrome?

Cadranel: That is what we thought at the beginning, that we were dealing with something here. Coeliac disease patients in childhood do, of course, have lowered immunity. Even if they have over-reactive immunity, they have an impaired immunity. And in all cases of malabsorption or malnutrition this is a very well known phenomenon. So we would have preferred to hypothesize that these children experienced colonization because of the coeliac disease. But this was not true, because all three of them were North Africans, and it may be due to ethnic origin more than to the disease itself.

Section 4

Diagnosis of *Campylobacter pylori* Infection

Monoclonal Antibodies Against *Campylobacter pylori*

L. ENGSTRAND, C. PÅHLSON, A. SCHWAN, and S. GUSTAVSSON

For many years gram-negative bacteria have been found to be attached to human gastric mucosa. S-shaped bacteria were seen closely associated with the surface epithelium, both within and between the gastric pits. The successful culture of these organisms from gastric biopsy material was reported in 1983 by Marshall and Warren [1]. Due to similarities to *Campylobacter* strains and frequent occurrence in the distal stomach the bacteria were termed *Campylobacter pyloridis* [2]. However, in 1987 the bacteria were renamed as *Campylobacter pylori* [3]. The organisms are found almost exclusively in connection with inflammatory changes of the gastric mucosa, and a proposed causal relation between *C. pylori*, gastritis and ulcer disease is under intense investigation throughout the world. This paper describes monoclonal antibodies for the detection of these bacteria, compared to culture and to another proposed method for rapid detection, namely direct inoculation of urea broth [4].

Hybridoma Production and Characterization

Immunization Protocol and Cell Fusion

As an antigen for immunization, in an attempt to achieve antibody-producing hybridomas [5], we used young colonies (72 h) of *Campylobacter pylori* (strain Canada 5437, obtained from Prof. D. Danielsson, Örebro, Sweden). The strain was grown on agar plates supplemented with 5% sheep blood. Cells from four plates were harvested in phosphate-buffered saline (PBS) and washed once in PBS. Approximately 400 µl packed cells were diluted in 400 µl PBS, and 800 µl Freund's complete adjuvants were added. The mixture was homogenized and vigorously emulgated for approximately 1 h by repeated aspiration with a syringe. Then 25 µl suspension was injected subcutaneously in each hind paw of five 8-week-old DBA/1J mice. Nine days after immunization the regional popliteal and inguinal lymph nodes were collected. The lymph nodes were ruptured by injection of PBS and the lymphocytes were centrifuged and prepared for fusion by washing once in PBS. Mouse myeloma cells X-63 were used as fusion partner. The cells were prepared for fusion by growth to blast stadium in Dulbecco's modified Eagle's medium (DMEM), supplemented with 10% fetal calf serum (FCS) glutamine and a mixture of penicillin and streptomycin. Before fusion X-63 cells were washed three times in PBS, 10×10^7 lymphocytes were mixed with 10×10^6 myeloma cells.

The fusion was carried out by addition of 500 μl polyetylene glycole (PEG) M_w 4000 for 90 s. The fusion was terminated by dilution in serum-free DMEM. The cells were spun down and resuspended in DMEM supplemented with 10% FCS, hypoxanthin and aminopterin (HAT-medium) and 10^9/ml rat thymocytes from a young Lewis rat. The mixture was distributed into five 96-well microtiter plates.

Hybrid Selection and Characterization of Monoclonal Antibodies

Supernatants from wells with growing cells were tested in ELISA and by indirect immunofluorescence (IF) as described elswhere [6] against the homologous strain. A strain of *C. jejuni* was used as negative control. A pure cultured strain stained by IF is shown in Fig. 1. Clones giving positive reaction were diluted into additional wells. Single clones were transferred into cell culture flasks and propagated in DMEM or in serum-free HL-1 medium (Ventrex Lab Inc., Portland, USA). The chosen clone was tested against forty clinical isolates of *C. pylori* and the unrelated bacteria shown in Table 1. The antibodies were concentrated by precipitation with an equal amount of saturated ammonium sulphate. This precipitate was diluted in water to approximately 5% of the original amount of cell culture medium. Isotype determination was performed by double immunodiffusion in 0.9% agarose gels. The diffusion precipitation was carried out against subspecific goat anti-mouse antibodies (Sigma chemical, St. Louis, Missouri, USA) and the antibodies were found to be of isotype IgG1.

SDS-PAGE gel electrophoresis of whole-cell lysate was performed in a midget electrophoresis cell (LKB, Bromma, Sweden) with myosin, β-galactosidase, phosphorylase, bovine albumin, egg albumin and carbonic anhydrase (Sigma chemical, St. Louis, Missouri, USA) as molecular weight markers. The gels were stained with Coomassie-blue or used for trans blotting of the proteins to nitrocellulose papers (NCM). In the blotting procedure the unbound sites on the NCM were blocked with 2% BSA. The protein reacting with the antibodies was detected by cell culture supernatant and visualized by addition of peroxidase-conjugated protein A, developed by the addition of carbazole and hydrogen peroxide. The antibodies reacted with a protein band migrating at approximately 25 kDa.

Table 1. Bacteria tested and found not to react with monoclonal antibodies directed against outer membrane protein from *Campylobacter pylori* as tested by ELISA

Acinetobacter anitratum	*K. pneumoniae*
Campylobacter jejuni	*Proteus mirabilis*
Citrobacter diversus	*Pseudomonas aeruginosa*
Enterobacter aerogenes	*Staphylococcus epidermidis*
Escherichia coli	*S. saprophyticus*
Klebsiella oxytoca	

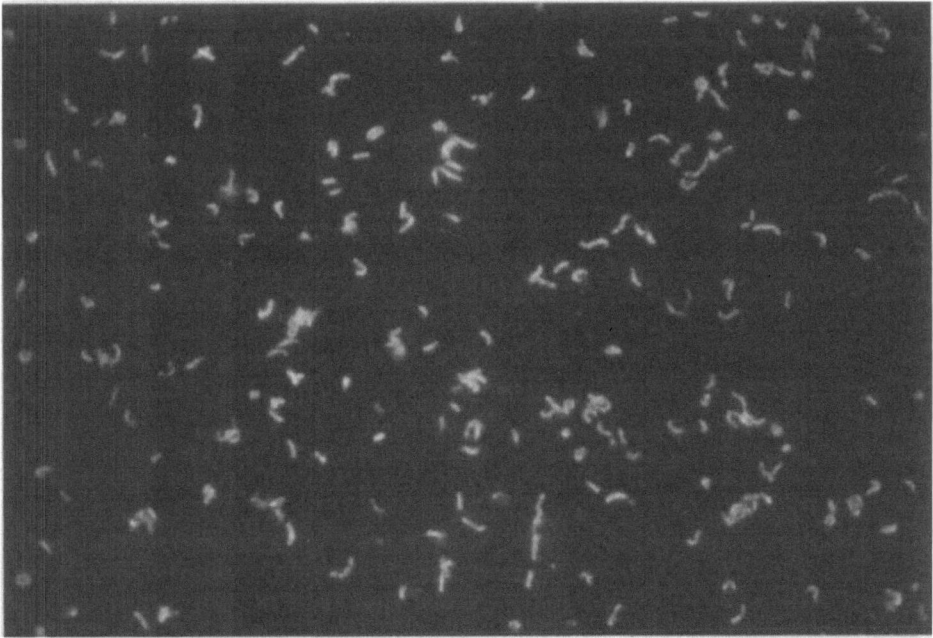

Fig. 1. Immunofluorescence of cultured cells of *Campylobacter pylori* after indirect staining with monoclonal antibodies (× 1000)

Clinical Studies of *Campylobacter pylori*

Microbiological Methods for Detection of *C. pylori*

Outpatients seen at the endoscopy room of the university hospital in Uppsala, Sweden, were studied. By endoscopy the presence of hyperemia, erosions and mucosal hypertrophy was noted. A biopsy was taken from the gastric antrum and immediately sent to the laboratory in sterile 0,9% saline. The biopsy was homogenized within 2 h and inoculated on blood agar plates with and without the addition of antibiotics. The following supplemented agar plates were used: 5% sheep blood agar with vancomycin, nalidixic acid, amphotericin B; and 5% sheep blood agar with vancomycin, trimethoprim, polymyxin B. The plates were incubated in anaerobic jars using the Campy Pak system (BBL) at 37°C for 7 days, with examination on the 3rd, 5th and 7th days. Suspected colonies were examined by Gram's stain and tested for the production of urease, catalase, oxidase and nitrate reductase. *C. pylori* colonies were positive for urease, catalase and oxidase and were negative for nitrate reductase. Biopsy homogenate was also inoculated into ureal broth which was examined every hour on the 1st day (4−7 h) and after 24 and 48 h. The results of culture and ureal broth testing are shown in Table 2.

Table 2. Detection of *Campylobacter pylori* with monoclonal antibodies and IF, compared to culture and detection by ureal hydrolysis in 30 persons with ulcer or gastritis or determined as healthy

Number of patients	Clinical observation	Culture	IF with Mabs	Urea test*
3	Ulcer	+	+	+2 h
1	Ulcer	+	+	+8 h
4	Ulcer	+	+	ND
3	Ulcer	+	+	−
2	Ulcer	−	−	+24 h
2	Ulcer	−	−	ND
1	Gastritis	+	+	+2 h
3	Gastritis	+	+	+24 h
1	Gastritis	−	−	+24 h
1	Gastritis	−	−	−
1	Gastritis	−	−	ND
1	Normal mucosa	−	−	+24 h
2	Normal mucosa	−	−	−
5	Normal mucosa	−	−	ND

ND, Not done; * positive within hours

Monoclonal Antibodies on Smears of Biopsy Homogenate

Glass slides were smeared with biopsy homogenate. The slides were air-dried and gently fixed in a flame. 50 µl cell culture supernatant was added for 20 min. The slides were washed in PBS for 10 min. Fluorescein isothiocyonate (FITC) conjugated rabbit anti-mouse antibodies (Dakopatts, Copenhagen, Denmark) were used as secondary antibodies for 20 min and the slides were washed in PBS for 10 min. The slides were mounted with PBS containing 10% glycerol and examined in a Nicon fluorescence microscope using Ploem optics and filters. A representative result is shown in Fig. 2. The results of the indirect microscopy are summarized in Table 2.

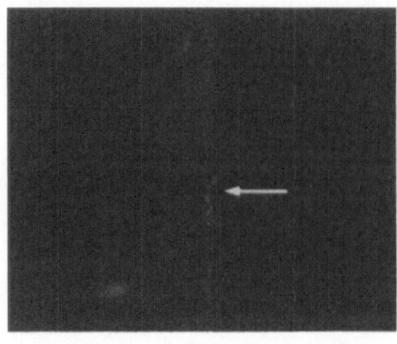

Fig. 2. Smear of gastric biopsy positive for *Campylobacter pylori* stained by monoclonal antibodies in indirect immunofluorescence (× 1000)

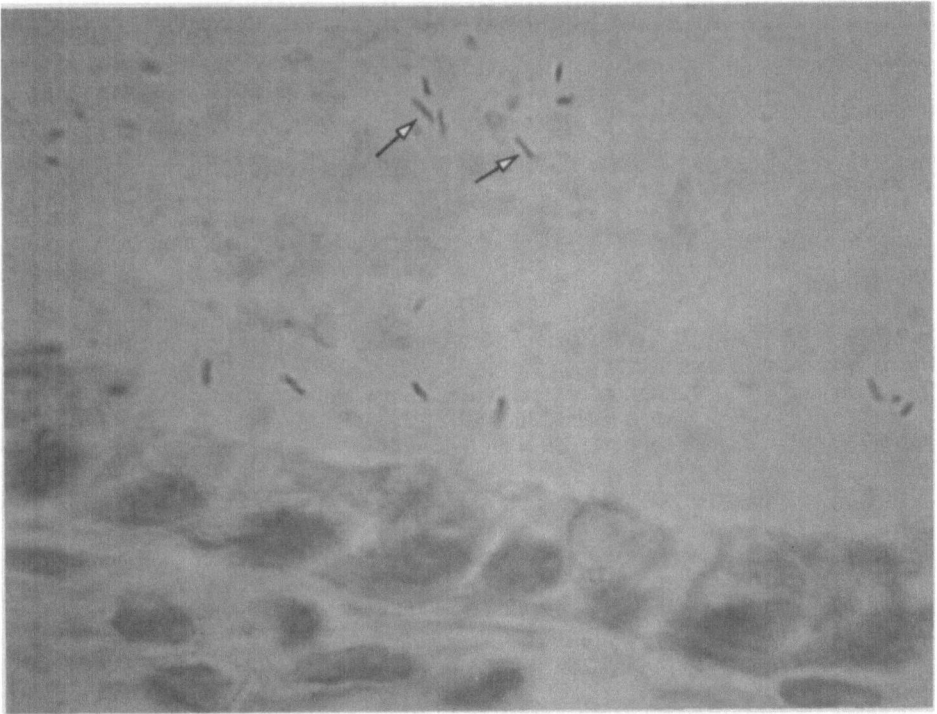

Fig. 3. Cryostat section of gastric mucosa stained by monoclonal antibodies and PAP; *Campylobacter pylori* stained brown, epithelial cells stained blue on the original picture (× 1000)

PAP Staining on Cryostat Sections

Cryostat sections, 4 µm thick, were processed for peroxidase-anti-peroxidase (PAP) staining according to the method of Sternberger [7]. Endogenic peroxidase was blocked by 0.3% hydrogen peroxidase and native swine serum diluted 1/10 for 15 min. The anti-*C. pylori* monoclonal antibodies were used as undiluted cell culture supernatant. As secondary antibody, rabbit anti-mouse Ig was used (diluted 1/40). Preformed complexes of horseradish peroxidase and mouse monoclonal anti-horseradish peroxidase antibody (diluted 1/250) were obtained from Dakopatts (Copenhagen, Denmark). The peroxidase reaction was developed with carbazole [8] and the sections counterstained with haematoxylin. Controls without the primary antibodies were included and gave no staining. Fig. 3 shows a stained cryostat section with *C. pylori*.

Conclusions and Prospects

We found that the direct detection of *C. pylori* by IF is in complete accordance with culture. The main advantage with the use of monoclonal antibodies is the short time needed for diagnosis: approximately 1 h as compared to several days for culture. PAP staining has proven possible to use. An advantage with this is that it requires only an ordinary light microscope.

We hope that monoclonal antibodies will contribute to the understanding of the role of these bacteria in diseases of the stomach and to the finding of the natural ecological niche of *C. pylori* and its transmission to humans.

References

1. Marshall BJ, Warren JR (1983) Unidentified curved bacilli on gastric epithelium in active chronic gastritis. Lancet I:1273–1275
2. Anonymous (1985) Validation of publication of new names and new combinations previously effectively published outside the IJSB. Int J Syst Bacteriol 85:223–225
3. Marshall BJ, Goodwin CS (1987) Revised nomenclature of Campylobacter pyloridis. Int J Syst Bacteriol 37:68
4. McNulty CAM, Wise R (1985) Rapid diagnosis of Campylobacter associated gastritis. Lancet I:1443–1444
5. Köhler G, Milstein C (1975) Continous cultures of fused cells secreting antibody of predefined specificity. Nature 256:495
6. Påhlson C, Hallén A, Forsum U (1986) Curver rods related to Mobiluncus-phenotypes as defined by monoclonal antibodies. Acta Pathol Microbiol Scand (B) 94:117
7. Sternberger LA (1979) Immunocytochemistry. Wiley Medical Publications, John Wiley & Sons, New York
8. Kaplow LS (1975) Substitute for benzidine in myeloperoxidase stains. Am J Clin Pathol 63:451

Production and Characterization of Monoclonal Antibodies Against *Campylobacter pylori*

M. GREGOR, M. WARRELMANN, A. NIEDER, H. MENGE, H. HAHN,
and E. O. RIECKEN

Introduction

In 1983 Warren and Marshall described the presence of bacteria in antral biopsies which were called *Campylobacter pylori* on the basis of their location, morphology, and microbiological characteristics [1]. In the years which followed there have been a number of reports, based on antral biopsies, about the association of *C. pylori* with antral gastritis (type B, nonimmune gastritis) as well as with peptic ulcers [1–13]. Culture techniques, urease tests, and various histological staining methods, as well as microscopic techniques have been used for diagnosis of antral colonization by *C. pylori* [1, 3, 4, 9, 13–18].

It was the purpose of our study to produce monoclonal antibodies against *C. pylori* and to compare the usefulness of such immunoreagents for immunocytochemical detection of *C. pylori* with the microbiological isolation of the bacterium in human antral biopsies.

Materials and Methods

Immunization

Whole cells of a strain of *C. pylori* (NCTC 11637) were used to immunize 6–8 week old female Balb/c mice (Bomholtgart, Denmark) by intraperitoneal injection with 10^7 cells on each occasion. Two booster injections were administered at weekly intervals and a final series of booster injections was given 2, 3, and 4 days before the fusion experiment.

Cell Fusion and Hybridoma Production

Mouse myeloma cells (2×10^7; P3-X63-Ag 8.653), which do not synthesize any antibody molecules, were fused with 5×10^5 mouse spleen cells by techniques which have been described elsewhere [19]. The plating medium was Dulbecco's modified Eagle's medium (Flow Laboratories) containing 20% fetal calf serum (Seromed). This was supplemented, during the first 2 weeks after the fusion experiment, by hypoxanthine (10^{-4} M), aminopterin (4×10^{-7} M), and thymidine

$(1.6 \times 10^{-5} M)$ (HAT, Sigma). After 2 weeks, culture supernatants were periodically tested for anti-*C. pylori* antibody production. Positive hybridomas were cloned over feeder layers of mouse peritoneal macrophages by the limiting dilution method. All selected subclones were routinely recloned and then grown to maximum density in 150-ml cultures.

Screening Assay

Culture fluids of growing hybridomas were tested for anti-*C. pylori* activity by an enzyme linked immunosorbent assay (ELISA). A whole cell preparation of a strain of *C. pylori* (NCTC 11637) was used as the antigen at a concentration of 2×10^6/well. Cell culture supernatants (100 µl) were incubated for 1 h at 37°C on prepared antigen coated, polyninyl chloride, "high activity" microtiter plates (Flow Laboratories). After washing, biotinylated antimouse Ig-F(ab')2 fragment (Amersham) from sheep was added at a dilution of 1/200 (100 µl). After repeated washing, biotinylated peroxidase streptavidin complex (Amersham) was added for 30 min at 37°C (100 µl). Then, 200 µl of substrate solution consisting of 2.2'-azino-di-(3-ethyl-benzthiazoline) sulfonate (1 mM) with 0.003% v/v hydrogen peroxide was added for 25 min at 37°C. The reaction was stopped with 50 µl of 0.001% w/v sodium azide in 0.1 M citric acid. The absorbance of the colored reaction was quantitated on an ELISA reader (Flow Laboratories) at 405 nm.

Immunohistochemistry

Immunoenzymatic studies were made using the alkaline phosphatase-anti-alkaline phosphatase (APAAP) method. Antral biopsies from 51 patients were taken during routine endoscopy, fixed in formol saline, and paraffin embedded. We have also used cryostat sections in a number of specimens, which gave almost identical results. For labelling of *C. pylori*-specific antigens the APAAP complex [calf intestine alkaline phosphatase, monoclonal mouse antibody against calf intestine alkaline phosphatase (Dianova)] was bound to the primary antibody via a rabbit anti-mouse IgG (H + L) and demonstrated with the new fuchsin development method. Endogenous alkaline phosphatase activity was blocked by the addition of levamisole to the enzyme substrate. The labelled sections were counterstained with hematoxylin.

Bacterial Cultures

Biopsy specimens were put into thioglycollate broth immediately after collection and kept at 4°C for up to 2 h after collection. These specimens were then put on Columbia chocolate agar with Skirrow supplement (vancomycin, trimethoprim, polymyxin B) with amphotericin B, and were incubated under microaerophilic conditions at 37°C for 5−7 days (Gas-Pac-System, Anaerocult-C). The appearance of small, translucent colonies consisting of typically gram-negative spiral rods with positive urease, catalase, and oxidase reactions was considered a positive result.

Results and Discussion

Three separate fusion experiments of mouse myeloma cells with spleen cells, from mice immunized with *C. pylori*, resulted in 720 wells containing viable hybridoma cells. Fourteen days after hybridization, initial screening revealed that 14 wells were positive for anti-*C. pylori* antibodies. A total of five stable cultures were cloned by the limiting dilution method. All antibodies tested were identified as IgG by immunoglobulin typing.

No cross-reactivity was found with *Campylobacter jejuni, Campylobacter coli*, or with a panel of unrelated bacteria (including *E. coli*) using ELISA and immunofluorescence as testing systems. Negative controls included the omission of primary as well as bridging antibody. To assess further the specificity of our monoclonal antibodies, preabsorption studies were carried out, showing a complete loss of immunoreactivity for ELISA as well as immunohistochemistry (see below) following the preabsorption onto *C. pylori* only.

Two monoclonal antibodies (87.4.4B2 and 87.3.9C6) were used for further studies. Figure 1 shows a typical antral biopsy specimen stained with the monoclonal antibody 87.4.4B2. *C. pylori* was identified by its characteristic morphology and position within the mucin layer of the antral mucosa. The bacterium was sometimes in close contact with the luminal surface of the epithelial cells of the mucosa. In accordance with other authors we could not detect any signs of tissue invasion. There was no further staining of *C. pylori* after the preabsorption of the monoclonal antibody 87.4.4B2 onto *C. pylori* strain NCTC 11637 (Fig. 2a, b). The results with the monoclonal antibody 87.3.9C6 closely resembled those obtained with 87.4.4B2 although staining was not consistent in all cases.

Table 1 shows the correlation between the immunohistochemical identification of *C. pylori* — using the monoclonal antibody 87.4.4B2 — and the microbiological isolation of *C. pylori* in corresponding antral biopsies. From the 51 patients in the study, *C. pylori* was detected by immunohistochemistry and culture in 14 of the patients and in 10 cases *C. pylori* was not detected by immunostaining nor by microbiological techniques. No correlation was found in 27 of the specimens. In this group of 27 patients, immunohistology failed to reveal the bacteria in 14 cases, but *C. pylori* was cultured from the biopsy specimen. In contrast, in 13 patients *C. pylori* was detected by immunohistochemistry but was not isolated by culture techniques.

There was no correlation between the prevalence or the activity of chronic gastritis and the identification of *C. pylori* as revealed by immunohistochemistry using the monoclonal antibody 87.4.4B2, although six out of seven cases of chronic atrophic gastritis did show colonization by *C. pylori*.

The lack of complete correlation between microbiological isolation of *C. pylori* and immunostaining by certain monoclonal antibodies is consistent

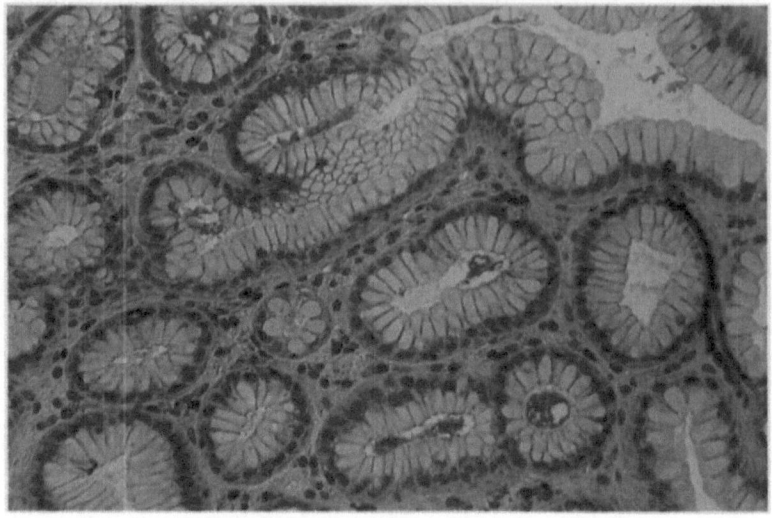

Fig. 1. Antral biopsy section immunostained with the monoclonal antibody 87.4.4B2 and counterstained with hematoxylin showing *C. pylori* colonization

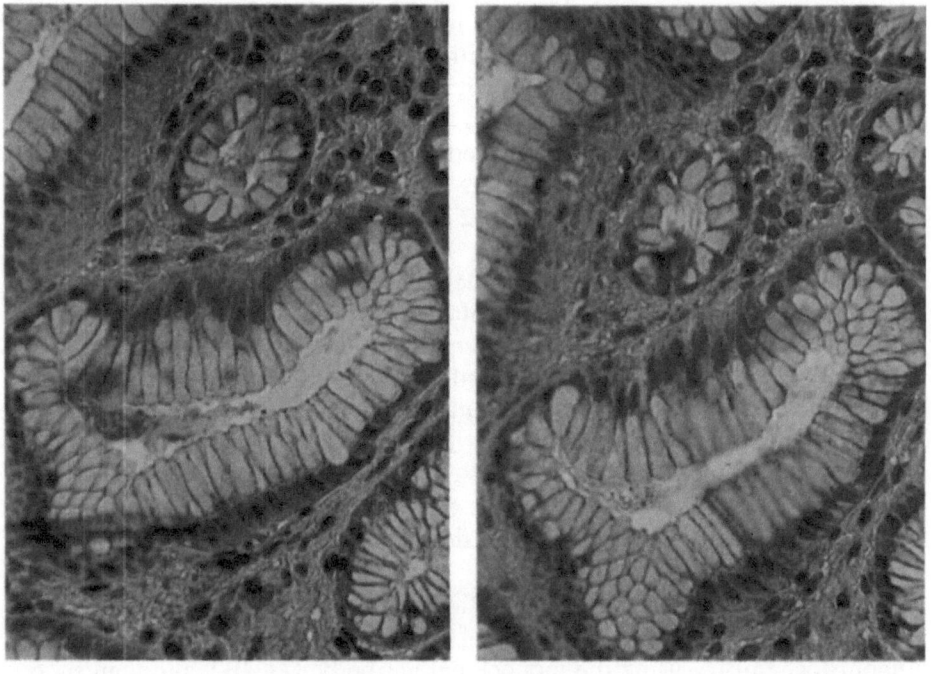

a   b

Fig. 2. a *C. pylori* in the antral mucosa immunostained with the monoclonal antibody 87.4.4B2. **b** Control incubation of the adjacent antral biopsy section following preabsorption of the monoclonal antibody 87.4.4B2 with 10^9 cells/ml of *C. pylori* (strain NCTC 11637)

Table 1. Immunohistochemical identification of *C. pylori* related to microbiological isolation of *C. pylori*

		Culture	
		+	−
87.4.4B2	+	14	13
	−	14	10

with the possibility that a single biopsy may not represent the stomach as a whole because of patchy colonization by *C. pylori*. Alternatively, it cannot be ruled out that more than one species included in the *C. pylori* group may be present. Finally, together with the heterogenous staining pattern of the monoclonal antibodies used, this lack of correlation may also indicate, as with *C. jejuni* [20], the existence of antigenic variability between different infecting strains of *C. pylori*. Further studies, using immunoblot analysis, are currently under way to identify the different antigenic determinants for the individual isolated monoclonal antibodies, and to distinguish antigenic heterogeneity in different isolates of *C. pylori* by their ability to react with certain antibodies. The demonstration of antigenic diversity in this species might be used in the analysis and identification of *C. pylori* in antral biopsies to form the basis of a serotyping system. Such a system may be relevant, in epidemiological and clinical studies of *C. pylori*- associated gastritis, to identify different pathogenic properties of the strains.

References

1. Warren JR, Marshall B (1983) Unidentified curved bacilli on gastric epithelium in active chronic gastritis. Lancet I:1273−1275
2. Kasper G, Dickgießer N (1984) Isolation of Campylobacter-like bacteria from gastric epithelium. Infection 12:179−180
3. Goodwin CS, Blincow ED, Warren JR, Waters TE, Sanderson CR, Easton L (1985) Evaluation of cultural techniques for isolating Campylobacter pyloridis from endoscopic biopsies of gastric mucosa. J Clin Pathol 38:1127−1131
4. Marshall BJ, McGechie DB, Rogers PA, Glancy RJ (1985) Pyloric Campylobacter and gastroduodenal disease. Med J Aust 142:439−444
5. Price AB, Levi J, Dolby JM, Dunscombe PL, Smith A, Clarke JC, Stephenson ML (1985) Campylobacter pyloridis in peptic ulcer disease. Microbiology, pathology, and scanning electron microscopy. Gut 26:1183−1188
6. Bayerdörffer E, Pirlet Th, Ottenjann R, Kasper G (1986) Peptisches Ulcus und Campylobacter pyloridis. Dtsch Med Wochenschr 111:1459−1461
7. Booth L, Holdstock G, Macbride H, Hatwin P, Gibson JR, Ireland A, Bamforth J, Duboulay CE, Lloy RS, Pearson AD (1986) Clinical importance of Campylobacter pyloridis and associated serum IgG and IgA antibody responses in patients undergoing upper gastrointestinal endoscopy. J Clin Pathol 39:215−219
8. Buck GE, Gourley WK, Lee WK, Subramanyan K, Latimer JM, DiNuzzo AR (1986) Relation of Campylobacter pyloridis to gastritis and peptic ulcer. J Infect Dis 153:664−669
9. Rathbone BJ, Wyatt JI, Heatley RV (1986) Campylobacter pyloridis − a new factor in peptic ulcer disease. Gut 27:635−641

10. von Wulffen H, Heesemann G, Bützow HG, Löning T, Laufs R (1986) Detection of Campylobacter pyloridis in patients with antrum gastritis and peptic ulcers by culture, complement fixation test, and immunoblot. J Clin Microbiol 24:716−720

11. Menge H, Warrelmann M, Loy V, Schmidt H, Gregor M, Skubis R, Hahn H, Riecken EO (1987) Erste prospektiv erhobene Befunde zum Vorkommen von Campylobacter pyloridis in der menschlichen Antrumschleimhaut in der Bundesrepublik Deutschland. Med Klin 82:23−25

12. Menge H, Warrelmann M, Loy V, Schmidt H, Gregor M, Skubis R, Hahn H, Riecken EO (1987) Campylobacter pylori in Magen, Duodenum und Kolon gastroenterologischer Patienten. Eine epidemiologische Studie an 120 Patienten. Dtsch Med Wochenschr 112:1403−1407

13. Niedobitek F, Grosse G, Taube F, Volkhemer G, Fehrenbach FJ, Werner E (1987) Untersuchungen zur Frage der bakteriellen Besiedlung der Magenschleimhaut. Z Gastroenterol 25:98−106

14. Langenberg ML, Tytgat GNJ, Schipper MEI, Rietra PJGM, Zanen HC (1984) Campylobacter-like organisms in the stomach of patients and healthy individuals. Lancet I:1348

15. Owen RJ, Martin SR, Bormann P (1985) Rapid urea hydrolysis by gastric campylobacters. Lancet I:111

16. Steer HW, Newell DG (1985) Immunological identification of Campylobacter pyloridis in gastric biopsy tissue. Lancet II:38

17. Pinkard KJ, Harrison B, Capstick JA, Medley G, Lambert JR (1986) Detection of Campylobacter pyloridis in gastric mucosa by phase contrast microscopy. J Clin Pathol 39:112−113

18. Marshall BJ, Warren JR, Francis GJ, Langton SR (1987) Rapid urease test in the management of Campylobacter pyloridis-associated gastritis. Am J Gastroenterol 82:200−210

19. Gregor M, Riecken EO (1985) Production and characterization of N-terminally and C-terminally directed monoclonal antibodies against pancreatic glucagon. Gastroenterology 89:571−580

20. Patton CM, Barett TJ, Morris GK (1985) Comparison of the Penne and Lior methods for serotyping Campylobacter sp. J Clin Microbiol 22:558−565

Discussion

Classen: You produce one monoclonal antibody against one *C. pylori* strain. How many different monoclonals should be made to find all important *C. pylori* strains?

Gregor: As an alternative you may start with a number of strains of *C. pylori*. The number of monoclonals you have to produce probably depends on your intention in the first place and then on the number of strains you are looking at.

Engstrand: Some papers describe the 25 kDa surface protein as homologous in several *C. pylori* strains. The monoclonal that we used immunolabelled this protein.

Rathbone: We have also been involved with monoclonals to *C. pylori*. We have one IgM monoclonal which only picks up half the strains we have tested it against. Although labelling *C. pylori* strains on smears, it does not identify them on cryostat sections. An interesting feature of this antibody is that it labels normal gastric epithelium and colonic carcinoma epithelium. I wonder if you have got any similar monoclonals?

Engstrand: No, we have not.

Gregor: Indeed, we found also one monoclonal antibody that stained only the epithelium of the gastric mucosa, but so far, this antibody has not been tested properly.

Riecken: As to the striking difference between the culture results and depicting the organisms by the monoclonal antibody, do you consider that the viability of the organism could be responsible for this difference, in addition to the other reasons which you have already mentioned?

Gregor: The biopsies were taken in a well standardized fashion: they were fixed in formalin immediately during the course of endoscopy or, alternatively, were placed into physiological saline solution and brought immediately to the Department of Bacteriology. I think that the number of negatives in culture and positives in monoclonal antibody staining reflects either the problem as to whether the biopsy taken for bacteriology has been representative of the whole stomach, or is a problem of detection limit. This may depend, for instance, upon whether you have done a homogenization before plating out the specimen.

Hahn: With reference to Dr. Riecken's question, one should consider that this bacterium might come in clusters, and that it is merely a matter of statistics as to whether one obtains such a cluster or not.

Langenberg: I want to ask why you use monoclonal antibodies rather than polyclonal antibodies in stomach, where there are very little other bacteria. I could see an advantage of using monoclonal antibodies when you want to pick up the *Campylobacter pylori* in throat smears or anything like that. But in the stomach I do not see any advantage.

Engstrand: Sometimes when we culture the homogenate, we find several Gram-negative bacteria, for example *Klebsiella* and *Proteus*. These bacteria could perhaps be found in Gram's staining, too. We have tested polyclonal antibodies in sera from mice immunized with *C. pylori*, and there are cross-reactions with *C. jejuni* and some other Gram-negative pools. So there are some other Gram-negative bacteria in the stomach especially after BI and BII surgery.

Gregor: If you try to define and to isolate antigenic determinants, it is extremely useful and efficient to use monoclonal antibodies as immunoreagents: this is what we are really looking for.

Rapid Identification of *Campylobacter pylori* in Gastric Biopsies

M. Deltenre, A. Burette, Y. Glupczinsky, E. Dekoster, C. de Prez, and C. Jonas

Since the initial report by Warren and Marshall in 1983 [25] and further description by the same authors [14] *Campylobacter pylori* (formerly *Campylobacter pyloridis*) or Gastric *Campylobacter*-like Organism type 1, GCLO-1 [18] has been detected through the world in antral mucosa of patients suffering from gastritis or peptic ulcer. Studies performed among a Belgian population of dyspeptic patients [4] revealed *Campylobacter pylori* (CP) in 53% of patients receiving routine endoscopies, primarily when duodenal ulcer or duodenitis was present. In a group of 552 patients with antral gastritis the activity and severity of inflammatory changes (evaluated according to modified Whitehead's classification [26]) strongly correlated with the presence of CP [3]. None of 42 patients with normal antral histology was found to have CP.

Despite the fact that the precise role of CP in peptic diseases is not yet fully understood, there is little doubt that this bacterium is more than a commensal, even if, as pointed by Axon [1], the clinical relevance of CP-associated gastritis may seem to be controversial, as gastritis may occur in symptom-free populations and has been described among normal volunteers [10]. In order to improve our knowledge of the etiopathogeny of gastritis and gastroduodenal ulcer, the accumulation of a great number of reliable data is necessary. And here a rapid, accurate and easy diagnostic test for presence of CP in antral mucosa would be of great help. Moreover, since long-term eradication of CP remains a problem, a routine and fast method to speed diagnosis of infection would allow easier inclusion of patients in therapeutic trials. In future, rapid diagnosis could be of great importance for prognosis, immediate therapeutic decision, and perhaps, prevention of so-called 'peptic' ulcer.

Many techniques for detection of CP have been described. Culture (on chocolate or horse blood agar) is usually considered a reference technique, but this method is time-consuming, requires special conditions for transportation of specimen incubation media and cannot give a rapid answer. Histology, chiefly with Warthin-Starry, hematoxylin-eosin, and recently acridine orange [24] stainings, does not provide a rapid diagnosis despite excellent accuracy. Serological tests [13, 21, 22] are certainly useful for epidemiological studies [21] but, once more, are not suitable for rapid identification of CP infection. Gram's staining of tissue smears [7] is reported to be efficient and, since the description by Langenberg et al. [10] of rapid ureal hydrolysis of *Campylobacter pylori*, home-made urease tests using Christensen's ureal broth have been widely used [15−17]. Both techniques seem to fulfill the desired condition of rapidity for diagnosis of CP infection in gastric mucosa.

Since the CLO test (Delta West, Canning Vale, Western Australia [17]) is not available in Belgium, a study was designed by our group to evaluate the accuracy of different modalities of urease test and to determine the best technique (or combination of techniques) for rapid, routine identification of CP.

Material and Method

Four antral biopsy specimens were systematically taken from 201 nonselected patients referred to endoscopy for various upper gastrointestinal complaints: two specimens were used for Gram's staining (GS) and for culture on chocolate agar under microaerophilic conditions (CU) and one was sent for histology by hematoxylin-eosin staining (H & E). The fourth specimen was inoculated into ureal broth (Table 1) within 3 h in the laboratory. Results were read 4 and 24 h after inoculation; these tests we term Late-inoculated Urease Tests 4 h and 24 h (LUT-4 and LUT-24). Tests were conducted on 201 patients.

In 112 patients a fifth biopsy was taken and immediately inoculated into the same ureal broth in the endoscopy unit (Immediately Inoculated Urease Tests 4 h and 24 h: IUT-4 and IUT-24).

IUT and LUT were considered to be positive when a characteristic pink colour appeared in the ureal broth within 4 or 24 h after inoculation. Patients were considered to be CP-positive when either culture, histology or Gram's staining revealed *Campylobacter pylori.*

Results

Of the 201 patients 133 (66%) were considered to have CP infection of antral mucosa; histology revealed gastritis in all cases. Culture was positive in 115/133 and this was the only reference test to be positive in 21 patients. Corresponding figures for Gram's staining were 58/133 and 3 patients, and for H & E staining 98/133 and 11 patients. Sensitivity of CU, GS and H & E were, respectively, 86%, 44% and 74%. Results of IUT and LUT are summarized in Table 2.

Specificity of Urease Tests. The specificity of all four techniques was excellent and ranged from 93% to 100%, with very high positive predictive values (96% − 100%).

Sensitivity and Accuracy of Urease Tests. IUT scores were significantly superior to those of LUT. Sensitivity of IUT-4 (54%) was higher than sensitivity of LUT-4 (31%) with $p < 0.02$. Accuracy rates (respectively, 63% and 55%) were not significantly different, but as regards 24-h tests the superiority of IUT was still more significant: sensitivity of IUT-24 was much higher than that of LUT-24 (77% versus 50%, $p < 0.00005$), and its accuracy (81% versus 67%) was also bet-

Table 1. Constituents of ureal broth

Peptone	1.0 g
Dextrose	1.0 g
Natrium Chloride	5.0 g
Monopotassium phosphate	0.4 g
Urea	20 g
Phenol red (1%)	0.1 ml
Tween 80	0.1 ml
Distilled water	1000 ml

(Steadhorn JE, J. Clin. Microbiol., 1979, 10:134−137)

Table 2. Respective value of immediately (IUT $n = 112$) versus late-incubated (LUT $n = 201$) urease tests (4 and 24 hours)

	IUT-4	IUT-24	LUT-4	LUT-24
Sensitivity	54% (45/84)	77% (65/84)	31% (41/131)	50% (65/131)
Specificity	93% (26/28)	93% (26/28)	100% (70/70)	99% (69/70)
Positive p.v.	96% (45/47)	97% (65/67)	100% (41/41)	98% (65/66)
Negative p.v.	40% (26/65)	58% (26/45)	44% (70/160)	51% (69/135)
Accuracy	63% (71/112)	81% (91/112)	55% (111/201)	67% (134/201)

Table 3: Respective value of cumulative IUT (4 and 24 h) and H & E biopsy staining versus biopsy specimen culture in 113 patients

	IUT-4 + IUT-24 + H & E		p	Culture	
Sensitivity	78/84	93%	NS	79/84	94%
Specificity	27/29	93%	NS	29/29	100%
Positive p.v.	78/80	98%	NS	79/79	100%
Negative p.v.	27/33	82%	NS	29/34	85%
Accuracy	105/113	93%	NS	108/113	96%

ter ($p < 0.0008$). The 24-h observation was clearly more accurate than the 4 h: 81% versus 63% for IUT and 67% versus 55% for LUT.

Comparison of IUT with Culture and Histology. In this study no significant difference in sensitivity nor in accuracy was found between IUT-24 and histology or culture. Sensitivity of IUT-24 was 77% compared to 74% for H & E and 86% for culture. Accuracy was respectively 81%, 83%, and 91%. Nevertheless, in terms of rapid identification, it must be stressed that IUT-4 had a lower sensitivity (54%) than histology (74%, $p < 0.005$) and culture (86%, $p < 0.0000002$). The same conclusion applies to accuracy: 63% for IUT-4 versus 83% for H & E and 91% for culture, which was tremendously more accurate ($p < 0.000000008$).

Can IUT and Histology Replace Culture? IUT-4 provided a correct and rapid diagnosis in 54% of cases with an acceptable specificity (93%), and IUT read after 24 h had the same accuracy and sensitivity as histology (using hematoxylin-eosin). Since culture of antral biopsy specimens may cause technical problems, particularly in small health centers, it seems, according to the results presented in Table 3, that a combination of IUT-4 and IUT-24 with H & E histology could make culture of biopsy specimens superfluous.

Discussion

Rapid diagnosis of infection with *Campylobacter pylori* is of great importance to progress in the physiopathology and management of gastritis and, probably, of gastroduodenal ulcer. The non-invasive 13C-urea breath test, recently proposed by Graham et al. [8] would provide an answer within 2 h but, until now, endoscopy and biopsy must be performed, at least when a patient is examined for the first time in order to obtain a precise diagnosis of possible gastroduodenal lesions. In future the breath test could be suitable for monitoring CP infection during and after antimicrobial management.

It takes more than 2 days for histology and 3–6 days to obtain culture results [17], and if Gram's stain of a biopsy smear is quicker, the result is usually not available before several hours. In our studies Gram's staining of biopsy specimens showed a low sensitivity (44%), which contrasts with the results reported by a group of investigators from Peru in 1986 [7]: sensitivity here was 67% (12/18 patients) and Gram-stained brush specimens were as efficient as silver-stained biopsies in detecting CP (21/23, or 93%).

Techniques using the remarkable urease activity of *Campylobacter pylori* [10] allow one to achieve an accurate and rapid diagnosis. In vitro experiments by Rathbone et al. [19] have shown that CP (1.7×10^9/ml), when inoculated with 10 mmol urea at 37° C, is able to produce more than 3 mg/ml ammonia within 3 min and induce a mean pH rise from 7.2 to 9.6. These findings have found some confirmation in vivo: Marshall and Langton [12], collecting gastric juice from 21 CP-positive patients, demonstrated a significant decrease in urea concentration: 0.45 ± 0.55 (SD) mmol/l versus 2.9 ± 0.98 mmol/l in uninfected patients. Moreover, urease activity seems to be a specific property of *Campylobacter pylori* as described by Owen et al. [18]. GCLO-2 is a single-flagellate, catalase- and oxidase-positive organism, isolated in 6 out of 328 patients by Kasper and Dickgiesser [9] and which could be closely related to *Campylobacter jejuni* [23]; it is urease-negative [18]. However, as reported by Fricker and Park [6], some nitrogen-fixing *Campylobacter* strains (e.g. *C. nitrofigilis*) are also urease-producing, but these have only been isolated from salt marshes – never in humans.

The commercially available CLO test [2, 11, 17], a mounted gel pellet containing urea and phenol red is an easy, quick and accurate diagnostic tool. The biopsy specimen is immediately pushed beneath the surface of the CLO test gel, and if *Campylobacter pylori* is present, the hydrolysis of urea produces ammonium, a rise in pH occurs and the gel turns pink. CLO test contains a bacteriostatic agent to prevent further production of urease by contaminating organisms and detects only preformed urease enzyme: *Campylobacter pylori* is the only organism living in gastric mucosa that contains enough preformed urease to be detected by rapid urease test [11].

Specificity of the CLO test is effectively 100% [11, 17], only one false positive has been reported by Borromeo et al. [2] in a series of 80 cases; sensitivity ranged from 90% [2] to 96% [17]. Recently Marshall et al. [11] reported only one false negative out of 79 patients; in this series 75% were positive after 20 min, 92% by 3 h, and 98% by 24 h. There is a correlation between the number of organisms seen on phase-contrast microscopy and the time required for CLO test to become positive [2]. Accuracy of the CLO test in the monitoring of treated patients is reported to be excellent [11], but more data are needed to confirm this finding.

The home-made urease test, as reported by McNulty and Wise [15], is a suitable alternative for rapid detection of CP when CLO test is not available. If the biopsy specimen is inoculated immediately in the endoscopy unit, the 24-h urease test is very sensitive, 91% [15] or 88% [16]. Of all the tests 80% were positive by 4 h and no false positive has been observed from 95 microscopically negative biopsy specimens [16]. Our results show a sensitivity of 77% for IUT-24 and 70% positive answers are obtained within 4 h. Crushing and grinding the specimen before inoculation may improve the sensitivity by releasing a greater number of organisms [16], since speed and depth of colour change are roughly proportional to the number of CP organisms present [15]. Sensitivity of the test has improved in our experience since biopsy specimens have begun to be crushed prior to inoculation.

Late-inoculated urease tests are less sensitive: 50% sensitivity for LUT-24 in our series and 75% in the series published by Morris et al. [17]. Late-inoculated tests can therefore be discarded in the diagnosis of CP infection.

Conclusions

For rapid identification of *Campylobacter pylori* in gastric biopsies the commercially available CLO test seems the easiest, quickest and most accurate method. The alternative of home-made urease test is interesting when CLO test is not available: if ureal broth is immediately inoculated with crushed biopsy specimen in the endoscopy unit, 80% of tests will be positive by 4 h, and sensitivity of the test read after 24 h is approximately 90% with virtually no false positive. In future, monoclonal antibodies as developped by Rathbone et al. [20], could play a role in diagnosis: Engstrand et al. [5] report 100% efficiency when compared to culture in a series of 17 patients (10 positive and 7 negative). The result was available within 1 h. However this expensive technique is not easily available for routine detection of *Campylobacter pylori*.

As far as final diagnosis of CP-associated gastritis is concerned, our study shows that culture is not mandatory: the immediately inoculated urease test after 4 h and that after 24 h, combined with routine Hematoxylin-Eosin staining of biopsy specimen reach the same accurracy as does culture: this point is of some interest for endoscopists who work alone or in small health centers in which sophisticated microbiological techniques are not available. However, culture should be performed when possible: the development of biochemical and/or immunological typing schemes would probably allow a better understanding of the epidemiology and the properties of this organism. Moreover, monitoring of the susceptibility to antimicrobial agents will probably be necessary in future, as more and more therapeutic trials with antibiotics are undertaken on large scale.

References

1. Axon ATR (1986) Campylobacter pyloridis: what role in gastritis and peptic ulcer? Br Med J 293:772
2. Borromeo M, Lambert JR, Pinkard KJ (1987) Evaluation of 'CLO-test' to detect Campylobacter pyloridis in gastric mucosa. J Clin Path 40:462–468
3. Burette A, Glupczynski Y, De Reuck M, Nyst JF, De Koster E, Deltenre M (1987) Campylobacter pylori: résultats d'une étude prospective. Gastroenterol Clin Biol 11:89 A
4. Burette A, Glupczynski Y, Van Gossum M, Jonas C, Deltenre M (1986) Campylobacter pyloridis in gastric antral biopsies: results of a prospective study on a serie of 212 patients. Dig Dis Sci 10:150 S
5. Engstrand L, Pahlson C, Gustavsson S, Schwan A (1986) Monoclonal antibodies for rapid identification of Campylobacter pyloridis. Lancet II:1402
6. Fricker CR, Park RWA (1985) Urease-positive campylobacters. Lancet I:394
7. Gastrointestinal Physiology Working Group (1986) Rapid identification of pyloric Campylobacter in Peruvians with gastritis. Dig Dis Sci 31:1089–1094
8. Graham DY, Klein PD, Evans DJ Jr., Evans DG, Alpert LC, Opekun AR, Boutton TW (1987) Campylobacter pylori detected noninvasively by the 13C-urea breath test. Lancet I:1174–1177
9. Kasper G, Dickgiesser N (1985) Isolation from gastric epithelium of campylobacter-like bacteria that are distinct from "Campylobacter pyloridis". Lancet I:111–112
10. Langenberg ML, Tytgat GNJ, Schipper MEI, Rietra PJGN, Zanen HC (1984) Campylobacter-like organisms in the stomach of patients and healthy individuals. Lancet I:1348
11. Marshall BJ, Warren JR, Francis GJ, Langton SR, Goodwin CS, Blincow ED (1987) Rapid Urease Test in the Mangement of Campylobacter pyloridis-Associated Gastritis. Am J Gastroenterol 82:200
12. Marshall BJ, Langton SR (1986) Urea hydrolysis in patients with Campylobacter pyloridis infection. Lancet I:965–966
13. Marshall BJ, McGechie DB, Francis GJ, Utley PJ (1984) Pyloric Campylobacter serology. Lancet I:281
14. Marshall BJ, Warren JR (1984) Unidentified curved bacilli in the stomach of patients with gastritis and peptic ulceration. Lancet I:1311–1314
15. McNulty CAH, Wise R (1985) Rapid diagnosis of Campylobacter-associated gastritis. Lancet I:1443–1444
16. McNulty CAM, Wise R (1986) Rapid diagnosis of Campylobacter pyloridis gastritis. Lancet I:387
17. Morris A, McIntyre D, Rose T, Nicholson G (1986) Rapid diagnosis of Campylobacter pyloridis infection. Lancet I:149
18. Owen RJ, Martin SR, Borman P (1985) Rapid urea hydrolysis by gastric Campylobacters. Lancet I:111

19. Rathbone BJ, Johnson AW, Tompkins D, Heatley RV, Losowsky MS (1986) Gastric ammonia production by Campylobacter pyloridis. Gut 27:A 1237
20. Rathbone BJ, Heatley RV, Losowsky MS, Trejdosiewicz LK (1986) Preparation of monoclonal antibodies to Campylobacter pyloridis. Gut 27:A 1238
21. Rathbone BJ, Wyatt JI, Worsley BW, Trejdosiewicz LK, Heatley RV, Losowsky MS (1985) Immune response to Campylobacter pyloridis. Lancet I:1217
22. Rathbone BJ, Wyatt JI, Tompkins D, Heatley RV, Losowsky MS (1986) Diagnostic IgG ELISA for gastric Campylobacter pyloridis infection using serum samples. Gut 27:A 607
23. Steele TW, Lanser JA, Sangster N (1985) Nitrate-negative Campylobacter-like organisms. Lancet I:394
24. Walters LL, Budin RE, Paull G (1986) Acridine-orange B identify Campylobacter pyloridis in formalin fixed, paraffin-embedded gastric biopsies. Lancet I:42
25. Warren JR, Marshall BJ (1983) Unidentified curved bacilli on gastric epithelium in active chronic gastritis. Lancet I:1273 – 1275
26. Whitehead R, Truelove SC, Gear MWL (1972) The histological diagnosis of chronic gastritis in fibreoptic gastroscope biopsy specimen. J Clin Path 25:1 – 11

Discussion

McNulty: I would like to make a series of comments about the biopsy urease test and the factors that alter the sensitivity and specificity of the test. First, transport of the biopsy specimen is important. If you transport the specimen in a saline or other transport media, urease will obviously diffuse in the fluid, and will decrease the urease concentration in the biopsy specimen. Secondly, the volume of broth used, is important. If you use 1 ml broth, you will get more false negatives than if you use 0.5 ml. Thirdly, you must crush or squash the biopsy specimen well in the broth. We now have modified our broth: we have removed peptone and glucose from it, and this may prevent the false positives that other workers describe. We have also increased the percentage of phenol red indicator, and our modified broth now has four times the amount of phenol red as in the method described by Deltenre. Lastly, the pH of the broth is extremely important; our pH is 6.8. If you use a lower pH, the phenol red indicator will obviously take longer to change colour. Using this modification, we have now analysed 600 biopsy specimens, achieving a specificity of 99.7% and a sensitivity of 96%. Also 72% of positive tests are positive within 2 h. If all researchers used the same biopsy urease broth, everybody would achieve this specificity and sensitivity.

Engstrand: Did you find any other unrelated Gram-negative bacteria which were positive for urea, when you cultured the biopsy homogenate? In Uppsala when we cultured some biopsies from patients with gastrectomy (BI, BII) we found strains of *Klebsiella* and *Proteus* also positive in the urea test. The urea tests were positive within 8 to 24 h and we found no *Campylobacter pylori*.

Deltenre: The first point is that endoscopes must be absolutely clean. They are cleaned before each procedure and perfused overnight. It is true that probably falsely positive results may be due to some *Klebsiella* or *Staphylococcus* as a contaminant in the biopsy. But it is a very rare instance, and to answer the comments of Dr. McNulty, I am not sure that the suppression of peptones and dextrose in the solution will make a big difference. Probably the difference is the pH, since our pH is much lower (5.8) than the pH of the broth you use, and also the volume of the biopsy sample, the volume of ureal broth, and of course the transportation. The transportation is indeed a problem; this is the reason why LUT is clearly inferior to IUT.

Marshall: One of the problems with the rapid urease test is that the person using it is often the gastroenterologist, and he is not necessarily thinking of taking a microbiological specimen. Dr. McNulty's revised test approaches the optimal results which you can obtain with a urease test. The CLO test perhaps has a slight advantage in that it is a gel, and therefore a very small amount of urease in close association with the mucosa must only change the pH in a very small volume, even smaller than, say, $0.5-1.0$ ml. But the other thing about these tests is that they will be affected by the drugs the patient takes. In my study of 350 CLO tests patients had their H2 blockers stopped the night before the test, so they did have acid in the stomach when they came to endoscopy. Secondly, I advised them to drink milk which has urea in it, which may potentiate the gastric urease activity. They drank a glass of milk at bedtime the night before the endoscopy. Secondly, I do not recommend that the biopsy be done on patients who have been treated with antibiotics or bismuth until 21 days after the end of antibacterial therapy. Thirdly, judging from Steward Hazell's recent data, it is useful to take a biopsy urease test from both the antrum and the body. The CLO test will be produced later this year with two wells for this purpose. Once you have performed a CLO test, if the test is positive in the endoscopy room, which is true in $70\%-80\%$ of cases, you do not need to do another test for *C. pylori* in urease-positive cases. So you can justify the cost on the basis of cancellation of other microbiological or histological studies. Finally, the CLO test should be kept in the shirt pocket and warmed to $30\degree$ C and then incubated in the pocket for another 3 h after insertion of the biopsy to speed the reaction.

Deltenre: Yes, I think that there is no question, according to the published papers, that the CLO test is clearly superior. The only problem is the price; this is why we tried to develop in my team a rapid identification. We perform 6000 upper GI endoscopies a year, one-half of them in the university and one-half of them in other health centers. So we need a rapid diagnosis, and the CLO test is probably the best for this. But the question of price is very important. Secondly, culture is not, according to my conclusions, routinely necessary. But it should be done each time that it is possible, because we must monitor the disease. Perhaps CP will change, and we had a bad experience, as you know, with ofloxacin. The in vitro susceptibility of CP in trials with ofloxacin was reduced $50-100$ fold after treatment without eradication. Ofloxacin-induced resistance was also observed for other fluoroquinolones, but fortunately not for amoxycillin. So from time to time, and in the university at least, you have to make cultures.

Tytgat: One question to Dr. McNulty: Could you explain why removal or lowering of the peptone and glucose content should decrease the falsely positive rate, and what the causes are of these false positives?

McNulty: We removed the peptone and glucose because at a previous meeting I attended I was told that I could get false positives. We actually have very little problem with false positives. Therefore we left these substances out, thinking that they were unnecessary additives.

Tytgat: But why should it decrease?

McNulty: If you incubate the ureal broth test at 37° C, organisms which utilize peptone and glucose would grow and produce urease; this could produce a false positive. If you remove these and have basically only urea, you should decrease the growth of other organisms and therefore lower the number of false positives. Since the test detects preformed enzyme, you do not need growth of *C. pylori* and therefore need no growth factors for this organism. We have also found that one does not need to incubate at 37° C.

Comparison Between Cultural and Histological Techniques in Diagnosis of *Campylobacter pylori* Colonization

H. MENGE, M. WARRELMANN, V. LOY, H. SCHMIDT, M. GREGOR, H. HAHN, and E. O. RIECKEN

During the 4 years which have passed since the detection of *Campylobacter pylori*, several techniques have been elaborated to demonstrate its presence in the human stomach. These methods provide either direct or indirect evidence for its existence on the gastric mucosa (Table 1). The bacterium itself can be traced directly by microbiological techniques or by its visualization in histological sections of the mucosa (Warren and Marshall 1983). Indirect evidence for its presence is obtained by the detection of serum antibodies or of preformed urease enzyme produced by *C. pylori* (Rathbone et al. 1986; McNulty and Wise 1986). Suitable methods to reveal this urease activity are the CLO test, the Christiansen urea medium (Warrelmann et al. 1987), and the urea breath test (Graham et al. 1987).

Studies comparing sensitivity and specificity of these different techniques in detecting the presence of *C. pylori* are sparse (Marshall et al. 1987; Borromeo et al. 1987), and they do not exist for the methods providing a direct proof of its presence. For this reason, we have performed a study comparing the effectiveness of the microbiological technique and of the silver staining method − applied to gastric biopsies (Warren and Marshall 1983) − in detecting *C. pylori* on the human antral mucosa.

Table 1. Methods providing direct or indirect evidence for the existence of *Campylobacter pylori* on the gastric mucosa

Direct evidence	
− microbiology	
− histology	
hematoxylin-eosin	− staining
silver	− staining
carbol-fuchsin	− staining
Gram	− staining
periodic acid Schiff (PAS)	− staining
Giemsa	− staining
toluidine blue	− staining
acridine-orange	− staining
Indirect evidence	
− CLO test	
− Christiansen urea medium	
− urea breath test	

Patients and Methods

One hundred and twenty unselected adult patients attending for diagnostic gastrointestinal endoscopy were included in this study. All were referred for the evaluation of abdominal pain, or for other upper abdominal complaints. Four antral biopsies were obtained from all patients. In each case, two specimens were fixed in 10% buffered formalin and processed routinely. Sections were stained with hematoxylin and eosin and using the Warthin-Starry technique (Warren and Marshall 1983). The two further biopsies from each patient were put on Columbia chocolate agar with Skirrow supplement (vancomycin, trimethoprim, polymyxin B) plus amphotericin B, and were incubated under microaerophilic conditions at 37°C for 5–7 days (Gas-Pac-System, Anaerocult-C) (Warren and Marshall 1983). The appearance of small (approx. 1 mm in diameter) translucent colonies consisting of typically gram-negative spiral rods with positive urease, catalase and oxidase reactions was considered a positive result. Strain CIP 101260 from the Pasteur Institute, Paris, was used as a reference strain.

Results

The histological sections of the antral biopsies of 10 patients (= 8.3%) did not permit a firm decision as to whether *C. pylori* was present or not (Table 2). In 20 persons, the antral biopsies revealed no colonization with *C. pylori* when using the histological technique, but in three of them the bacterium was demonstrated microbiologically (Table 2). Using the histological sections, stained according to Warthin-Starry, *C. pylori* was detected in the antral mucosa of 90 persons, whereas in only 51 patients was its presence exhibited under microaerophilic conditions. Even when the pathologist saw numerous bacteria, culturing was not always successful (Table 2).

Table 2. Evaluation of *Campylobacter pylori* colonization by histology and its parallel detection by microbiology in antral biopsies of 120 persons

Detection by histology		Detection by microbiology	
		+	−
Uncertain:	10	2	8
Negative:	20	3	17
Positive:	90	51	39
Few:	37	13	24
Moderate:	6	5	1
Numerous:	47	33	14

−, no growth; +, growth of *Campylobacter pylori*

Discussion

From the results obtained, three main conclusions can be drawn. In 8.3% of the biopsies the pathologist could not decide with certainty as to whether *C. pylori* was present or not. Obviously, this problem is inherent in all qualitative histological investigations, at least when borderline results are obtained. Yet it is rarely considered or discussed in relevant publications, though it can hardly be imagined that all other pathologists are always capable of deciding on firm grounds about the presence or absence of this bacterium. For this reason, the percentage of antral *C. pylori* colonization in a given population, as revealed by light microscopic examination of histological sections, must be regarded with reservation if this uncertainty is not mentioned. Microbiological techniques applied in parallel showed that in these doubtful cases, *C. pylori* is mostly absent.

In 20 patients no *Campylobacter pylori* colonization could be detected by light microscopy and in only three of them could the presence of the bacterium be demonstrated by the microbiological technique. This shows a correlation of results from both methods, when the histological sections do not reveal colonization of the antral mucosa by *C. pylori*. The three positive microbiological results in this series may be due to the sometimes patchy distribution of the bacterium in the human antrum.

Such a patchy distribution of the bacterium can hardly be responsible for the great diversity of the results obtained in the remaining 90 patients. It is more likely that the Warthin-Starry technique leads to an overestimation of the *C. pylori* colonization, and that other bacteria of similar shape (or staining artefacts) are equally detected in histological sections stained according to this method. It may be argued against this interpretation of our data that the microbiological technique hitherto applied is not as sensitive as the histological method in detecting *C. pylori*. Yet, up to now, microbiological growth has been the only tool for detecting this bacterium with certainty. Therefore this technique should be used nowadays as a reference detection method for *C. pylori* in antral biopsies, as only future investigations with monoclonal antibodies directed against this bacterium will establish the reliability of the direct visualization of *C. pylori* in histological sections.

References

1. Borromeo M, Lambert JR, Pinkard KJ (1987) Evaluation of "CLO-test" to detect Campylobacter pyloridis in gastric mucosa. J Clin Pathol 40:462–468
2. Graham DY, Klein PD, Evans DJ, Evans DG, Alpert LC, Opekum AR, Boutton TW (1987) Campylobacter pylori detection noninvasively by the ^{13}C-urea breath test. Lancet I:1174–1177
3. Marshall BJ, Warren JR, Francis GJ, Langton SR, Goodwin CS, Blincow ED (1987) Rapid urease test in the management of Campylobacter pyloridis-associated gastritis. Am J Gastroenterol 83:200–210
4. McNulty CAM, Wise R (1986) Rapid diagnosis of Campylobacter pyloridis gastritis. Lancet I:387

5. Rathbone BJ, Wyatt JI, Worsley BW, Shires SE, Trejdos-Iewicz LK, Heatley RV, Losowsky MS (1986) Systemic and local antibody responses to gastric Campylobacter pyloridis in non-ulcer disease. Gut 27:642 – 647
6. Warrelmann M, Hahn H, Menge H, Schmidt H (1987) Campylobacter pylori: Nach-weisverfahren. Dtsch Med Wochenschr 112:821 – 822
7. Warren JR, Marshall B (1983) Unidentified curved bacilli on gastric epithelium in active chronic gastritis. Lancet I:1273 – 1275

Discussion

Börsch: I wish to comment on the problem of a higher positive rate with histology versus with microbiology. We did a formal study in 149 patients comparing biopsy urease tests and histology, and we found the same thing in antral biopsies. We had 48% positive CLO tests and 62% positive histologies by modified Giemsa stain. We considered some of the latter to be false positives. After grading the histologic density of bacteria, we found these "false" positives predominantly to be grade 1 according to Marshall's grading. So we came to the conclusion that our histological examination gave false positives among the 1 gradings, but we did not have cultures to really rectify this assumption.

Tytgat: I think it is important to stress that quite a few factors can turn the cultures negative as Marshall summarized in one of his papers. There is a recent abstract in *Gastroenterology* (which was not accepted for the AGA Meeting) where investigators looked at the kind of anesthetic used for throat anesthesia. Apparently benzocaine interferes with culturing techniques and if you use lidocaine as an anesthetic, no interference with the cultures is seen. So there are a lot of factors to be considered if you take biopsies in these patients.

Menge: We hope that we are as good as you in endoscopy and do not need these anesthetics.

Hahn: Rather than relying on microscopic observations alone, I think the proof of the pudding still lies in cultivation of the organism. I am satisfied with our coincidence of 80%.

Houthoff: My experience is that in some cases where *C. pylori* cannot be demonstrated you can almost certainly infer, by the histological appearance of the mucosa, that the organism is present. And I think it would be justified to treat patients with the classic histologic changes of active chronic gastritis, even if the biopsies were negative on culture. What does everybody else think about that?

Furthermore, I would like to comment on the uncertainty of microorganisms in the mucosa being campylobacters in histological specimens. In my experience, if there is any doubt, it is not a campylobacter. If you take that as a starting point, the number of false positives decreases very rapidly. Also, if you have to look for a long time you are inclined to see a dubious campylobacter in the end, so the screening should not be too meticulous and time-consuming. In fact, in our study we used this as a guideline and then we didn't have false positives. But I was astonished by the fact that you had so many cases with a lot of bacteria in histology, and negative bacterial cultures. I think that a possible solution to this problem might be that the culturing conditions were not optimal.

Menge: If you compare our data with the data of other authors, the percentages of positive cultures are similar. That means that our culture techniques are as good as the international standard.

Wyatt: I would like to agree with Professor Houthoff that the appearance of *Campylobacter* in sections is so characteristic, when you are used to seeing them, that I do not feel that there is any risk of misidentifying another bacterium as a *C. pylori*. I would just like to ask you, if you feel you are getting the histological false positives because there are actually other bacteria in the stomach: can you speculate what those other bacteria might be?

Menge: I would not like to speculate about that.

Engstrand: In some cultured homogenates we found a gram-negative rod with similar morphology to *C. pylori*. In gram stains they looked nearly the same as *C. pylori*, but they were longer (approx. $8-10$ µm). They were cultured at $37°$ C in anaerobic jars. The monoclonals we used did not cross-react with these bacteria.

Menge: And might this contribute to the over-estimation using the histological technique?

Engstrand: If the bacteria look nearly the same in Gram staining you might see them in histological sections, too.

Hahn: We have to be quite careful about the possibility that this might just be transient flora which comes into the stomach by way of food uptake. Is your observation a consistent finding in the same patients with repeatedly taken specimens or is it just one single finding?

Engstrand: We have found this bacteria in three or four patients, and only in culture, not in histological sections. I do not know if it is an unrelated bacteria and have not compared our findings to histological sections.

Goodwin: I think the longer one cultures these organisms, the closer one comes to getting positive cultures. I would encourage everybody to encourage their microbiologists to try different isolation media and selective media. You can include colistin and can compare several media, and you will find you can get your culture rate up, until we find 100% positive cultures, in contrast to histology.

Experience with ^{14}C-Urea Breath Test in Detecting *Campylobacter pylori*

E. A. J. Rauws, G. N. J. Tytgat, W. Langenberg, and E. v. Royen

Campylobacter pylori has been isolated world-wide from gastric mucosal biopsies of patients with non-ulcer dyspepsia, duodenal or gastric ulcer and those of asymptomatic individuals, virtually exclusively when chronic active gastritis was present [1 – 10]. Although the precise role of *C. pylori* in any of these conditions remains unclear, there is growing evidence for a direct causal relationship to gastritis [11 – 14].

Until now *C. pylori* colonization can only be detected by culture of antral mucosal biopsies [15], by histological investigation of these biopsies or by an urease test [10, 16 – 20]. Recently Graham [21] described a non-invasive breath test with carbon-13 labelled urea. This breath test is based on our finding of a remarkably high urease activity of *C. pylori* [10]. When carbon-labelled urea is administered orally, urea-derived labelled carbon dioxide appears in the respiratory CO_2 of infected individuals.

In the present paper we describe our experience with carbon-14-labelled urea as a sensitive, inexpensive, non-invasive, reproducible breath-test to detect *C. pylori* colonization.

The urea breath test was performed after a overnight fast. Baseline samples of respiratory CO_2 were obtained. After ingestion of a liquid test meal to slow gastric emptying, 110 kBq (3 µCi) ^{14}C-urea mixed with ^{12}C urea was administered. Breath samples were collected in a trapping solution at 10-min intervals for 90 min and analysis from this solution for labelled CO_2 content was then made [22 – 25].

Materials and Methods

Patient group. A total of 68 non-ulcer dyspepsia patients referred for upper gastrointestinal endoscopy entered the study. Patients were not entered if they used any medication except antacids during the previous 4 weeks, or if they had previous gastric surgery or malignancy.

Endoscopy and biopsy. Upper gastrointestinal endoscopy was performed after an overnight fast. Antral mucosa biopsy specimens were taken using a sterilized biopsy forceps. Two specimens were placed in 2 ml of phosphate-buffered saline at 4° C for bacteriological examination. Two specimens were fixed in 10% buffered formalin for histological evaluation.

Study protocol. Upper gastrointestinal endoscopy was performed after an overnight fast and within 48 h; before the results of bacteriologic or histologic examination were known, the ^{14}C-urea breath test was performed.

Results

The urea breath test was performed on 68 non-ulcer dyspepsia patients, and in all patients endoscopy with antral mucosal biopsies for culture was performed to validate the results of the breath test. In all 38 *C. pylori* culture positive patients, a rapid rise in $^{14}CO_2$ occurred within 20 min after ingestion of ^{14}C-urea. In 30 patients with negative cultures no $^{14}CO_2$ could be detected in the exhaled breath for at least 90 min. The reproducibility of the urea breath test was evaluated in 7 patients by repetition of the breath test within 24 h; this revealed the same curves of $^{14}CO_2$ excretion. The bacterial load was assessed semiquantitatively and correlated with the amount of $^{14}CO_2$ excreted over time, also when only few colonies could be cultured.

Conclusion

The carbon-14 urea breath test is a simple, sensitive, inexpensive test to detect *C. pylori* colonization on gastric mucosa, to assess semiquantitatively the bacterial load, and can be used to perform epidemiologic and therapeutic trials without endoscopy or need for culture. In this $^{14}CO_2$ breath test not more than 3 µCi of radioactive isotopes with long half-life and emitting beta particles is administered, but the total body irradiation is small at about 5 mrad, compared with a natural and cosmic radiation dose of 1200 mrads. In one carbon-14 urea breath test, 1/10 of the radiation dose of a chest x-ray is used.

References

1. Warren JR, Marshall BJ (1983) Unidentified curved bacilli on gastric epithelium in active chronic gastritis. Lancet I: 1273–1275
2. Marshall BJ, Warren JR (1984) Unidentified curved bacilli in the stomach of patients with gastritis and peptic ulceration. Lancet I: 1311–1315
3. Meyrick Thomas J, Poynter D, Gooding C et al. (1984) Gastric spiral bacteria. Lancet II: 100
4. Rollason TP, Stone J, Rhodes JM (1984) Spiral organisms in endoscopic biopsies of the human stomach. J Clin Pathol 37: 23–26
5. Jones DM, Lessells AM, Eldridge J (1984) *Campylobacter* like organisms on the gastric mucosa: culture, histological, and serological studies. J Clin Pathol 37: 1002–1006
6. McNulty CAM, Watson DM (1984) Spiral bacteria of the gastric antrum. Lancet I: 1068–1069
7. Price AB, Levi J, Dolby et al. (1985) *Campylobacter pyloridis* in peptic ulcer disease: microbiology, pathology and scanning electron microscopy. Gut 26: 1183–1188

8. Buck GE, Gourley WK, Lee WK et al. (1986) Relation of *Campylobacter pyloridis* to gastritis and peptic ulcer. J Inf Dis 153:664–669
9. Marshall BJ, McGechie OB, Rogers PA, Glanchy RJ (1985) *Pyloric campylobacter* infection and gastroduodenal disease. Med J Austr 142:439–444
10. Langenberg ML, Tytgat GNJ, Schipper MEI, Rietra PJGM, Zanen HC (1984) *Campylobacter-like* organisms in the stomach of patients and healthy individuals. Lancet I:1348
11. Marshall BJ, Armstrong JA, McGechie DB, Glancy RJ (1985) Attempt to fulfil Koch's postulates for *pyloric campylobacter*. Med J Austr 142:436–439
12. Morris A, Nicholson G (1986) *Campylobacter pyloridis* ingestion causing gastritis and hypochlorhydria. Austral Microbiol 7:206
13. Anonymus (1985) *Pyloric Campylobacter* finds a volunteer. Lancet I:1021–1022
14. Langenberg ML, Rauws EAJ, Schipper MEI et al. (1985) The pathogenic role of gastric *Campylobacter*-like organisms (GCLO's) in GCLO-associated gastritis, studied by attempts to eliminate these organisms (abstract 98). In: Pearson AD, Skirrow MB et al. (eds) Campylobacter III; Proceedings of the Third International Workshop on Campylobacter Infections. Public Health Laboratory Service, London, 162–163
15. Goodwin CS, Blincow ED, Warren JR et al. (1985) Evaluation of culture techniques for isolating *Campylobacter pyloridis* from endoscopic biopsies of gastric mucosa. J Clin Pathol 38:1127–1311
16. Owen RJ, Martin SR, Borman P (1985) Rapid urea hydrolysis by gastric *campylobacters*. Lancet I:111
17. McNulty CAM, Wise R (1985) Rapid diagnosis of *Campylobacter* associated gastritis. Lancet I:1443–1444
18. Marshall BJ, Langton SR (1986) Urea hydrolysis in patients with *Campylobacter pyloridis* infection. Lancet I:965–966
19. Morris A, McIntyre D, Rose T et al. (1986) Rapid diagnosis of *Campylobacter pyloridis* infection. Lancet I:149
20. Hazell SL, Borody TJ, Gal A, Lee A (1987) *Campylobacter pyloridis* gastritis I: Detection of Urease as a Marker of bacterial Colonization and gastritis. Am J Gastroenterol 82:292–296
21. Graham DY, Evans DJ, Alpert LC et al. (1987) *Campylobacter pylori* detected noninvasively by the ¹³C-urea breath test. Lancet I:1174–1177
22. Abt AF, von Schuching SL (1966) Fat utilization test in disorders of fat metabolism. Bulletin of the Johns Hopkins Hospital 119:316–330
23. Newman A (1974) Breath-analysis tests in gastroenterology. Gut 15:308–323
24. Hepner GW (1974) Breath analysis: Gastroenterological applications. Gastroenterology 67:1250–1256
25. King CE, Toskes PP (1981) Alteration of CO_2 production during nonfasting isotopic CO_2 breath tests: concise communication. J Nucl Med 22:955–958

Discussion

Goodwin: I would just like to ask a couple of questions about the slides. On one of the slides you did write down three results with the word "some" at the bottom; was that some bacteria but a negative test?

Rauws: No, in these 11 patients there were some colonies detected on culture by the bacteriologist and we found a small rise in carbon-14 O_2 excretion in these patients in the exhaled air.

Goodwin: At the very end of the line?

Rauws: Yes.

Goodwin: And you regarded that as positively different from the negative tests?

Rauws: Well, these slides and also the results were obtained last week. We have to do a lot of statistical work to whether or not it represents a real difference.

Goodwin: Is it possible that could be within the range of the negative results?

Rauws: Yes, that is possible.

Marshall: We are using C14 breath which we give on an empty stomach, and we get 90% sensitivity and specificity with a sample taken at 15-min intervals with peak values about 10 times higher than yours because you have given your isotope within a meal. Just a comment about the radiation dose: most of these patients have had a barium meal X-ray which equals $10-20$ times the dose of radiation from one of the breath tests, so it is not really necessary to use a non-radioactive isotope.

Classen: Can you imagine that we could replace the isotope C14 with its long halflife time by another isotope, because I would find it very difficult to get this kind of breath test for application in humans through our X-ray or ethical authorities in West Germany?

Rauws: Certainly you can use carbon-13 urea and I think you would obtain the same results. We are also busy with carbon-13 urea at the moment, but it is very expensive. In Holland it costs 500 guilders per patient and you need a very expensive mass spectrometer to analyse the breath samples.

Cadranel: I think it is a very interesting test, of course, but I am worried about using ^{14}C in children, could you comment on the halflife of ^{14}C.

Rauws: The halflife time of ^{14}C is about 6000 years, so that it is very long, but it is also produced every day by the diesel motor of a car, nobody cares about that.

Flemström: I cannot help adding one point to your historical remarks. Gastric urease was an issue of gastric physiology at the beginning of the 1950s. It was then proposed by the Irishmen Fitzgerald and Conway that it was part of the H^+ ion transport process. Those papers are in the physiological literature and not in the literature on gastric ulcer.

Rauws: Well, I raised it, but I did not want to talk about all this history, so I glossed over it.

Rathbone: Your results following the bismuth compound were very interesting in that you decreased the $^{14}CO_2$ production by about 50% in 2 h, is that because bismuth has a direct effect on the urease?

Rauws: Well, I cannot answer that question. The electron-microscopy slide you saw already shows very severe destructive abnormalities two hours after bismuth ingestion. You could also expect, because of cell death, an enormous release of urease and you would then expect a higher peak in exhaled $^{14}CO_2$.

McNulty: I believe that the Procter and Gamble group in the USA has shown that bismuth salts are urease inhibitors, so that might explain the rapid decrease after two hours.

Pearson: Is it possible that the bacterial flora of the mouth some of which are urease positive may give you false positives?

Rauws: All patients were also endoscoped and biopsies for culture were obtained. We did not find any false positive nor false negative breath test in the patients.

Goodwin: We have done a lot more breath tests since Barry Marshall left us; if you look at the early part of the curve, in other words, the first 2 min, you get some higher counts but they dropped very rapidly. But I do think the five minute test we found is quite important and in our negatives we do not get positive results at 5 min and there is some drop after that. We get false negatives rather than false positives.

O'Morain: With this method you can make a dose response curve; you showed us that with one tablet of CBS 2 h later the test was negative, does the patient become positive the next day or can you titrate your dose of CBS?

Rauws: Well, we cannot answer that question yet because this was the result with the first patient. We have investigated several patients since then, but I do not know those results yet.

Systemic Immune Responses to *Campylobacter pylori* Colonization

H. VON WULFFEN

The correlation of detected *C. pylori* with antrum gastritis and peptic ulcers has generated much interest in the possibility of a *C. pylori* serology. The successful culturing of *C. pylori* by Marshall [11] opened the way for conducting serological studies using this organism as antigen. It is not surprising therefore that numerous studies employing a variety of serologic methods have appeared during the relatively short period that has elapsed since the first reports on this exciting organism by Warren [17] and Marshall [12]. Serology offers itself as a tool that is easier practically to utilize in epidemiological studies than histological or cultural methods can possibly be. It may also complement these methods and possibly even replace them when endoscopy is not feasible. Also, the study of systemic immune response may shed some light on the host-parasite relationship and, at least, offer some circumstantial evidence for the pathogenic role of *C. pylori*.

Previous Studies

Various serologic test methods have been employed, including complement fixation test [4, 15], agglutination test [4], passive haemagglutination assay [10], enzyme-linked immunosorbent assays [6, 13, 1, 2] and immunoblot techniques [7, 15]. All of these studies have clearly shown that sera from patients positive for *C. pylori* on culture usually displayed much higher titres or reactivities than those from patients with negative *C. pylori* findings. Also, the tests were usually negative for patients with normal antrum mucosa and positive for patients with antrum gastritis and/or peptic lesions. Most studies show an increasing prevalence of antibodies to *C. pylori* with increasing age, indicating that *C. pylori* is usually acquired later in life. This accords with the observation that the incidence of gastritis also is known to increase with age.

Serologic screening may also give some clues regarding the source and route of infection. Marshall [10] has presented data on women attending a venereal disease clinic and found that patients with a positive *Treponema*-passive haemagglutination test (TPHA) had a much higher prevalence (38%) of antibodies to *C. pylori* than those with a negative TPHA (3%). Jones [3], in a recent study using a complement fixation test, could not find an increased prevalence of antibodies to *C. pylori* in household contacts of infected patients, either in blood relatives nor among spouses.

Studies dealing with the differentiation of immune response in respect to the various immunoglobulin classes agree on a predominant IgG-type response and, to a lesser extent, IgA immune response. IgM does not seem to play a major role.

Results of Immunoblot Study

For a preliminary screening of about 100 patients we employed a complement fixation (CF) test [15] and found that patients with severe gastritis and those with duodenal ulcer had the highest incidence of CF reactivity (both with 79%). However, titres generally were quite low and rarely exceeded a value of 20.

Thus, to increase sensitivity and to find out more about the immune response to *C. pylori*, we made use of the immunoblot technique. By this method distinct patterns of immune response to various protein antigens can be differentiated. Furthermore, the patterns gained for IgG, IgM, and IgA can be compared with one another. To investigate the possibility that differences in seroreactivity may be due to antigenic differences between infecting *C. pylori* strains we studied [14] protein profiles of various *C. pylori* isolates by sodium dodecyl sulfate-polyacrylamide gel electrophoresis (SDS-PAGE) according to Laemmli [8].

Even *C. pylori* isolates that differed in respect to urea hydrolysis and plasmid content showed little interstrain variation in their protein profiles as judged from the Coomassie-blue stained gels. In contrast to these observations, immunoblot analysis did reveal some interstrain variations. For example, a high-molecular protein band of about 110-kDa that appears to be quite characteristic for *C. pylori* was missing in three of eight tested strains on both the IgG and the IgA immunoblot.

Regarding possible cross-reactivity with other *Campylobacter* species, SDS-PAGE revealed that the major protein bands of *C. pylori* are very distinct from those of *C. jejuni* and *C. coli*. Also, a positive *C. pylori* patient serum reacted very little with either *C. jejuni* or *C. coli* either on the IgG or the IgA immunoblots in comparison with the strong reaction with the proteins of all tested *C. pylori* strains.

DNA-DNA hybridization studies [14] underline these findings: blotted DNAs of various *C. pylori* strains hybridize strongly while no positive hybridization signals are seen between chromosomal DNAs of different *Campylobacter* species by the blot hybridization method.

Fig. 1 displays typical examples of IgG and IgA immunoblots that were obtained using a single *C. pylori* strain (CLO 185) as antigen. As can be seen, blots from patients with either severe or moderate antrum gastritis reveal a much denser set of reactive protein bands than any of those from patients with normal antrum mucosa. IgM immunoblots are not shown because 40 sera that were tested reacted only with a single band at about 60 kDa. Longer substrate incubation and dilution of sera at 1:50 instead of 1:100 increased the reactivity of protein bands sharply, but no differences could be observed between sera from

IgG Immunoblot

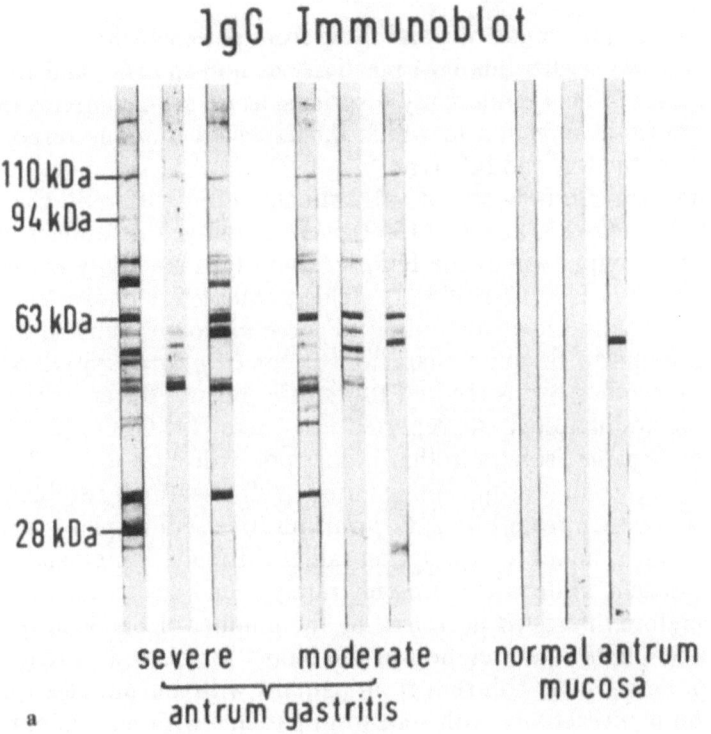

IgA Immunoblot

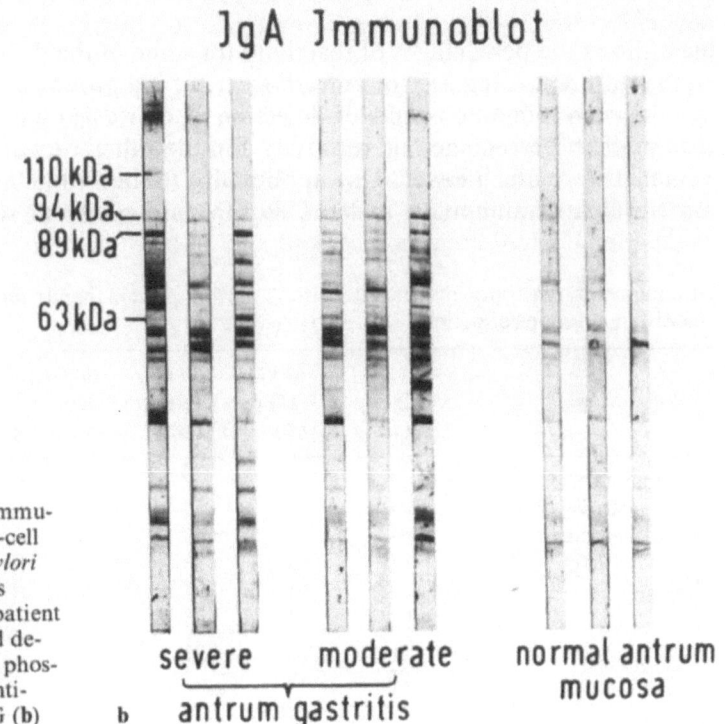

Fig. 1a, b. *C. pylori* immunoblots using a whole-cell lysate of a single *C. pylori* strain as antigen. Blots were incubated with patient sera diluted 1:100 and developed with alkaline phosphatase conjugated anti-human IgG (**a**) or IgG (**b**)

patients with antrum gastritis and those from patients with normal antrum mucosa. Thus, we regard this IgM reactivity as non-specific, and further probing for IgM ceased. This is not really surprising as we are apparently dealing with a chronic mucosal infection to which the expected immune response would be primarily of the IgA and IgG type.

Using sera from a set of 40 patients three different *C. pylori* strains (CLO 162, CLO 185, and CLO 232) were employed as antigen and tested in parallel for comparison of the IgG, IgA, and IgM reactivity patterns achieved. Two of these (CLO 162 and 185) yielded completely equivalent results while CLO 232 was discarded for failing to show a protein band of about 110 kDa that was found to be quite characteristic for *C. pylori* positive patients. In respect to the other bands studied this strain did not differ markedly from the other two strains tested. As reported elsewhere [14] CLO 232 differs from all our other *C. pylori* isolates in that it does not hydrolyze urea. CLO 185, a plasmid-carrying strain, was the antigen used in all tests finally evaluated.

As can be seen from Fig. 1, *C. pylori* positive sera display a variety of band patterns which makes interpretation rather difficult. Some bands appear to be quite consistent while others are only rarely found or are not very specific. We were therefore interested in restricting the number of bands to be evaluated in order to facilitate interpretation of the blots. Correlation of reactivity of individual protein bands with sera from patients with antrum gastritis, on the one hand, and non-reactivity with sera from patients with normal antrum mucosa, on the other, resulted in the selection of four protein bands for the IgG immunoblot: 110 kDa, 94 kDa, 63 kDa, and 28 kDa. For evaluation of the IgA immunoblots the 28-kDa band was omitted and a 89-kDa band was included instead.

Table 1 shows the percentages of reactivity for some of the different protein bands in the different categories of antrum gastritis and groups of patients and also gives the corresponding results of detection of *C. pylori* on culture and/or Gram's stain. The percentages of reactivity for the other protein bands that were evaluated were much lower. This applies also to the 110-kDa and 63-kDa bands on the IgA immunoblot, and the 89-kDa protein band was not even

Table 1. Immunoblot reactivity of characteristic *C. pylori* protein bands and detection of *C. pylori* in different groups of patients

Group	n	110 kDa IgG pos (%)	63 kDa IgG pos (%)	89 kDa IgA pos (%)	IgG + IgA-Score ≧ 1.5 (%)	*C. pylori* pos (%)
Normal antrum mucosa	37	11	25	8	27	8
Slight antrum gastritis	61	47	74	52	72	57
Moderate antrum gastritis	41	47	81	59	83	68
Severe antrum gastritis	29	81	88	88	100	88
Duodenal ulcer	35	59	91	71	94	97
Gastric ulcer	36	67	81	58	86	64
Blood donors	129	21	22	22	32	–
Children	96	15	18	7	19	–

evaluated for the IgG immunoblot due to its infrequent reactivity. Although the 63-kDa band alone was already positive for IgG in 88% of all sera from patients with severe antrum gastritis, an evaluation that took into account the reactivities for the other bands as well yielded even better results. Therefore, a semiquantitative grading system was introduced, whereby one point was assigned to each reactive band and one-half point to a weakly reactive band. This resulted in a maximum score of 4 for each tested serum for IgG or IgA and a maximum combined score of 8. Table 1 also gives the results achieved for the various groups of patients using a combined IgG + IgA score of 1.5 as cut-off value. It is obvious from this table that there is a clear correlation between test scores, on the one hand, and detection of *C. pylori*, antrum gastritis and peptic lesions, on the other.

Results for blood donors are in the range of the results that Langenberg et al. [9] obtained when they performed endoscopy on 24 healthy volunteers and found six of them to reveal *C. pylori* on culture and antrum gastritis on histopathology. It is also in agreement with the probable life-cycle prevalence of peptic lesions in the general population as reported in the literature [5].

The results achieved for the group of patients with normal antrum mucosa appear to be somewhat unsatisfactory at first glance. However, not all patients with normal antrum mucosa are negative for *C. pylori*. It is known that antrum gastritis may occur in a patchy distribution, and we have even seen patients with normal antrum mucosa, although very few, who show superficial gastritis of the corpus and were also positive for *C. pylori* on Gram's stain.

The results in Table 1 also suggest that there is a correlation between the degree of antrum gastritis and the achieved immunoblot scores. These differences, however, are not significant. In this respect we gain a somewhat clearer picture when we look at the median scores in Table 2, which shows that the different gastritis groups have median scores in the same range.

Also, we could not find a difference in the humoural immune response between those patients with antrum gastritis who had developed peptic lesions and those who had not. In particular, we could not detect an "ulcer band" nor could we find any difference in respect to the various immunoglobulin classes. In general, the IgA response was more or less complementary to the IgG response and did not allow any particular conclusions on its own.

Table 2. IgG + IgA median scores on *C. pylori* immunoblot test in various groups of patients

Group	n	IgG + IgA median score	Range
Normal antrum mucosa	37	0	0−5
Slight antrum gastritis	61	2.5	0−6
Moderate antrum gastritis	41	3.0	0.5−6.5
Severe antrum gastritis	29	3.0	1.5−8.0
Duodenal ulcer	35	3.0	0−6
Gastric ulcer	36	4.0	0−7.5
Blood donors	129	0	0−5.5
Children	96	0	0−4

Conclusions

What, then, may be the clinical applications for a *C. pylori* serology? First, it may be used in a confirmatory manner in addition to histologic and cultural findings. Secondly, and probably of more importance, it may turn out to be very useful in monitoring the long-term outcome of therapeutic trials. As we have only just begun to conduct therapeutic trials, we cannot report on own experiences here. Reports in the literature [10] on this are very limited but do point in the direction that significant reduction in titre may be expected within 3 months of successful eradication of *C. pylori*. A third application may be serologic screening of certain high-risk patients. In a preliminary retrospective study [16] we have looked at sera from patients before and after renal transplantation. Some patients who were clearly positive for *C. pylori* on immunoblot 2 years prior to transplantation but did not show a history of gastritis or peptic ulcers, developed peptic ulcers and even gastrointestinal haemorrhage soon after renal transplantation. Their *C. pylori* immunoblot patterns had not changed. Apparently, one might speculate, the change that possibly precipitated the development of peptic lesions occurred in the cell-mediated immunity of these patients.

Summary

The correlation of detected *C. pylori* with antrum gastritis and peptic ulcers has generated much interest in the possibility of a *C. pylori* serology. Numerous studies have appeared during the past three years employing a variety of serologic methods, including complement fixation tests, agglutination tests, passive haemagglutination assays, enzyme-linked immunosorbent assays, and immunoblot techniques. All these studies have demonstrated basically an excellent correlation of higher titres or reactivities with positive detection of *C. pylori* as well as with antrum gastritis and peptic lesions. There appears to be an increasing prevalence of antibodies to *C. pylori* with increasing age, which accords with the observation that the incidence of gastritis also increases with age. Thus far, seroepidemiologic studies have not solved the question of source and route of infection with *C. pylori*.

Studies dealing with the differentiation of the immune response in respect to the different immunoglobulin classes agree on a predominant IgG-type response and, to a lesser degree, IgA immune response. IgM does not seem to play a major role. This is in accordance with previous notions regarding the humoural immune response in chronic mucosal infections.

A *C. pylori* immunoblot study that we have recently conducted is presented and discussed in detail. A 110-kDa and a 63-kDa protein band on the IgG immunoblot and a 89-kDa protein band on the IgA immunoblot appeared to yield the best results. A semiquantitative scoring system was introduced to facilitate interpretation of the immunoblots. Possible applications for *C. pylori* serology are discussed.

References

1. Booth L, Holdstock G, MacBride H, Hawtin P, Gibson JR, Ireland A, Bamforth J, DuBoulay CE, Lloyd RS, Pearson A (1986) Clinical importance of *Campylobacter pyloridis* and associated serum IgG and IgA antibody responses in patients undergoing upper gastrointestinal endoscopy. J Clin Pathol 39:215–219
2. Goodwin CS, Blincow E, Peterson G, Sanderson C, Cheng W, Marshall BJ, Warren JR, McCulloch R (1987) Enzyme-linked immunosorbent assay for *Campylobacter pyloridis:* correlation with presence of *C. pyloridis* in the gastric mucosa. J Infec Dis 155:488–494
3. Jones DM, Eldridge J, Whorwell PJ (1987) Antibodies to *Campylobacter pyloridis* in household contacts of infected patients. B Med J 294:615
4. Jones DM, Lessells AM, Eldridge J (1984) Campylobacter like organisms on the gastric mucosa: culture, histological and serological studies. J Clin Pathol 37:1002–1006
5. Jorde R, Burhol PG (1987) Review: Asymptomatic peptic ulcer disease. Scand J Gastroenterol 22:129–134
6. Kaldor J, Tee W, McCarthy P, Watson J, Owyer B (1985) Immune response to *Campylobacter pyloridis* in patients with peptic ulceration. Lancet I:921
7. Kaldor J, Tee W, Nicolacopolous L, Demirtzoglou K, Noonan D, Dwyer B (1986) Immunoblot confirmation of immune response to *Campylobacter pyloridis* in patients with duodenal ulcers. Med J Australia 145:133–135
8. Laemmli UK (1970) Cleavage of structural proteins during the assembly of the head of bacteriophage T4. Nature 227:680–685
9. Langenberg ML, Tytgat GNJ, Schipper MEJ, Rietra PJG, Zanen HC (1984) Campylobacter-like organisms in the stomach of patients and healthy individuals. Lancet I:1348
10. Marshall BJ, McGechie DB, Francis GJ, Utley PG (1984) Pyloric campylobacter serology. Lancet II:281
11. Marshall BJ, Royce H, Annear DJ, Goodwin CS, Pearman JW, Warren JR, Armstrong JA (1984) Original isolation of *Campylobacter pyloridis* from human gastric mucosa. Microbios 25:83–88
12. Marshall BJ, Warren JR (1984) Unidentified curved bacilli in the stomach of patients with gastritis and peptic ulceration. Lancet I:1311–1314
13. Rathbone BJ, Wyatt JJ, Worsley BW, Trejdosiewicz LK, Heatley RV, Losowsky MS (1985) Immune response to *Campylobacter pyloridis.* Lancet I:1217
14. von Wulffen H (1987) Low degree of relatedness between *Campylobacter pyloridis* and enteropathogenic Campylobacter species as revealed by DNA-DNA blot hybridization and immunoblot studies. FEMS Letters 42:129–133
15. von Wulffen H, Heesemann J, Bützow GH, Löning T, Laufs R (1986) Detection of *Campylobacter pyloridis* in patients with antrum gastritis and peptic ulcers by culture, complement fixation test, and immunoblot. J Clin Microbiol 24:716–720
16. von Wulffen H, Grote HJ, Krämer-Hansen H (1987) Serological screening for *Campylobacter pylori* in candidates for renal transplantation. Lancet I:1140–1141
17. Warren JR (1983) Unidentified curved bacilli on gastric epithelium in active chronic gastritis. Lancet I:1273

Local Immune Responses to *Campylobacter pylori* Colonisation

J. I. WYATT and B. J. RATHBONE

Introduction

Chronic gastritis is a histological diagnosis which cannot be accurately predicted on the basis of gastroscopic appearances. The diagnosis rests on the presence of a mononuclear inflammatory cell infiltrate in the lamina propria of the stomach. Chronic gastritis defined in this way is so common and so inconsistently related to symptoms that its pathological significance is debated. Its prevalence increased with age to approximately 50% in elderly persons, and it has thus been considered by some to be a 'normal' aging phenomenon rather than a pathological abnormality.

The distribution of inflammation within the stomach forms the basis for classification of chronic gastritis. In type A chronic gastritis inflammation and glandular loss affect the acid-secreting body-type mucosa, sparing the antrum. This is the lesion associated with pernicious anaemia and is believed to be of autoimmune pathogenesis. Type B chronic gastritis involves the antrum (with or without body-mucosal inflammation) and is at least ten times as common. This previously 'idiopathic' chronic gastritis shows a remarkably close association with colonisation by *Campylobacter pylori*.

Normally the stomach is sterile, except for a transient flora ingested with meals. Its thick surface blanket of mucus is believed to protect the epithelium from contact with antigenic stimuli. The more distal gut has a prominent population of mucosal immunocompetent cells which mediate antibody responses to bacterial and other antigens present in the lumen. Such cells are relatively sparse in the normal stomach, and an increase in their number constitutes the lesion of chronic gastritis.

Type B Chronic Gastritis: Histology

Histological classification of chronic gastritis is commonly based on the distribution of the inflammatory infiltrate, as in the classification proposed by Whitehead [1]. Chronic superficial gastritis is present when the inflammation involves only the superficial portion of the mucosa. This is believed to progress to chronic atrophic gastritis, in which the inflammation extends more deeply into the glandular mucosa, associated with loss of glandular tissue. Foci of metaplasia to intestinal-type epithelium may occur in chronic atrophic gastritis. Chronic gastritis is histologically 'active' when acute inflammatory cells (neutrophils) are also present, infiltrating the gastric epithelium.

Because of their characteristic morphology, *C. pylori* can be readily recognised histologically in gastric biopsies [2]. We have observed *C. pylori* in 95% of antral biopsies showing chronic gastritis [3], which may be either superficial or atrophic, in keeping with the chronicity of colonisation. The presence of *C. pylori* in the antrum is always associated with some increase in inflammatory cells, although this may be slight. *C. pylori* usually colonises the body mucosa in type B gastritis whether it is morphologically normal or inflamed [4].

Most researchers have found a significant correlation between *C. pylori* and the presence of intraepithelial neutrophils [4–6]. In our experience the prevalence of *C. pylori* in biopsies showing active gastritis is 95%, and in inactive chronic gastritis 60%. An important characteristic of *C. pylori* colonisation is its sparing of intestinal metaplasia, showing the specificity of this organism for gastric-type epithelium. This is also seen in duodenitis, where *C. pylori* only colonises foci of metaplastic gastric epithelium [7].

Non-specific Mucosal Defenses

An increase in secretory component in inflamed gastric epithelium has been demonstrated by immunofluorescence [8] and immunoperoxidase techniques [9], implying enhanced transportation of dimeric IgA across the epithelium in chronic gastritis.

Lysozyme and lactoferrin are non-specific antimicrobial compounds, present in increased amounts in the gastric juice of subjects with chronic gastritis [8, 9]. Reduction in intracellular mucin occurs in chronic gastritis [10]; this may represent an increased rate of release of cytoplasmic mucin into the lumen during inflammation.

Specific Immune Response to *C. pylori*

High levels of *C. pylori* specific IgG and IgA are present in the serum in *Campylobacter*-associated gastritis. These can be detected by ELISA techniques and provide a sensitive and specific means of identifying colonised subjects [11]. Using the same technique, IgA and IgM classes of antibody recognising *C. pylori* were detected in gastric juice in a proportion of patients with C. pylori gastritis, but not in those with normal gastric mucosa [10].

To determine whether the anti-*Campylobacter* antibodies in gastric juice were produced locally by mucosal plasma cells, antral biopsies from normal and gastritic patients were maintained in organ culture for 6 days, and ELISA assay was performed on the pooled supernatant [12]. Preliminary results have shown *C. pylori* specific IgG and IgA in all seven cases of *Campylobacter*-associated gastritis, and from one of eight normals. Some IgM was detected from most biopsies, high levels were occasionally present (2/7 gastritics). Thus gastric lamina propria plasma cells in chronic gastritis synthesise antibodies to *C. pylori*.

Additional antral biopsies from these cases were obtained for histology, and were stained by the immunoperoxidase technique for IgG, IgA, and IgM. Numbers of plasma cells of each class per unit area of mucosa were counted, and compared with the in vitro antibody production. This demonstrated a correlation between the plasma cell numbers in the lamina propria and the presence of *C. pylori* specific antibody obtained during organ culture.

A study was performed to investigate the presence of anti-*C. pylori* antibody by histological techniques. *C. pylori* colonised antral and body biopsies from 27 patients were stained by immunoperoxidase for IgA, IgG, and IgM. These were studied for presence and distribution of peroxidase-positive *C. pylori*. Positive staining was interpreted as indicating the presence of host immunoglobulin adsorbed in vivo onto the surface of the organism. Results were related to the activity of inflammation in the biopsy. The results have been published in detail elsewhere [4]. Briefly, *C. pylori* positive for IgA were identified in all 29 biopsies of active gastritis and in most (60%) of those without neutrophils. IgG- and IgM-positive bacteria were present in 86% of active gastritis biopsies and in 24% of those showing inactive gastritis or colonised normal body mucosa. The association between IgG- and IgM-labelling and the presence of neutrophils was significant. In all cases bacteria unstained by peroxidase (i.e. having undetectable amounts of adsorbed antibody) were present, especially in the depths of the gastric pits.

T-cell Changes in Chronic Gastritis

T-lymphocytes in the gastric mucosa, unlike in the more distal gut, have received little attention in the literature. Using double-label immunofluorescence techniques, our preliminary data suggests a CD4:CD8 (helper:suppressor) ratio approximating to 1:1 in the normal stomach. In *C. pylori* associated gastritis there is an increase in numbers of the helper/inducer subset within both lamina propria and epithelium. There is also increased expression of the CD7 antigen which is associated with lymphocyte stimulation. Thus T-lymphocyte changes also contribute to the histological picture of chronic gastritis, although their significance is at present uncertain.

Conclusions

The principal diagnostic criterion for type B chronic gastritis is an increase in the mononuclear cell population in the gastric antrum. *C. pylori* are nearly always present in this condition. We have shown that the plasma cell component of chronic gastritis includes cells producing *C. pylori* specific immunoglobulin. Such antibody is produced by the antral mucosa in amounts which broadly correlate with the density of plasma cell infiltrate. In addition, the neutrophil infiltration in active chronic gastritis is associated with the presence of IgG- and IgM-coated *C. pylori* on the mucosal surface. These classes of antibody, unlike IgA, are mediators of neutrophil activity, suggesting that active inflammation is in response to the opsonised surface bacteria.

The non-specific defense mechanisms of the gastric mucosa are also appropriate to the combat of a bacterial pathogen. The histopathological features which characterise type B chronic gastritis suggest, as a pathogenetic basis, an immune response to a luminal antigen, rather than the effect of damage caused by postulated injurious chemical or physical agents. The antigenic stimulus is, at least in part, provided by the presence of *C. pylori*.

References

1. Whitehead R (1984) Mucosal biopsy of the upper gastrointestinal tract, 3rd edn. Saunders, Philadelphia
2. Marshall BJ, Warren JR (1984) Unidentified curved bacilli in the stomach of patients with gastritis and peptic ulceration. Lancet I:1311−1314
3. Rathbone BJ, Wyatt JI, Heatley RV (1986) Campylobacter pyloridis − a new factor in peptic ulcer disease? Gut 27:635−641
4. Wyatt JI, Rathbone BJ, Heatley RV (1986) Local immune response to gastric Campylobacter in non-ulcer dyspepsia. J Clin Pathol 39:863−870
5. Warren JR, Marshall BJ (1983) Unidentified curved bacilli on gastric epithelium in active chronic gastritis. Lancet I:1273−1275
6. Steer HW (1985) The gastro-duodenal epithelium in peptic ulceration. J Pathol 146:355−362
7. Wyatt JI, Rathbone BJ, Dixon MF, Heatley RV (1987) Campylobacter-associated gastritis and acid-induced gastric metaplasia in the pathogenesis of duodenitis. J Clin Pathol 40:841
8. Valnes K, Brandtzaeg P, Elgjo K, Stave R (1984) Specific and non-specific humoral defence factors in the epithelium of normal and inflamed gastric mucosa. Gastroenterology 86:402−412
9. Isaacson P (1982) Immunoperoxidase study of the secretory immunoglobulin system and lysozyme in normal and diseased gastric mucosa. Gut 23:578−588
10. Goodwin CS, Armstrong JA, Marshall BJ (1986) *Campylobacter pyloridis*, gastritis, and peptic ulceration. J Clin Pathol 39:353−365
11. Rathbone BJ, Wyatt JI, Worsley BW, Shires SE, Trejdosiewicz LK, Heatley RV, Losowsky MS (1986) Systemic and local antibody response to gastric *Campylobacter pyloridis* in non-ulcer dyspepsia. Gut 27:642−647
12. Rathbone BJ, Wyatt JI, Tompkins D, Heatley RV, Losowsky MS (1986) in vitro production of *Campylobacter pyloridis* specific antibodies by gastric mucosal biopsies. Gut 27:A607

Discussion

Tytgat: Suppose *C. pylori* is a commensal, what kind of an immune response would you expect, if any?

Wyatt: If we compare this to the situation in the colon, where the mucosa is in contact with plenty of commensal bacteria, the plasma cell infiltrate (which is normally present in the colon) is composed mainly of cells producing immunoglobulins against various species of *E. coli*. And so I think we may expect to see some sort of plasma cell response to *C. pylori* even if it is just a commensal and not causing the damage. I think that whether chronic gastritis is a pathological or physiological state, we can understand the bacteria and the plasma cells as being causally related to each other.

Pearson: I think Dr. Tytgat's point is possibly related to the fact that dead *E. coli* produce an antibody response.

Hahn: Having also monoclonal cells around in the picture, I wonder whether specific T cells are around.

Wyatt: Clearly we would expect there to be a T-cell component operating here as well, if this is an immune response against bacteria. We have looked at this to some extent and have some preliminary data. We found that the T cells are certainly increased in chronic gastritis compared with normal, both within the lamina propria and also within the epithelium. We suggest that the T-cell subset ratio (the helper-inducer to the suppressor ratio) seems to be about 1:1 in the normal stomach. In chronic gastritis the helper to suppressor ratio increases to 2–3:1, and this is seen both in the lamina propria and in the epithelium. The CD7 antigen, which is a marker of T-cell stimulation by T helper cells, also shows an increase in chronic gastritis. So, there is a T-cell component reaction, but its significance is at present unclear.

Hahn: One might also try proliferation of T cells.

Wyatt: Yes, that is right.

Tytgat: Does the presence of immunoglobulins around microorganisms prevent adherence to the epithelial cell membrane?

Wyatt: It has been suggested that IgA reduces colonization because it reduces the ability of bacteria to adhere onto epithelial cells and therefore allows the organism to be shed into the lumen of the gastrointestinal tract.

Riecken: I wonder whether you could give us again your definition of "inactive" gastritis?

Wyatt: Inactive gastritis is a chronic gastritis with mononuclear cells in the lamina propria, but without neutrophils passing through the epithelium. In an active gastritis the neutrophils are present in the epithelium as well as in the other components.

Tytgat: How reproducible is the finding that microorganisms deep in the pits or foveoli are not coated with immunoglobulins in contrast to those at the surface?

Wyatt: It was certainly something which was very apparent looking at all of these sections. The problem is how to interpret it. It was very rare to see a positive bacteria down within the pit, using immunoperoxidase for the immunoglobulins but not by immunoperoxidase with polyclonal anti-*C. pylori*, and so therefore it is not an artefact where the position in the mucosa is in some way interfering with the immunoperoxidase reaction. I think it is a reproducible feature which possibly represents a way in which the bacteria escapes host immunoglobulin.

Tytgat: But the results suggest that there is preferential IgA secretion at the luminal surface, and not in the pits?

Wyatt: No, that would be at variance with work which has been done on secretory components and transport of IgA. One explanation might be that IgA-coated organisms are not able to adhere, and therefore they have been passed out onto the surface of the mucosa, and we see them more there.

Ottenjann: Is there really a clear-cut order between inactive and active gastritis? And how many particles do you need to make the estimation of the activity or nonactivity? Two or three or four or five?

Wyatt: It is clear that there is a spectrum of the number of polymorphs within the epithelium, and quite often you are in the situation of looking at a sizable biopsy and seeing one or two polymorphs. Personally I call that active, but I am sure that there is a sampling defect. In very active cases then there is no doubt.

Deltenre: We studied the correlation between gastritis and the presence or frequency of *C. pylori*, grading, I think the gastritis according to the same criteria as yours, with Whitehead's criteria. There were two groups: G1 to G3 nonactive, mild, moderate, severe, and active gastritis from G4 to G6, mild, moderate, severe and we found a strong correlation between the frequency of *C. pylori* and grade of gastritis. My question is: from an immunological point of view, would you consider that active gastritis is in the early stages of the disease, or a more severe stage, or both?

Wyatt: It is very difficult to know what the changes with time are on the basis of one biopsy. When we have looked at people biopsied at six-week intervals, the severity of gastritis appeared to fluctuate. My concept is that the chronic gastritis persists with a waxing and waning of the degree of activity with time.

Section 5

Treatment of Chronic Gastritis and Peptic Ulcer with Bismuth Salts

Therapeutic Strategies in Medical Management of Peptic Ulcer Disease

M. GREGOR

Introduction

So far, all speakers in this symposium have focussed mainly on the harmful effects of gastric acidity on the gastric and duodenal mucosa. On the other hand, the assumed pathogenicity of *Campylobacter pylori* has opened a new perspective in the treatment of peptic ulcer disease. It may well be that the combined treatment of gastric acidity of *C. pylori*-colonization will display a synergistic effect in ulcer healing. However, since all the following presentations will give more details about *C. pylori*-colonization and eradication, we feel it is still necessary to highlight briefly the hitherto and conventional treatment of peptic ulcer disease.

The first question to be answered is:

What Do We Treat?

We treat the symptom, i.e., peptic ulcer, of an underlying disease which is multifactorial with respect to its etiology and pathophysiology [1]. This symptom shows a spontaneous healing rate within 4−6 weeks, which is regionally different, sometimes being very high as in the Federal Republic of Germany (duodenal ulcer, DU 79%) and Switzerland (DU 73%; gastric ulcer, GU 83%), sometimes less so, as in England (DU 29%) [2−5]. Furthermore, we treat a symptom with an annual recurrence rate of about 75% [6]. If 100 ulcer patients are followed up for 12 months after the initial healing of a peptic ulcer, 37% would have had one symptomatic attack, 27%, two or more attacks, and 36%, none [7]. For those patients with recurrent ulcer episodes we have to consider some type of long-term treatment.

A further characteristic feature in ulcer disease is the fact that the so-called characteristic symptoms provide only a poor indication of the presence or absence of an ulcer. About 50% of patients with "dyspepsia" will have an ulcer, and only 50% of patients with an ulcer will have "dyspepsia" [8]. In chronic ulcer disease about 15% of patients may have recurrent persistent ulcer without any symptoms. Therefore, it is mandatory to perform diagnostic upper endoscopy for evaluation of clinical studies as well as adequate medical management in peptic ulcer disease.

The second question to be answered is:

Why Do We Treat?

Peptic ulcer disease is of considerable socioeconomic impact: The annual peptic ulcer incidence was 0.18% in Denmark (1963–1968) and 0.29% in the USA (1975) [9]. The 1-year period prevalence of active ulcer disease is about 1.7% and the total lifetime prevalence is roughly 5%–10% [9]. Furthermore, ulcer disease is the cause of death in 1.4% of the patients during the first 9 years after diagnosis and constitutes a 20%, life-long, age-dependent risk of serious complications such as bleeding, perforation or obstruction [10–12].

The main treatment objectives in acute ulcer disease are to improve symptoms of pain, to prevent ulcer-related complications, and to accelerate ulcer healing which is probably the least important of all, although it is the endpoint in most clinical studies. The main treatment objectives in chronic ulcer disease are to prevent ulcer recurrence and ulcer-related complications, to maintain pain relief, and to restore normal social life. Overall, the primary treatment goal in chronic ulcer disease will be to cure the ulcer disease but, unfortunately, we are still far away from this.

The third question which should be answered is:

How Do We Treat?

The therapeutic targets are acid neutralization, acid suppression, and cytoprotection. Acid neutralization has been achieved using antacids, although in recent studies it has been shown that antacids even in very low doses are effective in relieving symptoms and accelerating ulcer healing probably via a cytoprotective effect rather than via their acid-neutralizing capacity [13]. The main therapeutic target, so far, is acid suppression by inhibition of the parietal cell. Such an inhibition may be achieved by blocking the stimulating histaminergic or cholinergic input at the receptor level, by inhibition of intracellular cyclic AMP generation, or by inhibition of the H^+/K^+-ATPase proton pump, the final common pathway of gastric acid secretion, using substituted benzimidazoles like omeprazole [14].

All these different therapeutic principles have been investigated in numerous clinical studies to evaluate their therapeutic effectiveness in peptic ulcer disease. Nevertheless, it is still difficult to draw a final conclusion as to which therapeutic regimen may be superior and should be recommended because a number of the criteria relevant for the evaluation of therapeutic trials have been ignored in the great majority of clinical studies. Most of these studies have at least a double-blind, randomized, and controlled design, but a definition of healing and relapse rate is mostly missing. What does it mean to consider the disappearance of an ulcer as a relevant definition of healing if an underlying disease still exists? What does it mean to argue about relapse rate if one considers only the symptomatic relapse as an indication for control endoscopy, bearing in mind the high percentage of patients who are asymptomatic but still have a peptic ulcer? Furthermore, the possible influence of other drugs like antacids, in addition to those under study, may be of importance because antacids, as already mentioned, have been effective in accelerating ulcer healing even in low doses [13]. So, the optional intake of antacids may well be relevant for the evaluation of therapeutic trials. Observer errors, comparability of groups, compliance check, and the so-called β-error based on an insufficient number of patients enrolled in the particular study are other important criteria for the evaluation of therapeutic trials. For instance, if one tries to find out the relevant and significant 10% difference between one treatment regimen and the other, let us say ranitidine and cimetidine, one would need at least 700 patients in one trial − a figure which has hardly been achieved by any of the clinical studies published up to now.

Despite such possible insufficiencies, Table 1 summarizes the pooled results of numerous clinical trials for the various treatment regimens in acute peptic ulcer healing [13 − 24]. In comparison with placebo all these therapeutic regimens show very similar healing rates for duodenal as well as gastric ulcers; they differ only with respect to the time needed for ulcer healing.

The criteria for drug selection, beside its effectiveness, are safety, acceptability, cost, scientific basis and practicability of treatment. With these criteria in mind, the various drug regimens are listed schematically in Table 2 to characterize their suitability for treatment of acute peptic ulcer.

Table 1. Summary of clinical trials comparing the efficacy (i. e., healing rate) of various drugs in patients with acute duodenal (DU) or gastric (GU) ulcers

	Healing rate [%]			
	DU		GU	
	Weeks of treatment		Weeks of treatment	
	4	8	4	8
Placebo	24 − 73		29 − 50	61 − 66
H$_2$-blocker	58 − 93	84 − 98	40 − 76	73 − 91
Omeprazole	92 − 97		81	95
Antacids	52 − 81		43	76
Pirenzepine	62 − 90			
PGE$_2$	59 − 80	77 − 89	32 − 54	68
Sucralfate	66 − 92	60 − 97 [a]	36 − 53	76 − 80
Bismuth (CBS)	50 − 89	67 − 93 [a]		70 − 85

[a] 6 weeks of treatment only.

Table 2. Summary of criteria for drug selection comparing various anti-ulcer drugs

	Acute healing	Pain relief	Convenience	Side effects	Scientific basis
Placebo	+/−	?	+	−	−
H₂-blocker	+	?	+	(+)	+
Antacid	+	?	−	(+)	−
Pirenzepine	+	?	(+)	(+)	(+)
PGE₂	+	?	−	(+)	−
Sucralfate	+	?	−	(+)	−
Bismuth	+	?	−	(+)	−

Placebo seems to be the drug of choice: It is quite effective (relative to the regional different spontaneous healing rates), and it has no side effects. It is very convenient to take and costs little; its pain relief, although critical to evaluate, is similar to other drugs. Unfortunately, it has no scientific basis. Therefore, histamine-blockers are still the treatment of choice for acute peptic ulcer. These H₂-blockers accelerate ulcer healing and are convenient to take. They have hardly any side effects, and are well-known for their good scientific basis. Alternatively, one may take any of the other drugs listed in Table 2 for treatment of acute peptic ulcer.

The most important question is:

How Do We Keep the Ulcer Healed?

Long-term treatment to reduce peptic ulcer recurrence rate after the acute ulcer has healed has been studied in a number of clinical trials [17−19, 22−24]. A significant decrease in annual relapse rate of duodenal ulcer has been reported following a maintenance therapy with H₂-blockers, pirenzepine, or sucralfate over a period of 12 months (Table 3). There were no significant differences between the various drug regimens in preventing duodenal ulcer relapses. The protection against relapse appears to remain only for as long as the drug is taken. The frequency of ulcer recurrences will be the same after maintenance therapy has been discontinued. The natural history of peptic ulcer disease is not influenced by such long-term medication.

Under these circumstances the disadvantages of a life-long maintenance therapy are of particular relevance: costs of treatment, lack of compliance, i.e., lack of efficiency, side effects, and loss of protection of the small intestine against invasion and colonization by ingested, potentially pathogenic organisms. The long-term impairment of the gastric acid-bactericidal barrier is one of the factors which predisposes to mixed infection with enteric pathogens causing diarrhea, such as typhoid, cholera, and various forms of salmonella

Table 3. Summary of comparative studies of long-term treatment with various drugs in the prevention of duodenal ulcer recurrence

Treatment (12 months)	Dose	Relapse rate (%)
Placebo		44 – 96
Cimetidine	400 mg	10 – 32
Ranitidine	150 mg	11 – 25
Famotidine	20 mg	24 – 36
Pirenzepine	50 mg	15 – 47
Sucralfate	2 – 2.5 g	44 – 47

dysentery, which form a major public health problem in Third World nations [25 – 29].

The most serious, although hypothetical, risk of long-term acid suppression may be the development of gastric cancer. Possible mechanisms of gastric carcinogenesis have been proposed [26, 28 – 34]:

1. Bacterial overgrowth of the stomach and subsequent intragastric production of potentially carcinogenic N-nitroso compounds from nitrates and nitrites in the diet.
2. Hypergastrinemia or stimulation of some other trophic agent during achlorhydria leading to hyperplasia and neoplasia of gastric mucosal endocrine cells. Such neoplastic change in gastric enterochromaffin-like (ECL) cells have been well documented in rats following long-term treatment with very high doses of omeprazole [26, 30 – 32].
   Further studies are needed to provide complete assurance about these concerns.

It has been shown that the subsequent relapse rate of duodenal ulcer is less in the 12 months after successful initial treatment with colloidal bismuth than with H_2-receptor antagonists [35 – 37]. These results imply that drug treatment with colloidal bismuth given for a short period in duodenal ulcer disease influences the progress of the disease and may alter the natural history of peptic ulceration. Therefore, infrequent intermittent short courses of colloidal bismuth may be a reasonable alternative to maintenance treatment with acid-suppressing drugs for prevention of duodenal ulcer recurrences [38].

Although, every uncomplicated peptic ulcer is primarily a problem for medical management, elective surgery should be considered in long-lasting peptic ulcer disease if there is a persistent failure to heal despite adequate medical measures or repeated recurrences under adequate maintenance therapy as well as no risk from the operation. In the great majority of cases, however, the most important reason for treatment failures is inadequate medical therapy caused by noncompliance of various types, i.e., errors of omission, errors of dosage, mistakes in timing, and taking additional medication like potentially ulcerogenic drugs not prescribed by the physicians.

Practical Therapeutic Approach in Peptic Ulcer Disease

Figure 1 shows a flow course of practical therapeutic approach to the patient with peptic ulcer disease which should certainly be adapted and individualized for each patient.

Upper endoscopy is performed in patients with persistent "dyspepsia". If gastric ulcer is seen, biopsy specimens need to be taken to exclude malignancy. In the case of a benign peptic ulcer a full course treatment is started for 4−6 weeks with a single, early evening dosis of H_2-blockers (i.e., ranitidine 300 mg) and an optional intake of antacids 1 h after the meal. Alternatively, the patient may be treated with sucralfate, pirenzepine, or colloidal bismuth. Control endoscopy should be performed after 6 weeks. If benign peptic ulcer is not healed and non-compliance is possibly not the cause for treatment failure,

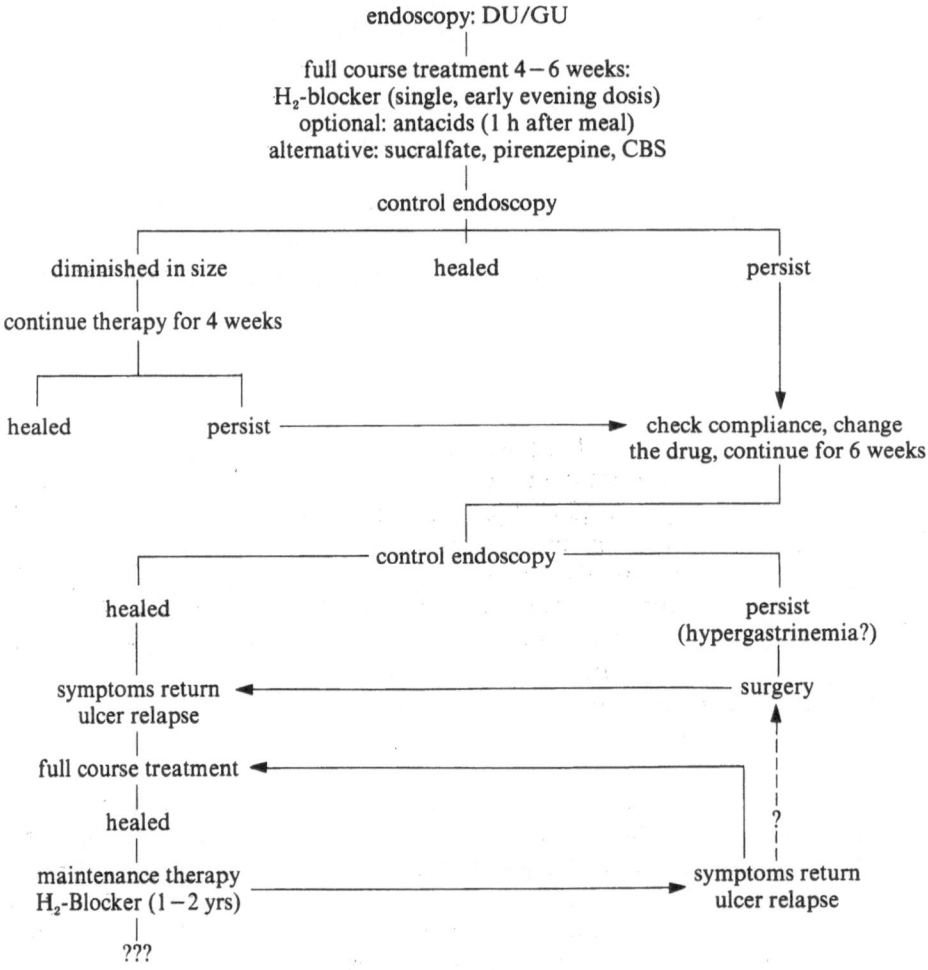

Fig. 1. Flow course of therapeutic approach to the patient with peptic ulcer disease

change the drug and continue for a further 6 weeks. Thereafter, control endoscopy is repeated. If the gastric ulcer still persists, unchanged in size, and hypergastrinemia is excluded surgery should be performed, not to overlook gastric carcinoma. After the peptic ulcer has healed, drug therapy is gradually reduced and then stopped. If symptoms return and a benign peptic ulcer relapse is documented by endoscopy, a full course of the acute therapeutic regimen is started again. Thereafter, maintenance therapy should be given with half the dosis of H_2-blocker at bedtime for at least $1-2$ years. In patients with a symptomatic ulcer relapse while on maintenance therapy, the maintenance medication may be augmented for $4-8$ weeks and should be restored to the lower maintenance dose level after the ulcer has healed.

In summary, short-term healing of acute peptic ulcer is usually not difficult to achieve with the various drug regimens available including acid-secreting inhibitors, antacids, or protective drugs. The main question still to be answered is: How do we keep the ulcer healed? This means also, in particular during this symposium, elucidating the role of microbiology in peptic ulcer disease. Perhaps, the current therapeutic approach to peptic ulcer disease may have to be changed at the end of this meeting.

References

1. Boyd EJS, Wormsley KG (1985) Etiology and pathogenesis of peptic ulcer. In: Berk JE (ed) Bockus Gastroenterology, vol 2. WB Saunders, Philadelphia, pp 1013−1059
2. Malchow H, Sewing K-F, Albinus M, Horn B, Schomerus H, Dölle W (1978) Cimetidin in der stationären Behandlung des peptischen Ulkus. I. Wirkung auf die Heilung des Ulcus duodeni. Dtsch Med Wochenschr 103:149−152
3. Scheurer U, Witzel L, Halter F, Keller HM, Huber R, Galaeazzi R (1977) Gastric and duodenal ulcer healing and placebo treatment. Gastroenterology 72:838−851
4. Multicentre trial: the effect of cimetidine on duodenal ulceration (1977) In: Burland WL, Simkins MA (eds) Cimetidine. Excerpta Medica, Amsterdam, pp 260−271
5. Dobrilla G (1983) Placebo in the evaluation of antiulcer drugs. Int J Tissue React 5:329−337
6. Pounder RE (1981) Model of medical treatment for duodenal ulcer. Lancet I:29−30
7. Bardhan KD (1980) Intermittent treatment of duodenal ulcer with cimetidine. Br Med J 281:20−22
8. Thompson ABR, Mahachai V (1985) Medical management of uncomplicated peptic ulcer disease. In: Berk JE (ed) Bockus Gastroenterology, vol 2. WB Saunders, Philadelphia, pp 1116−1154
9. Kurata JH, Haile BM (1984) Epidemiology of peptic ulcer disease. In: Isenberg JI, Johansson C (eds) Peptic ulcer disease. WB Saunders, London, pp 289−308 (Clinics in Gastroenterology, vol 13:2)
10. Bonnevie O (1977) Causes of death in duodenal and gastric ulcer. Gastroenterology 73:1000−1004
11. Bonnevie O (1978) Survival in peptic ulcer. Gastroenterology 75:1055−1060
12. Pulvertraft CN (1968) Comments on the incidence and natural history of gastric and duodenal ulcer. Postgrad Med J 44:597−602
13. Berstad A, Weberg R (1986) Antacids in the treatment of gastroduodenal ulcer. Scand J Gastroenterol 21:385−391
14. Friedman G (1987) Omeprazole. Am J Gastroenterol 83:188−191
15. Clissold SP, Campli-Richards DM (1986) Omeprazole. A preliminary review of its pharmacodynamic and pharmacokinetic properties, and therapeutic potential in peptic ulcer disease and Zollinger-Ellison syndrome. Drugs 32:15−47

16. Walan A (1984) Antacids and anticholinergics in the treatment of duodenal ulcer. In: Isenberg JI, Johansson C (eds) Peptic ulcer disease. WB Saunders, London, pp 473−499 (Clinics in Gastroenterology, vol 13:2)
17. Brogden RN, Heel RC, Speight TM, Avery GS (1984) Sucralfate. A review of its pharmacodynamic properties and therapeutic use in peptic ulcer disease. Drugs 27:194−209
18. Carmine AA, Brogden RN (1985) Pirenzepine. A review of its pharmacodynamic and pharmacokinetic properties and therapeutic efficacy in peptic ulcer disease and other allied diseases. Drugs 30:85−126
19. Tytgat GNJ, Hameeteman W, Van Olffen GH (1984) Sucralfate, bismuth compounds, substituted benzimidazoles, trimipramine and pirenzepine in the short- and long-term treatment of duodenal ulcer. In: Isenberg JI, Johansson C (eds) Peptic ulcer disease. WB Saunders, London, pp 543−568 (Clinics in Gastroenterology, vol 13:2)
20. Monk JP, Clissold SP (1987) Misoprostol. A preliminary review of its pharmacodynamic and pharmacokinetic properties and therapeutic efficacy in the treatment of peptic ulcer disease. Drugs 33:1−30
21. Thompson ABR (ed) (1986) Protective and therapeutic effects of gastrointestinal prostaglandins. Enprostil: a new modality. Am J Med 81 (2A):1−88
22. Campoli-Richards DM, Clissold SP (1986) Famotidine. Pharmacodynamic and pharmacokinetic properties and a preliminary review of its therapeutic use in peptic ulcer disease and Zollinger-Ellison syndrome. Drugs 32:197−221
23. Brogden RN, Carmine AA, Heel RC, Speight TM, Avery GS (1982) Ranitidine: a review of its pharmacology and therapeutic use in peptic ulcer disease and other allied diseases. Drugs 24:267−303
24. Meyrick TJ, Misiewicz G (1984) Histamine H_2-receptor antagonists in the short- and long-term treatment of duodenal ulcer. In: Isenberg JI, Johansson C (eds) Peptic ulcer disease. WB Saunders, London, pp 501−543 (Clinics in Gastroenterology, vol 13:2)
25. Ruddell WSJ, Axon ATR, Findlay JM, Bartholomew BA, Hill MJ (1980) Effect of cimetidine on the gastric bacterial flora. Lancet I:672−674
26. Sharma BK, Santana JA, Wood EC, Walt RP, Pereira M, Noone P, Smith PLR, Walters CL, Pounder RE (1984) Intragastric bacterial activity and nitrosation before, during and after treatment with omeprazole. Br Med J 289:717−719
27. Merson MH, Ouchterlony O, Holmgren J (eds) (1980) In: Cholera and related diarrhoeas. Karger, Basel, pp 34−45
28. Milton-Thompson GJ, Lightfoot NF, Ahmet L (1982) Intragastric acidity, bacteria, nitrite and N-nitroso compounds before, during and after cimetidine treatment. Lancet I:1091−1095
29. Howden CW, Hunt RH (1987) Relationship between gastric secretion and infection. Gut 28:96−107
30. Stockmann R, Fölsch UR, Bonatz G, Wulfrath M, Creutzfeldt W (1984) Influence of a substituted benzimidazole (omeprazole) on rat gastric endocrine cells. Dig Dis Sci 29:83S
31. Ekman L, Hansson E, Havu N, Carlsson E, Lundberg C (1985) Toxicological studies on omeprazole. Scand J Gastroenterol [Suppl] 108:53−69
32. Hakanson R, Sundler F, Carlsson E, Mattson H, Larsson H (1986) Proliferation of enterochromaffin-like (ECL) cells in the rat stomach following omeprazole treatment. Hepatogastroenterol 32:48−49
33. Wormsley KG (1984) Assessing the safety of drugs for the long-term treatment of peptic ulcer. Gut 25:1416−1423
34. Penston J, Wormsley KG (1987) Achlorhydria: hypergastrinaemia: carcinoids − a flawed hypothesis? Gut 28:488−505
35. Martin DF, Hollanders D, May SJ, Ravenscroft MM, Tweedle DEF, Miller JP (1981) Difference in relapse rates of duodenal ulcer after healing with cimetidine or tripotassium dicitrato bismuthate. Lancet I:7−10
36. Hamilton I, O'Connor HJ, Wood NC, Bradbury I, Axon ATR (1986) Healing and recurrence of duodenal ulcer after treatment with tripotassium dicitrato bismuthate (TDB) tablets or cimetidine. Gut 27:106−110
37. Tytgat GNJ (1987) Colloidal bismuth subcitrate in peptic ulcer − a review. Digestion 37 [Suppl 2]:31−41
38. Colin-Jones DG (1986) There is more to healing ulcers than suppressing acid. Gut 27:475−480

Discussion

Halter: Are you still sending patients with simple peptic ulcer for surgical treatment, and if so, why?

Gregor: No, we are not sending the patients with a simple peptic ulcer for surgical treatment. We call for the surgeon only if there is an apparent lack of efficiency of medical therapy over a period of several months, i.e., a persistent failure to heal. We ask also for surgical therapy of gastric ulcer in case of continuous suspicion of malignancy.

Halter: But not with your large endoscopic experience.

Gregor: Sometimes, we all meet those patients with nonhealing gastric ulcer where we have taken an adequate number of biopsies even a second or third time and we still end up suspecting malignancy.

Halter: Would you, under such circumstances, not be ready to change the medication and use the more potent acid inhibitor? Would you ever consider Omeprazole?

Gregor: Yes, we certainly change the medication in case of a persistent peptic ulcer as shown on my second slide summarizing our current strategy in management of peptic ulcer disease, and that means: change the drug. We have not used Omeprazole so far because of this unresolved argument about Omeprazole possibly inducing gastric carcinoids as shown at least in rats.

von Wulffen: Of course you often have the problem that the ulcer has healed and a patient still has pain independent of whether you treated him with H2 blockers or with bismuth or antibiotics. You look into the stomach and the ulcer is gone, but the patient still complains. So I was quite intrigued reading a paper, unfortunately I cannot remember the name of the journal or the author or the substance used, but anyway, the idea was that they looked at the nonulcer dyspepsia and did a placebo controlled study with one group receiving placebo and the other group a motility increasing substance and they found relief, significantly increased relief in the group receiving the motility drug versus the placebo group. Since I am a microbiologist, it was just by chance that I read this paper because it was not dealing with *C. pylori* at all, or with any infectious etiology, but I was just wondering whether possibly motility problems of the stomach have something to do with the pain and with the disease itself. As a bacteriologist, of course, I know the saying that where there is stasis there is infection and if there is a stomach with reduced motility, there might be a better chance that the infection by *C. pylori* could spread, and if you relieve this symptom and increase motility then the infection might possibly be contained.

Gregor: In face of the symptoms of nonulcer dyspepsia I would first look for *C. pylori*. In case of a positive diagnosis I would then start treatment using either bismuth alone or in combination with an antibiotic not worrying about a possible but so far unproven pathophysiological relationship between gastric motility and *C. pylori* colonization. Nevertheless we should keep in mind the possible existence of such a relationship and perhaps there will be some studies in the near future trying to answer this question positively.

Halter: I think Dr. von Wulffen was alluding to a paper on Cisapride recently published in *Gut* (28:300, 1987) by Prof. L. Barbri's group from Bologne, Italy.

Axon: You have stated what is commonly believed that treatment should start with an H2 receptor antagonist to reduce acid. I would like to ask why you still advocate this when you have already demonstrated that there is an increased recurrent rate also, the healing rate is no higher and you run certain risks by reducing acid, why don't you start, with, say CBS first, and then use an H2 receptor antagonist, if that is ineffective?

Gregor: The main topic of my presentation was to focus on conventional therapy of peptic ulcer disease and that means up to now to reduce gastric acid secretion. It will certainly be the subject of all the following presentations and in fact of the whole meeting to discuss alternative therapeutic strategies and in particular the possible role of bismuth compounds. At the end of this meeting it may well be that we all agree to use bismuth in the first place for treatment in peptic ulcer disease.

Halter: I know that you are not only an excellent clinician but also a physiologist or at least an ex-physiologist and we have not discussed the question whether prolonged inhibition of gastric acid secretion modulates the receptors on the parietal cells. Is there enough evidence in your opinion that the receptors on the parietal cells are modulated after prolonged inhibition of acid secretion. Could this be a reason for the high recurrence rate?

Gregor: I do not know of any direct experimental evidence for an increased sensitivity of the parietal cells at the receptor level following prolonged acid suppression using for instance the isolated parietal cell model developed by A. Soll and his colleagues. But there may well be some indirect evidence for such receptor modulation on the parietal cell following prolonged acid inhibition which I can not remember at the moment.

Halter: There are studies by Dr. Berstad's group in Oslo which suggest that there is an increased sensitivity of the receptor on the parietal cells to histamine and pentagastrin following prolonged treatment with histamine H2 receptor antagonists.

Brunner: I do not want to leave this meeting without mentioning the well known results on ulcer therapy with Omeprazole. Dr. Tytgat, who is sitting beside me here, has already published his results on Ranitidine-resistant ulcers. We have treated almost 100 such patients successfully with Omeprazole and you all know that when you have a Ranitidine-resistant ulcer you can just write to Astra in Germany and they will send Omeprazole for your patient. We have sent patients who did not respond to ranitidin to surgeons and the results were extremely bad. Those patients who do not respond to 600 mg Ranitidine and also have very poor results in surgery, respond excellently to the therapy with Omeprazole. Omeprazole is a very potent drug and very effective. Until we have something better, we should include Omeprazole on the list of therapeutics for peptic ulcer disease.

Gregor: Omeprazole certainly is a potent acid inhibitor and very effective in peptic ulcer healing even in such cases which do not respond favorably to other drugs like H2 blockers in the first place. But you still face the problem of treating the symptoms of an underlying disease which implicates an unresolved high recurrence rate when you stop treatment with Omeprazole. Again, so far the implications of a longterm treatment using Omeprazole in terms of possible side effects are not fully understood and to my knowledge this issue has not been addressed so far.

Halter: I must warn you, Dr. Gregor, that what Professor Brunner mentioned is absolutely true, but you have to fill out very time-consuming detailed forms for each patient you treat with this new drug.

Classen: How do these patients progress when their ulcers have healed? In other words, do you control these patients after short-term therapy with Omeprazole endoscopically and what are the results?

Brunner: Since we are just preparing this publication I can talk about it already. We have been making a five year study on Omeprazole therapy for Ranitidine-resistant ulcers. The longest patient has been taking the drug for four years already. All patients are on 40 mg daily. It is a joint study between Hannover and Göttingen. No clinical, laboratory or morpholic abnormalities have been observed to date.

Gregor: Well, when you have finished your study and if the finalized results indeed have the relevance you just mentioned I may have to change some of my slides on therapeutic strategies in management of peptic ulcer disease and I am quite willing to do so.

Gastroprotective and Ulcer Healing Properties of Bismuth Salts

S. J. KONTUREK, T. BRZOZOWSKI, D. DROZDOWICZ, and W. BIELANSKI

Introduction

Bismuth compounds have been used over two centuries for the treatment of various gastrointestinal disorders due to their local protective, demulcent, and antacid properties. Some of the bismuth salts, particularly subnitrates, subgallates, phosphates, or aluminates, used in large doses (15 – 20 g/day) were reported to cause intoxication involving the central nervous system (encephalopathy) that occurred in France in the last decade in the form of a toxicological epidemic (Bader 1986). This limited the clinical use of bismuth salts in some countries but more recently the preparation of colloidal bismuth subcitrate (De-Nol) was developed and this offered a new approach in ulcer therapy due to the selective binding of the drug to the ulcer base, the formation of a protection barrier against acid-pepsin attack and its activity against Campylobacter pylori (Lee 1982; Marshall et al. 1985). With the successful clinical application of De-Nol in ulcer therapy (Tytgat et al. 1984) no single report of bismuth intoxication has appeared probably due to the low dosage (below 0.5 g/day) of bismuth used and its application in the colloidal form that reduced its absorption from the gut and excluded potential neurotoxicity. It should be mentioned, however, that no side effects have been reported with bismuth subsalicylate (Pepto Bismol) which has been used for stomach discomfort in noncolloidal form but also at low dosage (up to about 2.0 g/day). In some countries bismuth subnitrate is still prescribed at low dosage by general practitioners in peptic ulcer therapy, also without reports of side effects.

De-Nol was found to be gastroprotective in experimental animals (Hall and Hoven 1987; Konturek et al. 1987d) and to enhance ulcer healing in humans (Tytgat et al. 1984). No study so far has been undertaken to compare the gastroprotective and ulcer healing properties of various bismuth salts. This report describes the gastroprotective effects of De-Nol, Pepta Bismol, and bismuth subnitrate against absolute ethanol and acidified aspirin (ASA) and the ulcer healing action of De-Nol in rats.

Material and Methods

Studies on Gastroprotection

Acute gastric ulcerations were induced in Wistar rats (180 – 200 g body weight) by intragastric administration of absolute ethanol or acidified aspirin (ASA).

Absolute ethanol was administered to 24 h fasted rats in a volume of 1 ml using a metal orogastric tube (Konturek et al. 1987). One hour later the animals were killed by a blow to the head, the stomach was removed and the area of gastric necrotic lesions was measured by planimetry (Morphomat 10, Zeiss, FRG).

Acidified ASA was administered in 24 h fasted rats in a bolus dose of 60 mg/kg followed by a dose of 42 mg/kg/h for a 3-h period. ASA was dissolved in 0.15 M HCl and instilled intragastrically via a plastic tube inserted surgically into the stomach 2 h before the start of the experiment as described in a previous publication (Konturek et al. 1981). After 3 h of ASA administration, the animals were killed and the area of gastric ulcerations was determined by planimetry. De-Nol (given by Dr D. W. R. Hall, Biological Research Department, Gist-brocades, Delft), Pepto Bismol (given by C. J. Klein, Roehm Pharma, FRG) or bismuth subnitrate (Polfa, Poland) were suspended in water and administered intragastrically (i.g.) in various doses about 30 min before the administration of 100% ethanol or acidified ASA. For comparison, 16,16-dimethyl-PGE$_2$ (given by Dr. J. Pike, Upjohn Co., Kalamazoo, Michigan) was used orally in a standard protective dose (10 µg/kg/h).

Determination of the Role of Prostaglandins (PG)
in Bismuth Salt-Treated Gastric Mucosa

The role of endogenous PG in the protection by bismuth salts was examined in two ways:

1) by direct measurement of mucosal generation of PGE$_2$ by radio-immunoassay of PGE$_2$ using commercially available kits (New England Nuclear, Dreieich, Germany),
2) by reversal of the gastroprotective effects of bismuth salts by pretreatment with indomethacin.

Gastric endogenous PG was measured in fasted animals immediately after killing. The abdomen was opened and the stomach was removed and cut. A large biopsy (about 50 mg) of the oxyntic mucosa was taken for the measurement of the capability of the mucosa to generate PGE$_2$ as described in a previous publication (Konturek et al. 1981). All experiments were carried out on 24 h fasted Wistar rats. Each series of experiments was repeated and each experimental group included 8 – 10 animals.

Studies on Healing of Chronic Gastric Ulcerations

Chronic gastric ulcerations were induced in 24 h fasted rats (weighing 180–200 g), which were anesthetized with ether, using the modification (Konturek et al. 1987e) of Okabe et al.'s method (1971). Briefly, after the rat was anesthetized, the abdomen was opened and the stomach exposed. A plastic mould of 4.2 mm in diameter was applied to the serosal surface of the distal portion of the stomach just proximal to the antral mucosa. Then 100% acetic acid was poured through the mould and kept on the serosal surface for about 20 s. This method was found to cause immediate necrosis of the entire thickness of the mucosa and submucosa, exactly within the area (about 13.8 mm²) of the application of the acetic acid. After removal of the acetic acid, the abdomen was closed and the animals were allowed to recover from the anesthesia and then fed normal chow diet and water *a libitum*. Animals were killed at 2 and 7 days after ulcer formation. The ulcer area was measured by planimetry (Morphomat). De-Nol, Pepto Bismol, bismuth subnitrate or 16,16-dimethyl-PGE₂ was added to the drinking water every day starting from the second day after ulcer formation. The results are expressed as means ($\pm$ SEM) of the ulcer area on killing.

Results

Effects of Bismuth Salts or Methylated PG on Acute Gastric Mucosal Lesions Induced by Absolute Ethanol and Acidified ASA

In control tests, absolute ethanol induced lesions in all animals; the mean lesion area was 72.3 ± 5.8 mm² and the number of lesions was 16.0 ± 2.2 (Table 1). De-Nol, Pepto Bismol and bismuth subnitrate reduced the number of ethanol-induced gastric necroses in relation to the dose; the doses reducing the mean ulcer number by 50% (ID50) were about 4, 52 and 37 mg/kg, respectively. Methylated PGE₂ at a standard dose of 10 µg/kg reduced the lesion area and number of lesions by about 80%. Acidified ASA without bismuth salts (control experiments) induced gastric ulcers in all 20 rats tested with a mean ulcer area of 62.2 ± 5.6 mm² and an ulcer number of 16.4 ± 2.3. All three bismuth salts prevented, in relation to the dose, the formation of ASA-induced lesions, the ID50 for De-Nol was about 25 mg/kg, that for Pepto Bismol 60 mg/kg, and for bismuth subnitrate 70 mg/kg. Methylated PGE₂ at a dose of 10 µg/kg almost completely prevented the production of ASA-induced ulcerations.

Effects of Bismuth Salts on mucosal Generation of PGE₂

Mucosal generation of PGE₂ in control experiments in intact stomachs averaged about 422 ± 60 ng/g wet tissue (Table 2). Intragastric administration of De-Nol at a dose of 40 mg/kg caused a significant increase in the mucosal generation of

Table 1. Effects of graded doses of De-Nol, Pepto-Bismol and Bismuth subnitrate given orally on mean area and mean number of gastric lesions induced by 100% ethanol. Mean ±SEM of 8–10 experiments on 8–10 rats

Type of test	No. of rats	Lesion area (mm^2)	Lesion number
100% Ethanol	12	72.3±5.8	16.0±2.2
100% Ethanol + De-Nol			
2.5 mg/kg	8	64.7±3.2	14.2±2.8
5.0 mg/kg	8	34.3±3.5[a]	6.5±2.5[a]
10.0 mg/kg	8	8.3±2.5[a]	3.1±0.7[a]
20.0 mg/kg	8	4.7±1.2[a]	2.8±0.5[a]
40.0 mg/kg	8	2.1±0.6[a]	1.8±0.3[a]
100% Ethanol + Pepto-Bismol			
10 mg/kg	8	63.2±6.2	15.5±2.8
20 mg/kg	9	50.3±5.1[a]	11.9±2.2[a]
40 mg/kg	9	41.6±4.2[a]	11.5±1.8[a]
80 mg/kg	8	25.1±2.8[a]	6.2±0.9[a]
160 mg/kg	8	16.2±4.2[a]	5.0±1.0[a]
100% Ethanol + Bismuth subnitrate			
10 mg/kg	10	56.9±4.5	12.4±2.8
20 mg/kg	8	48.7±4.0[a]	8.6±1.8[a]
40 mg/kg	8	30.2±4.8[a]	6.2±1.4[a]
80 mg/kg	8	22.4±3.6[a]	5.0±2.0[a]
100% Ethanol + 16,16 dm PGE$_2$			
10 µg/kg	10	3.5±1.0[a]	2.4±0.5[a]

[a] Significant ($P < 0.05$) decrease below the control value was only obtained with 100% ethanol

Table 2. Effects of De-Nol, Pepto-Bismol and Bismuth subnitrate on mucosal generation of PGE$_2$ in rats with intact stomach and after mucosal injury with 100% ethanol or acidified ASA

Type of test	Mucosal generation of PGE$_2$ (ng/g)
Intact stomach (Control)	422±60
De-Nol (40 mg/kg)	530±46[a]
Pepto-Bismol (40 mg/kg)	480±62
Bismuth subnitrate (40 mg/kg)	473±58
100% Ethanol	648±76[a]
De-Nol + 100% Ethanol	672±54[a]
Pepto-Bismol + 100% Ethanol	710±81[a]
Bismuth subnitrate + 100% Ethanol	675±64[a]
ASA alone (60 mg/kg + 42 mg/kg/h for 3 h)	52±14[a]
De-Nol + ASA	48±12[a]
Pepto-Bismol + ASA	34±16[a]
Bismuth subnitrate + ASA	49±12[a]

[a] Significant ($P < 0.05$) change from control values obtained from intact stomach

PGE$_2$. No significant change in PG generation was observed when Pepto Bismol or bismuth subnitrate was used at the same dosage (40 mg/kg). Following the administration of 100% ethanol, mucosal generation of PGE$_2$ was increased by about 50% above control and the addition of any of the bismuth salts did not significantly affect this increased generation of PGE$_2$. Following the administration of acidified ASA at a dose that induced gastric ulcerations, mucosal PGE$_2$ was reduced by about 90% and the addition of any of the bismuth salts did not influence this suppressed PGE generation.

Effects of Indomethacin on the Protective Effects of Bismuth Salts Against Ethanol-induced Gastric Lesions

After 90-min exposure to indomethacin (5 mg/kg) given orally, only single and small mucosal erosions were produced (Table 3). When administered 90 min before absolute ethanol, pre-exposure to indomethacin produced a small and

Table 3. Reversal of gastroprotective effects of De-Nol, Pepto-Bismol and Bismuth subnitrate by pretreatment with indomethacin given intragastrically (5 mg/kg)

Type of test	No. of rats	Mean lesion area (mm²)	Mean lesion number
Indo (5 mg/kg)	10	3.1 ± 1.0	4.7 ± 1.2
100% Ethanol (Control)	12	72.3 ± 5.8	16.0 ± 2.2
Indo (5 mg/kg) + 100% Ethanol	10	79.8 + 4.7	18.3 ± 3.5
De-Nol (40 mg/kg) + 100% Ethanol	10	5.2 ± 1.8 [a]	6.0 ± 1.1 [a]
Indo (5 mg/kg) + De-Nol + 100% Ethanol	8	34.1 ± 8.2 [b]	15.3 ± 3.1 [b]
Pepto-Bismol (40 mg/kg) + 100% Ethanol	10	44.6 ± 5.2 [a]	12.4 ± 1.6
Indo (5 mg/kg) + Pepto-Bismol + 100% Ethanol	8	86.8 ± 9.2 [b]	18.1 ± 3.3
Bismuth subnitrate + 100% Ethanol	8	53.4 ± 6.1 [a]	14.2 ± 2.4
Indo (5mg/kg) + Bismuth subnitrate + 100% Ethanol	8	81.2 ± 8.3 [b]	17.2 ± 3.9

[a] Significant ($P < 0.05$) decrease below the control value obtained in 100% ethanol-treated rats
[b] Significant ($P < 0.05$) increase above the value obtained with bismuth salt plus 100% ethanol

Table 4. Mean area of gastric ulcerations induced by serosal application of acetic acid in control rats and in those treated with bismuth salts or 16,16 dimethyl PGE$_2$ administered po for 7 days. Mean ± SEM of 8 − 20 rats

Type of test	No. of rats	Area of ulcers (mm²)	
		2nd day	7th day
Control	20	14.2 ± 1.6	8.1 ± 0.9
De-Nol (100 mg/kg)	20	13.8 ± 1.4	3.6 ± 0.8 [a]
Bismuth subnitrate (400 mg/kg)	10	13.9 ± 2.4	5.8 ± 0.6 [a]
16,16dmPGE$_2$ (10 µg/kg)	10	14.6 ± 1.8	7.8 ± 1.2

[a] Significant ($P < 0.05$) decrease below the value obtained in control untreated rats.

statistically insignificant increase in the ulcer area from 72.3 ± 5.8 to 79.8 ± 4.7 mm^2 and in the ulcer number from 16.0 ± 2.2 to 18.3 ± 3.5. De-Nol (40 mg/kg) administered intragastrically 30 min before absolute ethanol, resulted in almost complete prevention of gastric ulcerations. Pretreatment with indomethacin followed by De-Nol resulted in a significant increase in the area and number of ethanol lesions but they did not reach the values obtained with ethanol alone. Pretreatment with Pepto Bismol or bismuth subnitrate at the same dose (40 mg/kg) resulted in a smaller but significant decrease in ethanol-induced gastric damage and this was also significantly increased following pretreatment with indomethacin (Table 3).

Effects of Bismuth Salts and Methylated PG on Healing of Chronic Gastric Ulcerations in Rats

De-Nol and bismuth subnitrate were administered daily in the approximate doses of 100 mg/kg and 400 mg/kg respectively by addition to the drinking water. The rate of spontaneous healing of chronic gastric ulcerations induced by acetic acid in the absence of bismuth salts is shown in Table 4. The initial area of gastric ulcers measured two days after ulcer induction averaged about 14.2 ± 1.6 mm^2. After 7 days the ulcer area declined to about 8.1 ± 0.9 mm^2. The treatment with bismuth salts significantly enhanced the rate of ulcer healing; the most effective in this respect was De-Nol but bismuth subnitrate was also effective. In constrast, 16,16 dmPGE$_2$ in a gastroprotective dose failed to effect the ulcer healing rate.

Discussion

This study provides evidence that all three bismuth salts, De-Nol, Pepto Bismol, and bismuth subnitrate, are effective in the prevention of acute gastric lesions and in the enhancement of healing of chronic gastric ulceration in rats.

As in previous studies (Hall and Hoven 1987; Konturek et al. 1987) we found that De-Nol was highly effective in the prevention of acute gastric lesions induced by 100% ethanol or acidified ASA. In addition, we observed that other bismuth salts such as Pepto Bismol or bismuth subnitrate also exhibited gastroprotective properties though 9—12 times larger doses of these salts were required to obtain a similar degree of protection to that obtained with De-Nol. This difference in gastroprotective activity between De-Nol and other bismuth salts could be attributed to the colloidal form of bismuth subcitrate as opposed to other bismuth salts employed in noncolloidal dispersion. The colloidal form probably provides better protection of the mucosa by forming a more effective protective barrier on the mucosal surface against acid-pepsin attack (Lee 1982). De-Nol appears to be a more active stimulant of the mucosal generation of PGE$_2$ than other bismuth salts which could also contribute to the increased gastroprotection afforded by this agent. It should be emphasized however, that the protection provided by Pepto Bismol or bismuth subnitrate may also involve increased mucosal biosynthesis of PG. This notion is supported by our present finding that the pretreatment with indomethacin (to block PG biosynthesis) reversed, in part, the gastroprotective action of each of the bismuth salts used. Thus, it may be assumed that all three tested bismuth salts exhibit a PG stimulation activity, possibly by acting on mucosal macrophages to release these protective mediators. It is likely that PG formed by bismuth salts is responsible for the strengthening of the mucosal barrier by stimulating mucus alkaline secretion (Konturek et al. 1987a), tightening of the mucosal barrier (Lee 1982), and increasing mucosal resistance and cell renewal (Tarnawski 1985).

The important role of PG in gastroprotection afforded by various bismuth salts is supported by the fact that similar gastroprotective effects can be induced by exogenous PGE_2 administered in a small nonantisecretory dose (10 µg/kg). However, the fact that bismuth salts also provide some protection against mucosal injury caused by aspirin, a potent inhibitor of PG cyclooxygenase, is a strong argument against stimulation of the PG mechanism being the sole protective mechanism of bismuth salts. Since aspirin may cause mucosal injury not only by the reduction in the biosynthesis of protective PG but also by stimulating increased formation of the harmful products of lipooxygenase pathway (Konturek et al. 1987b), it is likely that the protection by bismuth salts may also involve suppression of the leukotriene biosynthesis. Further studies are needed to determine the exact mechanism of gastroprotective effects of bismuth salts.

The major finding of this report is that De-Nol and to certain extent Pepto Bismol and bismuth subnitrate enhance the healing rate of chronic gastric ulceration induced by serosal application of acetic acid. Although De-Nol and other colloidal bismuth preparations were reported to speed the healing and to delay the recurrence of chronic duodenal ulcerations in men (Tytgat et al. 1984; Hamilton et al. 1986) this is the first experimental study showing that De-Nol as well as other noncolloidal bismuth preparations are effective in the healing of the standardized model of chronic ulcers in rats. A noncolloidal bismuth salt such as bismuth subnitrate appears to be several times less potent on a weight basis in ulcer healing than colloidal bismuth subcitrate, but the difference in the ulcer healing potency between De-Nol and this noncolloidal bismuth salt is much smaller than that in the gastroprotective potency. It remains to be determined whether Pepto Bismol exhibits any influence on ulcer healing.

The mechanism of the ulcer healing efficacy of bismuth salts is not obvious but there is little doubt that the PG mechanism plays little role in this respect. Indeed, exogenous PGE_2 administered in a nonantisecretory dose failed to affect the healing rate of our chronic ulcerations. Our recent studies (Konturek et al. 1987c) with De-Nol indicate that this agent is capable of binding pH-dependently epidermal growth factor (EGF) and of accumulating this potent mitogenic peptide in the area of ulceration to promote reepithelialization and tissue repair. It remains to be determined whether this interaction between bismuth salts and EGF is specific for De-Nol or whether other bismuth salts share similar properties.

Summary

We compared the gastroprotective effects of colloidal bismuth subcitrate (De-Nol) with those of noncolloidal bismuth salts including bismuth subsalicylate (Pepto Bismol) and bismuth subnitrate. All three bismuth preparations used prevented the formation of acute gastric damage caused by absolute ethanol and acidified aspirin (ASA). The dose of De-Nol, Pepto Bismol and bismuth subnitrate reducing by about 50% the area of ethanol-induced damage was 4.2, 52 and 40 mg/kg, and that reducing by 50% the ASA-induced area of damage was 25, 60 and 70 mg/kg. The prevention by bismuth salts of ethanol-induced damage was accompanied by an increase in the mucosal generation of PGE_2 (prostaglandin E2) which was reversed, in part, by pretreatment with indomethacin suggesting the involvement of prostaglandin (PG) in this protection. De-Nol was also effective in the enhancement of healing of chronic gastric ulcerations induced by serosal application of acetic acid and this effect was unrelated to PG but probably involved epidermal growth factor (EGF). This report provides evidence that various bismuth salts exhibit gastroprotective effects probably mediated by PG, and enhance healing of chronic gastric ulcerations via the EGF mechanism.

References

1. Bader JP (1986) A review of clinical evidence on side effects of bismuth derivatives: the French experience. In: Gibinski K (ed) Non-systemic ulcer therapy with De-nol: efficacy and tolerance. Excerpta Medica, Amsterdam
2. Hall DWR, Hoven WE (1987) Gastric mucosal protection by prostaglandin E2 generation in rats by colloidal bismuth subcitrate (De-Nol). Arch Int Pharmacodyn 2297:420−427
3. Hamilton I, O'Connor HJ, Wood WC, Bradbury I, Axon ATR (1986) Healing and recurrence of duodenal ulcer after treatment with tripotassium dicitrato bismuthate (TDB) tablets or cimetidine. Gut 27:106−110
4. Konturek SJ, Radecki T, Brzozowski T, Piastucki I, Dembinski A, Dembinska-Kiec A, Zmuda A and Gryglewski R (1981) Gastric cytoprotection by epidermal growth factor. Role of endogenous prostaglandins and DNA synthesis. Gastroenterology 81:438−443
5. Konturek SJ, Bilski J, Kwiecien N, Obutlowicz W, Kopp B, Oleksy J (1987a) De-Nol stimulates gastric and duodenal alkaline secretion via prostaglandin dependent mechanism. Gut (in press)
6. Konturek SJ, Brzozowski T, Radecki T, Drozdowicz D (1987b) Role of leukotrienes in acute gastric lesions induced by ethanol, taurocholate, aspirin and stress in rats. Dig Dis Sci (in press)
7. Konturek SJ, Dembinski A, Warzecha Z (1987c) Epidermal growth factor (EGF) in the gastroprotective and ulcer healing actions of colloidal bismuth subcitrate. Gut (in press)
8. Konturek SJ, Radecki T, Piastucki I, Brzozowski T, Drozdowicz D (1987d) Gastroprotection by colloidal bismuth subcitrate (De-Nol) and sucralfate. Role of endogenous prostaglandins. Gut 28:201−205
9. Konturek SJ, Stachura J, Radecki T, Drozdowicz D, Brzozowski T (1987e) Cytoprotective and ulcer healing properties of prostaglandin E2 colloidal bismuth and sucralfate in rats. Digestion (in press)
10. Lee SP (1982) A potential mechanism of action of bismuth subcitrate: diffusion barrier to hydrochloric acid. Scand J Gastroenterol 17 [Suppl 80]:17−21

11. Marshall BJ, McGechie DB, Rogers PA, Gaancy RJ (1985) Pyloric campylobacter infection and gastroduodenal disease. Med J Aust 142:439 – 444
12. Okabe S, Pfiffer CJ, Roth JLA (1971) A method for experimental penetrating gastric and duodenal ulcers in rats. Am J Dig Dis 16:277 – 284
13. Tarnawski A (1985) Prevention and treatment of gastrointestinal mucosal injury with cytoprotective agents. Med J Aust 142:S13 – S17
14. Tytgat GNJ, Hameeteman W, van Olffen GH (1984) Sucralfate, bismuth compounds, substituted benzimidazoles, trimipramine and pirenzepine in the short- and long-term treatment of duodenal ulcer. Clin Gastroenterol 13:543 – 568

Discussion

Halter: You have used the term "cytoprotection" numerous times. Does "cytoprotection" or mucosal protection really work for humans? Can we really extrapolate from animal models to humans?

Konturek: That is a good point. But I am not a clinician; I can only refer to studies which have been performed by other investigators, and there is no doubt that, for example prostaglandins, sucralfate, and De-Nol are protective in humans against acute damage, induced both by aspirin and by ethanol. But whether it has any meaning in terms of healing of chronic ulcer, that is difficult to say at this time. In fact, in our model we tried to use a small dose of prostaglandin, 10 μg per kg body weight three times daily, the dose which, as you know, does not affect gastric acid secretion and that is cytoprotective. But we found no evidence for it increasing the healing rate of chronic ulcer. So, prevention of acute damage and healing of chronic ulcerations are probably two different processes, and you cannot make conclusions from the protection results and extrapolate them to the healing studies.

Halter: Well, we actually did a similar study and we even had the impression that in the rat, prostaglandin even slightly delayed healing of experimental ulcers.

Flemström: Just out of curiosity, what would the binding force between the drug and the ulcer crater be, and in case it is some protein binding, why is it the drug does not bind to food and is just swept away?

Konturek: I believe that EFG receptors are in the mucosa along the gut. As you know, EGF binds to the receptors and then is internalized into the cell. And I think that when the mucosa is damaged, I mean because of exposure to the ulcerogen, the number of receptors may be increased as new epithelial cells and fibroblasts appear. There is no mucus cover but just new cells around the ulcer area and more receptor sites. EGF by itself, without any drug, already binds in larger amounts to the eroded area. This may stimulate the growth of new epithelial cells and fibroblasts. Bismuth salts increase the amounts of EGF in the ulcer area.

Flemström: Does the drug also stick to the ulcer crater?

Konturek: In that case it is quite well known that both De-Nol and sucralfate have this ability to bind to the eroded area to the protein by a chelating process, I do not know, how it works, but probably, by complexing of the bismuth salt and also of the sucralfate to the proteins of the eroded area. Why they do not bind to the proteins in the food, I do not know, they may be different proteins, I mean partly degraded.

Ottenjann: Do you think in human beings, when they have a peptic ulcer and we start to treat this ulcer, there are also more receptors than in other situations?

Konturek: I am just waiting for some volunteers with peptic ulcers for such studies. But it is actually very simple to test the ulcer area for the presence of EGF receptors. I do not think that EGF would be a good drug. It is very expensive though it is produced by gene technology in large amounts, so it may become less expensive, and thus could then be useful for ulcer therapy. It works when given orally though it is more potent when given parenterally, but it also works orally.

Börsch: I am interested in your statement on the accumulation of bismuth in the ulcer area. Is this luminal bismuth, or is it intramucosal bismuth? If it is intraepithelial or intramucosal bismuth, how does it get there – via bloodstream or via direct absorption?

Konturek: From what I understand, the accumulation of bismuth is mostly in macrophages. According to some Japanese studies, even a single dose of bismuth salt may result in a flushing of the macrophages into the ulcer area where the bismuth salts are accumulated. How bismuth salts get into macrophages, I do not know, but these are mostly macrophages which accumulate bismuth salt. I believe that prostaglandins are also released in response to bismuth salts by these cells.

Treatment of Peptic Ulcer Disease with Bismuth Preparations

G. N. J. TYTGAT, C. Y. NIO, and B. T. J. VAN DEN BERG

The purpose of this overview is to analyze the therapeutic possibilities of the mucosal protective agent, colloidal bismuth subcitrate (CBS), in both duodenal (DU) and gastric ulcer (GU) and to put its healing potential into proper perspective.

Mechanism of Action

Colloidal bismuth subcitrate (tripotassium dicitratobismuthate) is a complex bismuth salt of citric acid. Trivalent $Bi(OH)_3$ and trivalent citric acid have many possibilities for salt formation, creating molecules of different structure and size. On average, the molecules are so large that an aqueous solution becomes colloidal. In an acid medium ($pH < 5$) bismuth citrate bonds open up, leading to the formation of various insoluble compounds, the smallest one being bismuth oxychloride. More complex structures containing free carboxyl groups and positively charged Bi^+ groups are also formed.

CBS selectively chelates with the proteinaceous material of an ulcer base, forming a coating that protects against the destructive activities of acid, pepsin and presumably bile. This rather specific ulcer coating in vivo can be illustrated by specific bismuth staining with brucine sulphate (Koo et al. 1982). Lee (1982) showed that bismuth was present in abundance in the crater and margins of human gastric ulcers, whereas only traces could be found in the surrounding mucosa. Colloidal bismuth subcitrate, complexed with gastric mucus, has been shown drastically to retard diffusion of hydrogen ions (Lee 1982). Furthermore colloidal bismuth subcitrate has been shown to bind pepsin. Therefore, colloidal bismuth complexed with proteins and mucoglycoproteins behaves as a barrier to HCl and pepsin, thereby preventing them from reaching the ulcer base. Furthermore, several studies have shown that CBS is capable of stimulating prostaglandin synthesis on release, both in animals and in man (Hall 1986; Konturek 1986; Estela 1984).

Clinical Efficacy in Duodenal Ulcer

In the vast majority of Studies CBS was administered at a dose of four coated or chewable tablets daily, one tablet given about 30 min before each of the

Table 1. Healing rates reported for duodenal ulcer after 4 weeks

		Colloidal bismuth subcitrate		Cimetidine	
		(*n*)	(%)	(*n*)	(%)
Martin	1981	25/38	66	22/37	60
Shreeve	1983	18/24	75	13/24	54
Paccini	1980	5/8	63	8/9	89
Gibinski	1983	50/55	91	44/61	72
Lazzaroni	1983	15/20	75	15/20	75
Vantrappen	1982	9/14	64	8/14	57
Harley	1983	23/28	82	15/26	58
Badial Acenes	1982	12/15	80	7/11	64
Oosthoek	1983	13/23	57	8/21	38
Bianchi Porro	1984	21/25	84	18/25	72
Anzures	1982	7/9	78	2/6	33
Baars	1984	16/16	100	10/18	56
		214/275	78	170/272	63
		$\chi^2 = 14,62$	$df = 1$	$p < 0.001$	

		Colloidal bismuth subcitrate		Ranitidine	
		(*n*)	(%)	(*n*)	(%)
Bianchi Porro	1984	40/49	82	34/50	68
Lee	1985	52/58	90	48/59	81
Ward	1984	25/33	76	28/32	87
		117/140	84 (Av)	110/141	78 (Av)
		$\chi^2 = 1.06$	$df = 1$	$p = 0.30$ (NS)	

three main meals and the fourth tablet 2 h after the evening meal. CBS has been evaluated in a double-blind fashion in various placebo-controlled duodenal ulcer trials and shows an average healing rate of 75% compared to 34% after placebo, indicating a highly significant difference (Tytgat et al. 1984).

CBS has also been compared directly to cimetidine and ranitidine. The average healing rate was 78% after 4 weeks therapy with CBS versus 63% with cimetidine (usually in a dose of 200 mg three times daily at meals and 400 mg at night): this is statistically a significant difference. When compared to ranitidine (usually 150 mg twice daily) the average healing rate was 84% with CBS versus 78% with ranitidine (not statistically significant) (Table 1). After 8 weeks treatment with CBS and that with cimetidine resulted in healing rates of 93% and 86%, respectively (non-significant). The results after 8 weeks treatment are identical for CBS (95%) and ranitidine (94%) (Table 2). When compared to other anti-ulcer drugs, the average therapeutic gain of 47% with CBS in treating duodenal ulcer (Table 3) is quite substantial and compares favourably with the gains of other pharmaceutical compounds. CBS leads to rapid symptomatic im-

Table 2. Healing rates reported for duodenal ulcer after 8 weeks

		Colloidal bismuth subcitrate		Cimetidine	
		(*n*)	(%)	(*n*)	(%)
Martin	1981	33/37	89	29/34	85
Gibinski	1983	52/55	95	54/61	89
Lazzaroni	1983	17/19	88	16/20	80
Bianchi Porro	1984	25/25	100	21/24	88
		127/136	93 (Av)	120/139	86 (Av)
		$\chi^2 = 3.01$	$df = 1$	$p = 0.08$	
		Colloidal bismuth subcitrate		Ranitidine	
		(*n*)	(%)	(*n*)	(%)
Bianchi Porro	1984	47/49	96	46/50	92
Lee	1985	56/58	97	57/59	97
Ward	1984	30/33	91	30/32	94
		133/140	95 (Av)	133/141	94 (Av)
		$\chi^2 = 0.00$	$df = 1$	$p > 0.9$ (NS)	

Table 3. Patients showing average therapeutic gains after 4 weeks of currently used therapies of duodenal ulcer

	Number of patients (*n*)	Percentage difference to placebo healing rate	
		(%)	(SD)
CBS	389	47	11
Sucralfate	560	29	9
Trimipramine	140	37	27
Pirenzepine	586	36	8
Ranitidine	923	43	11
Cimetidine	1087	34	17
Prostaglandins	755	31	10

provement. The overall pain scores are indistinguishable from the scores seen after cimetidine. The same holds true for other studies comparing CBS with ranitidine (Moshal et al. 1981). Very recently 600 mg t.i.d. bismuth subsalicylate (Pepto-Bismol) was evaluated in duodenal ulcer disease. The four-weeks healing rate with bismuth subsalicylate was 70% versus 62% for that with cimetidine (Eberhardt et al. 1987).

Two studies need to be discussed separately. Lam compared CBS and high-dose cimetidine in 25 of 212 patients whose DU had not responded to 4 weeks therapy with 1 g cimetidine/day. Overall CBS healed 85% of cimetidine-resistant ulcers whereas a higher dose of cimetidine healed only 40%, which was a significant difference (Lam et al. 1984). This has recently been confirmed by Bianchi Porro et al. (1986) who compared the efficacy of CBS with that of two different cimetidine dosages (1.2 and 2.0 g/day) in the treatment of 43 DU patients who failed to respond to an 8-week therapy with H_2-blockers. CBS treatment resulted in a healing rate of 85.7% after 4 weeks treatment, showing a statistically significant difference ($p < 0.05$) to healing rates after cimetidine treatment (46.7% and 42.9% respectively).

Recently Salmon (1987) conducted a single-blind multicentre study to investigate the probable benefit of combined therapy with CBS and cimetidine in the treatment of duodenal ulcer. The healing rates after 4 weeks treatment were 75% ($n = 12$) for CBS alone, 68.8% ($n = 16$) for cimetidine alone and 84.6% ($n = 13$) for the combined treatment. The healing rates after 8 weeks treatment were 91.7%, 93.8%, and 84.6%, respectively. These interim results raise the possibility of increased early (4 weeks) healing with the combination therapy. The numbers however are too small to draw firm conclusions.

Four studies (Crowe 1985; Danilewitz 1986; Hollanders 1986; Lazzaroni et al. 1986) have evaluated b.i.d. administration versus q.i.d. administration of CBS in duodenal ulcer. The 4-week CBS healing ratio for b.i.d. and q.i.d. were, respectively, 64% and 71%. The healing ratios after 8 weeks were 91% (b.i.d.) versus 83% (q.i.d.). Thus, the results obtained in these 150 patients were roughly comparable to those reported by Salmon.

Relapse Rate and Maintenance Therapy in Duodenal Ulcer

Most intriguing in all the DU studies is that it has been clearly shown that the percentage of patients with DU in prolonged remission after healing with CBS is substantially higher, close to 60%, after 1 year of follow-up, as compared to roughly 30% with cimetidine patients. The same relationship is seen when CBS is compared to ranitidine. Only very recently has an evaluation of maintenance therapy with a low dose of CBS begun (Bianchi Porro et al. 1987). In this study, after an initial 4-week treatment with 480 mg CBS (four tablets) resulting in endoscopically proven healing of the ulcer, 28 patients entered the 6-month maintenance phase, during which they were randomly allocated to receive either 120 mg CBS (one tablet) or a placebo. After 6 months interim results have revealed that 38.5% of the CBS-treated patients showed an endoscopically confirmed duodenal ulcer relapse versus 80% of the placebo-treated patients. In a previous trial by Bianchi Porro et al. (1984) there was no difference between the relapse rate after CBS-induced healing and *without* maintenance therapy and the relapse rate which can be observed after cimetidine-induced healing and *with* maintenance therapy of 400 mg cimetidine nightly. Therefore we may conclude that a short-term course of CBS therapy induces long-term protection against relapse.

Clinical Efficacy in Gastric Ulcer

CBS was evaluated in a double-blind fashion in ten controlled gastric ulcer trials and showed an average healing rate of 72% compared to 33% with placebo, a highly significant difference (Tytgat et al. 1984). CBS has also been compared directly to cimetidine in various trials (Table 4). The average 4-week healing rate is 68% with CBS versus 54% with cimetidine. This difference is statistically significant. After 8 weeks of treatment the healing rates are 81% and 71% respectively, numerically but not statistically significant in favour of CBS (Gibinski et al. 1983; Kisfalvi 1986). Parente et al. observed a healing rate of 70% after 4 weeks treatment with CBS ($n = 40$) as compared to 63% after treatment with ranitidine ($n = 40$). After 8 weeks therapy the healing rates had risen to 88% and 79% respectively. Both differences were statistically significant. The average therapeutic gain of 47% after CBS in gastric ulcer is again quite substantial and compares very favourably with the results obtained with the other drugs, and may even be superior (Table 5). Also in gastric ulcer CBS leads to rapid symptomatic improvement.

Table 4. Healing rates reported for gastric ulcer after 4 weeks

		Colloidal bismuth subcitrate		Cimetidine	
		(n)	(%)	(n)	(%)
Paccini	1980	3/4	75	0/3	0
Gibinski	1983	32/47	68	17/36	47
Baars	1984	12/21	57	10/17	59
Kisfalvi	1986	19/28	68	12/22	55
Tytgat	1982	17/28	61	13/30	43
Søltoft	1984	22/27	81	20/27	74
Anzures	1982	1/2	50	3/3	100
		106/157	68 (Av)	75/138	54 (Av)
		$\chi^2 = 4.83$	$df = 1$	$p = 0.03$	

Table 5. Average therapeutic gains after 4 weeks of currently used therapies of gastric ulcer

	Number of patients (n)	Percentage difference to placebo healing rate	
		(%)	(SD)
CBS	291	47	13
Sucralfate	157	33	6
Trimipramine	341	21	12
Pirenzepine	78	23	
Ranitidine	310	33	17
Cimetidine	336	23	9

Most intriguing has been the finding that also in gastric ulcer, remission after healing with CBS is more prolonged than after healing with H_2-blockers. The numbers however are still too small to reach statistical significance (Pickard 1985).

Side Effects

For almost two centuries bismuth salts have been used in medicine, mainly for the treatment of various common gastrointestinal disorders, for instance, irritable colon, constipation, and prevention of traveller's diarrhoea. The most plausible explanation for cases of intoxication, that is, encephalopathy, which have been seen in France are the high daily doses and long periods during which bismuth-containing preparations other than CBS were ingested. Very often blood levels were 20 times as high as today's safety limit of 100 mcg/l.

Side effects have since been trivial, consisting of transient darkening of the tongue and dentures and blackening of stool, which the unaware could mistake for melena. Oral and dental staining does not occur with the more recently introduced coated tablet (to be swallowed), which has been shown to be equally as effective as the chewable tablet. During short-term studies at present blood bismuth levels may rise slightly but always remain well below the safety limit of 0.48 mmol/l (100 mcg/l). Urine levels of bismuth rise with the dose, indicating some intestinal absorption. Therefore it is recommended to have a 2-month bismuth-free interval after each course of treatment with CBS (Bader 1987).

Conclusion

The major role of CBS in the treatment of peptic ulcer disease is its mucosal protective action, which centers upon coating of the ulcer base and strengthening of the mucus barrier against further acid attack and upon reducing peptic activity. By stimulating endogenous prostaglandin synthesis CBS could possibly exert a protective effect at a cellular level.

It is obvious from the data presented here, that mucosa protectors are to be considered as valid alternatives in the treatment of duodenal and gastric ulcers. CBS is either equal to or (for genuine, non-drug-induced GU) superior to other anti-ulcer agents currently in use for the treatment of peptic disease. CBS should be the first choice in the treatment of resistant ulcers.

The most remarkable finding is the retardation of the occurrence of relapse of both DU and GU after initial healing with CBS. The question as to why an ulcer, healed after treatment with an acid-suppressing drug, relapses faster than one which healed after treatment with a mucosal-protective drug such as CBS remains unanswered. Perhaps newly available data concerning the activity of CBS against *Campylobacter pylori* and the improvement of gastroduodenal morphology thus brought about could provide an explanation for the better resistance to recurrent ulceration of the mucosal lining.

It is now generally accepted that the presence of *C. pylori* is associated with active chronic gastritis. CBS is the only ulcer-healing drug which has in vitro and in vivo efficacy against *C. pylori* (Tytgat et al. 1986, Rauws et al. 1987). A German clinical trial performed by Eberhardt et al. (1987) and published very recently in abstract form revealed that oral bismuth subsalicylate (Pepto-Bismol tablets) in a dose of 600 mg t.i.d. for 4 weeks reduced the number of *C. pylori* positive patients by 75% in comparison with 40% reduction in the (400 mg b.i.d.) cimetidine-treated group. Before therapy the number of *C. pylori* positive cases were identical for both treatment groups.

If future studies can prove beyond doubt that underlying gastrobulbitis is the main factor responsible for the recurrent nature of peptic ulcer disease, physicians will then have to concentrate on ways of eradicating this microorganism. According to the available information, colloidal bismuth subcitrate appears to be of vital importance in this regard. Another explanation for the relapse phenomenon may be connected with the effects of CBS upon endogenous prostaglandin synthesis. Preliminary studies have shown that ulcer recurrence after exogenous prostaglandin administration may also be delayed (O'Keefe et al. 1985). However, more experience is necessary to evaluate these findings.

More studies will be needed in the near future to elucidate the mode of action of CBS in relation to both *C. pylori* and the prostaglandin synthesis.

References

1. Anzures ME, Murguia D (1982) Resultados preliminares del estudio doblo ciego en 30 pacientes con ulcera peptica tratados con subcitrato de bismuto, cimetidina o placebo. Compend Invest Clin Latinoam 2 (suppl 1):51
2. Baars H, Boekhorst JC, van Dommelen CKV, et al. (1984) De Nol versus cimetidine (Tagamet), een vergelijkend onderzoek bij peptisch ulcus bij de internistenpraktijk. J Drug Res 9:187
3. Bader JP (1987) The safety Profile of De-Nol. Digestion 37 (suppl 2):53−59
4. Badial Acenes F, Morako PO, Ramos HR, Saénz VF (1982) Subcitrato de bismutho vs cimetidina en el tratamiento de la ulcera peptica. Compend Invest Clin Latinoam 2 (suppl 1), 55
5. Bianchi Porro G, Barbara L, Cheli R, et al. (1984) Comparison of tripotassium dicitrato bismuthate (TDB) tablets and ranitidine in the healing and relapse of duodenal ulcers. Gut 25:565
6. Bianchi Porro G, Lazzaroni M, Petrillo M, De Nicola C (1984) Relapse rates in duodenal ulcer patients formerly treated with bismuth subcitrate or maintained with cimetidine. Lancet II:698
7. Bianchi Porro G, Petrillo M, De Nichola C, Lazzaroni M (1984) A double blind endoscopic study with De-Nol tablets and cimetidine for duodenal ulcer. Scand J Gastroent 19:905−908
8. Bianchi Porro G, Parente F, Lazzaroni M, Pace F (1986) Colloidal bismuth subcitrate and two different dosages of cimetidine in the treatment of resistant duodenal ulcer. Scand J Gastroenterol 21 (suppl 122):39−41
9. Bianchi Porro G, Lazzaroni M, Cortvriendt WRE (1987) Colloidal bismuth subcitrate in duodenal ulcer disease. Digestion 37 (suppl 22):47−52
10. Crowe J, Hollanders D (1985) Results from two studies in duodenal ulcer patients to assess the relative efficacy of two regimens of De-Nol chewable tablets; one tablet 4 times a day (qds) against two tablets taken twice daily (bd). Intern Rep Gist-brocades

11. Danilewitz MD, Bank L (1986) A study to compare the therapeutic efficacy of two regimens of De-Nol swallow tablets in the treatment of duodenal ulceration: two tablets given twice daily against the usual 4 times daily regimen. S Afr med J 70:57
12. Eberhardt R, Kaspar G, Dettmer A et al (1987) Effect of oral bismuth subsalicylate on Campylobacter pyloridis and on duodenal ulcer. Gastroenterology 92 (5):1379
13. Estella R, Feller A, Backhouse C, Castro R, Ugarte G (1984) Effects of colloidal bismuth subcitrate and aluminiumhydroxide on gastric and duodenal levels of prostagladin E2. Rev Med Chile 112:975−981
14. Gibinski K, Gabryelewicz A, Marlicz K, Dzieniszewsie J (1983) A double-blind multi-center trial comparing De-Nol and cimetidine for healing and relapse rate over 12 months in the treatment of peptic ulcers. Intern Rep Gist-brocades
15. Hall DWR, Van den Hoven WE (1986) Protective properties of colloidal bismuth subcitrate on gastric mucosa. Scand J Gastroenterol 21 (suppl 122):11−13
16. Harley H, Alp MH (1983) Treatment of chronic duodenal ulceration, effectiveness of colloidal bismuth subcitrate tablets compared with cimetidine. Med J Aust 2:627
17. Hollanders D (1986) Twice daily tripotassium dicitrato bismuthate in the treatment of duodenal ulceration. Postgrad Med J 62:19−21
18. Kisfalvi I (1986) A comparative trial with De-Nol, cimetidine and carbenoxolone in the healing of benign gastric ulceration. In: Gibinsky K (ed) Proc Symp at 3rd Congr Pol Gastroenterol Soc Lublin 1985. Excerpta Medica, Amsterdam, pp 26−32
19. Konturek SJ, Radecki T, Piastucki I, Dorzdowicz D (1986) Advances in the understanding of mechanism of cytoprotective action by colloidal bismuth subcitrate. Scan J Gastroenterol 21 (suppl 122):6−10
20. Koo J, Ho J, Lam SK, et al. (1982) Selective coating of gastric ulcer by tripotassium dicitratobismuthate in the rat. Gastroenterology 82:864−870
21. Lam SK, Lee NW, Koo J, Hui WM, Fok KH (1984) Randomised crossover trial of tripotassium dicitrato bismuthate versus high dose cimetidine for duodenal ulcers resistant to standard dose of cimetidine. Gut 25:703−706
22. Lazzaroni M, Petrillo M, De Nicola C, Bianchi Porro G (1983) De-Nol liquid and cimetidine twice daily in the treatment of duodenal ulcer. A preliminary study. Br J Clin Pract 37:379−381
23. Lazzaroni M, Parente F, Prada A, Bianchi Porro G (1986) Colloidal bismuth subcitrate as coated tablets: four times versus twice daily dosage in duodenal ulcer. Scand J Gastroenterol 21 (suppl 122):51−53
24. Lee SP (1982) A potential mechanism of action of colloidal bismuth subcitrate: diffusion barrier to hydrochloric acid. Scand J Gastroenterol 17 (suppl 80):17−21
25. Lee FI, Samloff IM, Hardman M (1985) Comparison of tripotassium dicitratobismuthate tablets with ranitidine in healing and relapse of duodenal ulcers. Lancet I:1299−1302
26. Martin DF, Hollanders D, May SJ et al. (1981) Difference in relapse rates of duodenal ulcer after healing with cimetidine or tripotassium dicitratobismuthate. Lancet I:7−10
27. Moshal MG, Spitaels JM, Khan F (1981) Tripotassium dicitratobismuthate chewing tablets and cimetidine tablets in the treatment of duodenal ulcers. S Afr med J 60:420−423
28. O'Keefe SJD, Spitaels JM, Mannion G, Naiher N (1985) Misoprostol, a synthetic prostaglandin E2 analogue, in the treatment of duodenal ulcers. S Afr med J 67:321−324
29. Oosthoek D, Wille JJ, Naber FB, Knaap KC (1983) De-Nol versus Tagamet, een vergelijkend onderzoek bij peptisch ulcus. J Drug Res 8:1555
30. Paccini J, Espejo H (1980) El subcitrato de bismuto colloidal y la cimetidina en el tratamiento de la ulcera peptica. Colloidal bismuth subcitrate and cimetidine in the treatment of peptic ulcers (Spanish and English). Trib Med 16:30
31. Parente F, Lazzaroni M, Bianchi Porro G (1986) Colloidal bismuth subcitrate and ranitidine in the short-term treatment of benign gastric ulcer. Scand J Gastroent 21 (suppl 122):42−45
32. Pickard R (1985) Clinical review of colloidal bismuth subcitrate. In: Axon ATR (ed) Proceedings of the International Symposium on Pathogenesis and the Treatment of Peptic Ulcer Disease, Cairo 1985. Excerpta Medica, Amsterdam pp 55−64
33. Rauws EAJ, Langenberg ML, Houthof HJ, Zanen HC, Tytgat GNJ (1988) Campylobacter pyloridis associated active chronic gastritis. A prospective study of the prevalence, and the effects of antibacterial and anti-ulcer treatment. Gastroenterology 94:33−40

34. Salmon PR (1987) Combination Treatment: Colloidal Bismuth Subcitrate with H_2-antagonists. Digestion 37 (suppl 2):42–46
35. Shreeve DR, Klass HJ, Jones PE (1983) Comparison of cimetidine and tripotassium dicitrato bismuthate in healing and relapse of duodenal ulcers. Digestion 28:96
37. Søltoft J, Iverson TO, Linde NC, Rahbeck I (1984) A double-blind, double dummy trial comparing De-Nol and cimetidine in the treatment of gastric ulcers. Intern Rep Gist-brocades
38. Tytgat GNJ, Van Bentem N, Olffen G, et al. (1982) Controlled trial comparing colloidal bismuth subcitrate tablets, cimetidine and placebo in the treatment of gastric ulceration. Scand J Gastroenterol 17 (suppl 80):31–38
39. Tytgat GNJ, Hameeteman W, Van Olffen GH (1984) Sucralfate, bismuth compounds, substituted benzimidazoles, trimipramine and pirenzepine in the short- and long-term treatment of duodenal ulcer. Clin Gastroenterol 13:543–568
40. Tytgat GNJ, Rauws EAJ, Langenberg ML (1986) The Campylobacter pyloridis story. Acta Endoscopica 16:141–144
41. Vantrappen G, Schuurman P, Rutgeerts P, Janssen J (1982) A comparative study of colloidal bismuth subcitrate and cimetidine on the healing and recurrence of duodenal ulcer. Scand J Gastroenterol 17 (suppl 80):23
42. Ward M, Cowen AE (1984) A double-blind trial comparing De-Nol tablets and ranitidine in the treatment of duodenal ulcers. Intern Rep Gist-brocades

Discussion

Börsch: I have seen the Eberhardt data (*Gastroenterology* 92:1379, 1987). I think they gave two tablets three times a day, which is three times 600 mg of Bismuth subsalicylate which adds up to 1800 mg per day. I suppose, with the De-Nol preparation you gave about 180 mg 4 times a day, which is less than half the dose. So there might be differences between these two preparations, since Eberhardt et al. gave a much higher dose.

Cadranel: Can you speculate on treatment with the bismuth salts in children because there are laws in certain countries of Europe forbidding it being given to patients below 5–12 years of age depending on the country. And the reason is that maybe there could be an absorption through the intercellular spaces. That is what is said. Can you comment on that?

Tytgat: I think that there is no doubt that some bismuth gets absorbed into the small intestine via micropinocytosis. That has been well studied. Once in the cell it enters the lysosomes and is bound to metallotheonine. If this metal-binding protein is saturated, then bismuth might enter the organism. Absorbed bismuth is then gradually excreted in the urine for several days after intake. I think the whole problem with bismuth is that the potential toxicity has been exaggerated due to the publications in French literature. In France they had patients taking enormous amounts of bismuth nitrate for 10, 20, 30 years and indeed they reacted with high blood levels and high levels in the brain. Bismuth is indeed a heavy metal and we should be careful. For now I think we should limit therapy to two or three months. There are some maintenance trials being prepared with a lower dose in Bianchi Porro's group and the bismuth levels in that study have remained quite low so far.

Ottenjann: I have another question. What about the discoloration of the teeth and the feces?

Tytgat: Discoloration of the teeth with the current tablets for swallowing is not a problem any more. Discoloration of the stool certainly remains, but this is of no clinical importance – you have to warn the patient that this is a phenomenon to be expected.

Classen: Do you study kidney and liver function etc. before you administer bismuth tablets?

Tytgat: No.

Ottenjann: Do you put bismuth at top of the list of ulcer healing substances?

Tytgat: I cannot answer you from the chemical point of view. I do not know. Perhaps Professor Konturek can answer this question.

Konturek: Bismuth salts form complexes with proteins of the ulcerated mucosa to form a protective barrier against further acid-pepsin damage. They also delay the diffusion of H^+ and interact with mucus glycoproteins to form the mucus less permeable for pepsin. They also decrease proteolytic activity of the gastric juice and inhibit pepsin secretion.

Tytgat: But what the true chemical nature is, I do not know. What I do know is that it certainly retards diffusion of hydrogen ions. That has been very well studied by a New Zealand group and confirmed by others. But what it specifically does to mucus, that I do not know.

Treatment of Campylobacter Gastritis with Bismuth Salts

C. A. M. McNulty

Bismuth compounds have been used for over two centuries for the treatment of various gastrointestinal disorders because of their local protective demulcent, antacid and antidiarrhoeal properties. Bismuth salts also have an antimicrobial effect against *Campylobacter pylori* (McNulty et al. 1985) and other gastrointestinal pathogens (Manhart 1984).

After completing a small prevalence study in 1984 (McNulty and Watson 1984), that confirmed the strong association of *C. pylori* with histologically proven gastritis, we planned a placebo-controlled treatment study. In vitro *C. pylori* is sensitive to many antimicrobial agents including erythromycin and bismuth salts (McNulty et al. 1985, Goodwin et al. 1986). Erythromycin was chosen because of its success in other *Campylobacter* infections. The aim of the treatment study was to evaluate the in vivo eradication of *C. pylori* with

a) bismuth subsalicylate, a locally acting antimicrobial agent,
b) erythromycin ethylsuccinate, a systemically acting antimicrobial agent,
c) placebo matched to bismuth subsalicylate.

The correlation between eradication of *C. pylori* and improvement in histologically proven gastritis, endoscopic appearances and symptoms was also assessed.

Patients were enrolled into the treatment study if they were positive for *C. pylori;* patients were excluded if they had oesophagitis or peptic ulceration, if they had recently received antimicrobial therapy, or if they were allergic to the medications. Patients were randomised to receive one of three treatments:

1) Bismuth subsalicylate (Pepto-Bismol, Procter and Gamble, Cincinnati, Ohio, USA) 30 ml four times per day, for 21 days.
2) Placebo matched to the bismuth subsalicylate 30 ml four times per day, for 21 days.
3) Placebo matched to erythromycin 10 ml for 1 week followed by erythromycin ethylsuccinate (Erythroped, Abbott Labs, Kent, UK) 10 ml (500 mg) four times per day, for 2 weeks.

Microbiology. The presence of *C. pylori* in antral biopsies was evaluated by three methods:

1) Gram's stain of biopsy smear.
2) Culture in microaerobic conditions at 37 ° C for up to 7 days.
3) Biopsy urease test (using Christensen's 2% urea broth).

A patient was considered positive for *C. pylori* if the Gram's stain, histological section or culture was positive.

Histopathology. Biopsy specimens were stained with haematoxylin and eosin stain and assessed blindly. Specimens were graded according to mononuclear and polymorphonuclear infiltration (0−4). Scores were summed, and if the summed score was 3 or greater, the patient was considered to have histologically confirmed gastritis. The presence or absence of spiral bacteria was noted.

Endoscopy. The presence of hyperaemia and erosions was noted before and after treatment.

Symptomatic assessment. Symptomatic improvement was evaluated by the investigator and by patient diaries. Four specific symptoms were evaluated: nausea or vomiting, heartburn, indigestion and belching.

Fifty patients complied completely with the protocol. Fifteen were cleared of *C. pylori* at 3 weeks: these were 14 of the 18 patients given bismuth (78%) and one of the 15 given erythromycin (7%). None of the 17 patients given placebo were cleared of *C. pylori*. Bismuth proved significantly better than placebo ($p < 0.001$) and erythromycin in clearing organisms (Fig. 1).

Of the 15 patients cleared of *C. pylori* 13 started treatment with histologically confirmed gastritis, which resolved in 12. Of the 35 patients with persistent infection gastritis was present before treatment in 32 and resolution occurred in only 4 (12.5%) ($p < 0.0001$). Gastritis resolved in 13 out of 16 patients (81%) treated with bismuth compared with only 3 of 13 receiving erythromycin ($p = 0.001$) and none of 16 given placebo ($p < 0.001$) (Fig. 2). The histological appearance of the gastric mucosa in patients with *C. pylori* was characterised by polymorphonuclear and mononuclear infiltration and by shortening of the

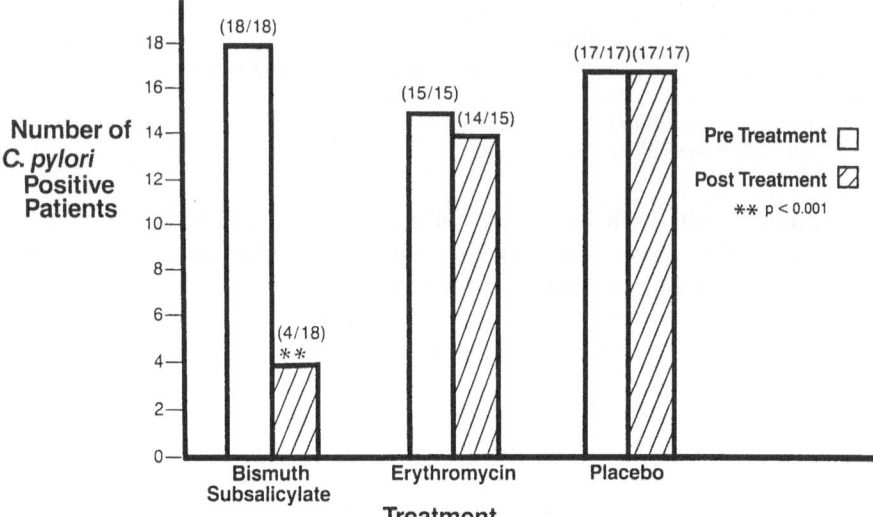

Fig. 1. Presence of *C. pylori* by treatment group

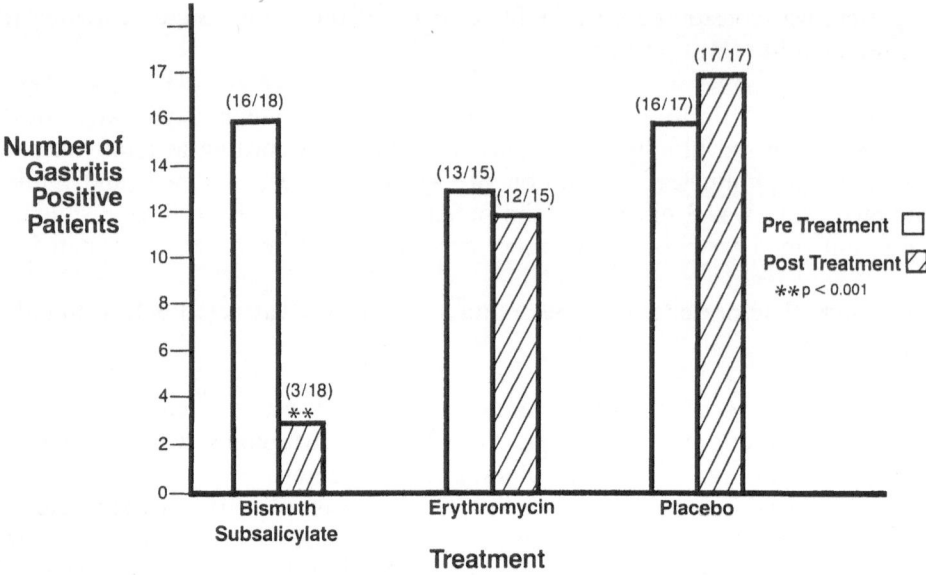

Fig. 2. Presence of gastritis by treatment group

Table 1. Correlation between clearance of *C. pylori* and patient improvement

		Patients cleared of organism ($n = 15$)	Patients not cleared of Organism ($n = 35$)	p value of χ^2
PMN score	Before	1.53	1.90	
	After	0.13[a]	1.97	
Monocyte score	Before	2.60	2.54	
	After	1.47[a]	2.54	
Improvement of endoscopic appearance antral/duodenal erosions		4/5 (80%)	1/4 (25%)[b]	< 0.001
Hyperaemia		3/4 (75%)	0/5 (0%)	

[a] $p < 0.0002$ compared to before treatment
[b] patients developed ulcers

longitudinal cells with increased nuclear activity and reduced mucin content. Clearance of *C. pylori* was associated with a significant reduction in this polymorphonuclear and mononuclear infiltration (Table 1).

At initial endoscopy 18 of the 50 patients had an abnormal endoscopic appearance of the stomach or duodenum. Improvement in appearances was associated with clearance of *C. pylori* (Table 1). There was significantly better improvement in endoscopic appearances in patients cleared of organisms than in those with persistent infection ($\chi^2 = 15.0$, $p < 0.001$). There was significantly greater improvement in endoscopic appearances in the bismuth group (7 of 18) than in the erythromycin group (none of 15, $\chi^2 = 5.2$, $p = 0.05$) or placebo group (none of 17 patients, $\chi^2 = 8.3$, $p < 0.01$).

Fifty-two of the 60 patients who started treatment had symptoms (44 indigestion, 35 belching, 34 heartburn, 25 nausea). Clearance of *C. pylori* was associated with improvement in symptoms. Using patient diaries, heartburn appeared significantly improved on bismuth (50%) and erythromycin (33%) compared to placebo (17%) ($p < 0.005$). Looking at the overall symptomatic improvement assessed by the investigator, 11 of 12 patients with symptoms (92%) in the group cleared of *C. pylori* reported improvement of symptoms, compared with 21 out of 32 patients with symptoms (66%) in the group with persistent infection ($0.05 < p < 0.1$).

This study confirms the strong correlation between the presence of *C. pylori* in the gastric antrum and histologically confirmed gastritis. Clearance of *C. pylori* was strongly associated with resolution of this gastritis and with greater improvement in endoscopic appearances than was observed in patients with persistent infection. Bismuth was more effective in clearing *Campylobacter* and in improving gastritis than either erythromycin of placebo.

Many investigators have now confirmed the success of bismuth salts in the treatment of histologically confirmed gastritis. Lanza et al. (1986) in a placebo-controlled study using bismuth subsalicylate found that the bismuth cleared 7 of 10 patients of *C. pylori* and gastritis. Placebo was ineffective. Other researchers have used colloidal bismuth subcitrate (CBS) (De Nol, Gist Brocades, Delft, The Netherlands). Tytgat et al. (Poster, IVth International Workshop on *Campylobacter* Infections, June 16−18, 1987) found that CBS (4×120 mg/day) cleared *C. pylori* from 35 of 84 patients treated for 8 weeks. Four weeks later only 8 of these patients were still seen to be *Campylobacter*-free. The combination of amoxycillin plus CBS was much more successful. In a placebo-controlled trial Lambert et al. (1986) found that CBS (4×108 mg/day) for 4 weeks cleared bacteria from 11 of 15 (73%) patients. None of the patients who received placebo were cleared of organisms. A significant improvement in both acute and chronic inflammatory infiltrate was seen in subjects with eradication.

In open-ended studies Jones et al. (1985) and Marshall et al. (1985) have also found CBS to be effective in clearing *C. pylori* and histologically confirmed gastritis.

The efficacy of bismuth may be explained either by its antimicrobial activity or by its mucosal-protective effect on the gastric mucosa. Minimum inhibitory concentrations of bismuth salts for *C. pylori* are in the range 4−32 mg/l (McNulty et al. 1985). These concentrations are probably achieved locally in the lumen of the stomach and in the gastric crypts. Using electron microscopy of gastric biopsy specimens, Marshall et al. (1985) have shown that coating of *C. pylori* present in the gastric crypts by bismuth salt is followed by swelling and lysis of the organisms. This confirms that bismuth salts penetrate the mucus layer of the stomach and reach the gastric crypts in sufficiently high concentration to kill *C. pylori*.

On the other hand studies have shown that bismuth salts, including bismuth subsalicylate, protect the gastric mucosa against the erosive properties of aspirin and alcohol (Holroyde et al. 1984). A mucosal coat of bismuth-protein chelate, as formed by tripotassium dicitratobismuthate, may protect the mucosa from gastric acid and allow resolution of gastritis with alteration of the gastric milieu so that *C. pylori* can no longer survive. Sucralfate, however, another mucosal-protective agent (Ligumsky et al. 1984) which has little in vitro activity against *C. pylori* (Marshall et al. 1985), does not eradicate *C. pylori* from the gastric mucosa and has no effect on histologically confirmed gastritis (Langenberg et al. 1985). The ineffectiveness of a solely mucosal protective agent in resolving gastritis suggests that it is the antimicrobial activity of the bismuth salt that is important.

Relapse has been a problem with the single agents used in trials so far. The organisms are obviously not being completely eradicated. The bismuth salts and antimicrobials used so far probably do not reach all areas colonised by *C. pylori*. The few bacteria remaining can then multiply and recolonise the whole of the gastric mucosa. More aggressive initial treatment is therefore needed. The most appropriate treatment to reduce this relapse rate could be a 4-week combination of a locally active bismuth salt and an antimicrobial such as amoxycillin or nitrofurantoin. Good in vitro activity of an antimicrobial agent against *C. pylori* does not necessarily lead to in vivo success. Erythromycin and the quinolones are highly active against *C. pylori* but neither have any effect in vivo (Glupczynski et al. 1987).

Should these organisms prove important in the aetiology of gastritis and duodenal ulceration, the current approach to treating these conditions may be incorrect. Although H_2-receptor antagonists produce symptomatic and endoscopic resolution of gastritis and peptic ulceration, ulcer relapse is higher with these agents than with bismuth salts (Miller and Faragher 1986). H_2-receptor antagonists have no effect on histologically confirmed gastritis (Fullman et al. 1985). Antacids and histamine H_2-receptor blockers decrease secretion of gastric acid and have no activity against *C. pylori* (Lambert et al. 1986; Goodwin et al. 1986). These allow increased colonisation of the stomach by bacteria and may also allow *C. pylori* to multiply.

The effect of *C. pylori* on gastritis needs to be investigated further but results thus far strongly suggest that *C. pylori* is important in the aetiology of these conditions and that eradication should improve therapeutic outcome.

References

1. Fullman H, Van Deventer G, Schaneidman D et al. (1985) "Healed" duodenal ulcers are histologically ill. Gastroenterology 88:1390
2. Glupczynski Y, Labbe M, Burette A, Delmee M, Avesani V, Bruck C (1987) Treatment failure of ofloxacin in *Campylobacter pylori* infection. Lancet I:1096
3. Goodwin CS, Blake P, Blincow E (1986) The minimum inhibitory and bactericidal concentrations of antibiotics and anti-ulcer agents against *Campylobacter pyloridis*. J Antimicrob Chemother 17:309–314
4. Holroyde MJ, Yeakle C, Pebble J (1984) Gastric cytoprotection by bismuth subsalicylate. Gastroenterology 86:1116
5. Jones DM, Eldridge J, Whorwell PJ, Miller JP (1985) The effects of various anti-ulcer regimens and antibiotics on the presence of *Campylobacter pyloridis* and its antibody. Cam-

pylobacter III: Proceedings of the Third International Workshop on Campylobacter Infections. Public Health Laboratory Service, London, 161–162

6. Lambert JR, Dunn KL, Turner H et al. (1986) Effect on histological gastritis following eradication of *Campylobacter pyloridis*. Gastroenterology 90:1509 (abstract)

7. Langenberg ML, Rauws EAJ, Schipper MEI et al. (1985) The pathogenic role of *Campylobacter pyloridis*, studied by attempts to eliminate these organisms. In: Pearson AD, Skirrow MB, Lior H, Rowe B (eds) Campylobacter III: Proceedings of the Third International Workshop on Campylobacter Infections, Ottawa, 1985. Public Health Laboratory Service, London, 162–163

8. Lanza FL, Rack MF, Peterson DF (1986) Eradication of *Campylobacter pyloridis* with Bismuth subsalicylate. Am J Gastroenterol 81:853

9. Ligumsky M, Karmeli F, Rachmilewitz D (1984) Sucralfate stimulation of gastric PGE_2 syntheses – possible mechanism to explain its effective cytoprotective properties. Gastroenterology 86:1164

10. Marshall BJ, Armstrong JA, McGeckie DB et al. (1985) The antimicrobial action of bismuth: early results of antibacterial regimens in the treatment of duodenal ulcer. Campylobacter III: Proceedings of the Third International Workshop on Campylobacter Infections. Public Health Laboratory Service, London, 161

11. McNulty CAM, Watson DM (1984) Spiral bacteria of the gastric antrum. Lancet I:1068–1069

12. McNulty CAM, Dent J, Wise R (1985) Susceptibility of clinical isolates of *Campylobacter pyloridis* to 11 antimicrobial agents. Antimicrob Agents Chemother 28:837–838

13. McNulty CAM, Gearty JC, Crump B et al. (1986) *Campylobacter pyloridis* and associated gastritis: investigator blind, placebo controlled trial of bismuth salicylate and erythromycin ethylsuccinate. Brit Med J 293:645–649

14. Miller JP, Faragher EB (1986) Relapse of duodenal ulcer: does it matter which drug is used in initial treatment. Brit Med J 293:1117–1118

Discussion

von Wulffen: In face of the dosages that you are presently using, do you see any clear contraindications in any patients, for example renal insufficiency or patients with CNS disease?

McNulty: We took serum concentrations of bismuth during treatment and the highest concentration was less than twelve parts per billion in all these patients. So we did not find any high concentrations at all. I think there are other studies with lower dosages underway, so I think probably this high dose is unnecessary. I cannot speculate on the reduced dosage that may be necessary in the presence of poor renal function as I have no experience of it.

von Wulffen: So far you have excluded them from therapy, or have you included them?

McNulty: In the study we did there were no patients with other medical problems included.

Ober: I am intellectually displeased by this discrepancy between nonclearing of symptoms on the one hand and clearing of histology and bacteriology on the other hand. What would you give as an explanation for that?

McNulty: You are right about the fact that symptoms do not improve in line with the histology, except for heartburn.

Ober: Just as histology and bacteriology do improve?

McNulty: In our study the questions about symptoms may not have been asked correctly. I think that in a future study you would have to be very careful about how you ask about symptoms. Our main criteria in the study was to see whether it cleared *C. pylori* histological gastritis. The symptoms were a secondary thing that we also looked into. In retrospect I would not use the same sort of patient diaries, they were far too complicated to fill in. I would agree that physicians are not going to be interested in this organism unless clearance is associated with symptomatic improvement.

Halter: I think you did not discuss possible effects of antacids on *Campylobacter*. To what degree do antacids influence *C. pylori* in vitro and in vivo?

McNulty: Campylobacters survive only in a pH of between 5 and 8. Antacids seem to have no effect on the organisms. In a large study we asked patients about antacid usage. Usage of antacids had no effect on recovery of the organisms from patients attending upper gastrointestinal endoscopy and sucralfate also had no effect.

Börsch: You have discussed the effect of ulcer-healing drugs on gastritis. Doing that you have excluded sucralfate from the list of agents that improve gastritis. Hui et al. from the Lam group have published a single-blind study on 140 patients in *Gastroenterology* (92:1442, 1987) and they have shown that sucralfate significantly improves the activity of chronic gastritis as compared with cimetidine. So we have to include sucralfate in this list.

McNulty: Is that histologically proven gastritis?

Börsch: Yes, it was active gastritis according to Whitehead classification, and the activity was reduced to nul or mild.

McNulty: Well, that is interesting. I did not know that. From the literature I have read, including work from Langenberg and Tytgat, sucralfate has no effect on histologically proven gastritis or on *C. pylori*. In our study, the patients who had been on sucralfate still had histologically proven gastritis.

Tytgat: Who did the study with antiacid in vivo, showing that it did not have any effect?

McNulty: On histologically proven gastritis? Or on symptoms?

Tytgat: On *C. pylori*.

McNulty: On *C. pylori* – in our present study the frequency of *C. pylori* in patients on antacids is the same as the frequency of *C. pylori* in patients on no medication.

Tytgat: But has that been published?

McNulty: No it has not.

Tytgat: There is something very interesting with the antacids. In the beginning it was said that they were ineffective, or that you had to use very high doses in peptic ulcer disease, and we are now in the range of 120 or 149 millimole neutralizing capacity which appears to be sufficient for full healing. And nobody understands why that is. Perhaps it has something to do with *C. pylori* and with inflammation in the stomach.

Goodwin: I would just like to make a comment on the symptoms, purely anecdotally with the patients that I have treated in West Australia. I was surprised how well the symptoms improved over a long period, rather than immediately after treatment. A year later, a group that I had treated, although they had not lost their symptoms immediately after treatment, seemed to be much better a year later, I think symptoms may well be a very difficult area in gastroenterology. I have not yet found a gastroenterologist who can tell me what pain is due to, and I do not know that they know the cause of any other symptoms. So, when they know what they are caused by, I will tell them how to get rid of them.

Ottenjann: May I ask you how many particles you use for judgment of clearing up and improvement of histology?

McNulty: How many biopsy specimens? We use two of them.

Ottenjann: Only two? And that is enough?

McNulty: Well that is what the histopathologist says. We have two for histopathology and two for microbiology.

Attempts to Eradicate *Campylobacter pylori* – Dutch Experiences

E. A. J. Rauws, W. Langenberg, H. J. Houthoff, and G. N. J. Tytgat

Introduction

Campylobacter pylori (C. pylori) was rediscovered by Warren and Marshall in 1983 [1]. The presence of these bacilli on the gastric mucosa is closely associated with histologically demonstrable gastritis [2–6]. The number of bacteria appears related to the severity of gastritis. *C. pylori* colonises the gastric mucosa in almost 100% of patients with peptic ulcer disease, in 70% of the non-ulcer dyspepsia patients and in 20% of a group asymptomatic volunteers. Marshall and Warren hypothesized that *C. pylori* causes acute gastritis and achlorhydria, which in some patients progresses to chronic gastritis, dyspeptic symptoms and eventually ulceration in some patients [7]. In order to determine whether *C. pylori* is aetiologically related to the gastric inflammatory changes, we have tried to eliminate the organisms by various therapeutic regimens and have studied the effect of these therapeutic attempts upon the gastric mucosa.

Microscopy and Culture

The organism can be seen on conventional histological section (H&E) or on a Warthin-Starry silver stained section. *C. pylori* is a curved or spiral-shaped Gram-negative bacillus, resembling *C. jejuni* by light microscopy and antibiotic sensitivity pattern. *C. pylori* is isolated on moist chocolate agar incubated at 37°C in a microaerophilic atmosphere, suitable for the growth of *C. jejuni*. These bacteria differ from other *Campylobacter* in their possession of multiple unipolar sheathed flagella and in their protein electrophoretic pattern [8, 9]. Colonies are oxidase-positive, catalase-positive, indole-negative, nitrate-negative, do not ferment glucose nor hydrolyse hippurate and are remarkable for their powerful urease activity [10].

Histology

C. pylori organisms are usually found in and beneath the mucus layer, in close association with the surface epithelium. The microclimate in the mucus gel seems to favour their growth, presumably because the pH is neutral in contrast with the acid pH of gastric lumen.

Hypothesis

The very high urease activity permits hydrolysis of urea resulting in alterations in the milieu of the gastric epithelium. Recently another unique property of *C. pylori* has been discovered. It was found that *C. pylori* produces a protease which is capable of rapid degradation of gastric mucin. Possibly, these degenerative changes induced in gastric mucosal defense by *C. pylori* are the determining factor in the pathogenesis of gastritis and peptic ulcer [11]. There is convincing evidence in the literature that the presence of *C. pylori* is associated with histological evidence of chronic active gastritis [2−7]. Most characteristic is the presence of acute and chronic inflammation in the lamina propria, polymorphonuclear leukocytes permeating between the epithelial cells, mucus depletion and superficial erosions. A close relationship between the number of intra-epithelial polymorphonuclear leukocytes and the number of microorganisms supports the pathogenetic significance for these bacteria in mucosal inflammation.

Natural History

We followed a large number of culture-positive and culture-negative patients over a 2-year period. During this time all culture-positive patients remained positive and all culture-negative patients remained negative. The absence of spontaneous disappearance is important when interpreting treatment results.

Attempts at Eradication of *C. pylori*

Several attempts have been made to eradicate *C. pylori* from the gastric mucosa [12−16]. The lack of concordance between in vitro sensitivity and in vivo efficacy in eradicating *C. pylori* is remarkable. In vitro *C. pylori* is sensitive to penicillin G, ampicillin, cephalothin, cefotaxim, kanamycin, tobramycin, streptomycin, erythromycin, but not susceptible to lincomycin, vancomycin, colistin and cefsulodin [17]. *C. pylori* is sensitive to erythromycin in vitro, but erythromycin ethylsuccinate has no effect in vivo [14]. The antibiotics successfully tested in vivo are amoxicillin and tinidazol, usually in combination with colloidal bismuth subcitrate [16−19]. We also tried to evaluate the efficacy of various therapeutic regimens normally used in peptic ulcer disease and various antibiotics which appear active in vitro against *C. pylori*. In addition we tried to ascertain whether these drugs had any influence upon gastric inflammatory changes. In summary H_2-receptor blockers, spiramycin and sucralphate are of no benefit as we have seen no eradication nor suppression of *C. pylori* colonization and also no histologic recovery was noted.

Colloidal bismuth subcitrate leads to disappearance of *C. pylori* when tested directly after a treatment course in about 50% of cases. Such clearance is paralleled by a decrease in inflammatory changes. Treatment with amoxicillin monotherapy leads to early disappearance of *C. pylori* in 70% of cases, also paralleled by disappearance of the inflammatory changes of the mucosa. The most promising results were obtained with combination therapy of colloidal bismuth subcitrate (local effect) plus amoxicillin (systemic antimicrobial effect). When tested directly after treatment with the combination of colloidal bismuth subcitrate and amoxicillin *C. pylori* could no longer be cultured in 90% of cases. There was concomitant improvement of the gastric mucosa. However, if one re-examines those patients who became *C. pylori* culture-negative 1 month later, one finds only 40% of the patients have remained culture-negative.

Through analysis of the DNA composition of the microorganisms in various patients it could be demonstrated that the reoccurring microorganisms had the same DNA pattern as cultured before initial treatment [20]. Thus, either re-infection from the same source or recrudescence from not fully eradicated microorganisms had occurred.

Presumably some microorganisms survive the apparently successful treatment and recolonize the gastric mucosa after cessation of therapy. If one succeeds in eradicating *C. pylori* from the stomach, as indicated by the fact that no microorganisms can be cultured from antral biopsies 1 month after cessation of treatment, recolonization seldom occurs during a follow-up of more than 1 year.

Conclusion

Many studies have confirmed the strong correlation between the presence of *C. pylori* on the gastric mucosa and histologically confirmed chronic active gastritis and peptic ulceration. In human volunteer ingestion studies, *C. pylori* ingestion was followed by epigastric discomfort, nausea and vomiting, increase in fasting gastric pH with histological gastritis [7, 21]. The evidence that *C. pylori* is important in the etiology of upper gastrointestinal disease is rapidly accumulating.

We have shown that eradication of *C. pylori* is possible with colloidal bismuth subcitrate, amoxicillin monotherapy or the combination of colloidal bismuth subcitrate and amoxicillin; nevertheless, recrudescence is common already within 4 weeks after the treatment period. Eradication and suppression of *C. pylori* is paralleled by disappearance of the inflammatory changes of the gastric mucosa. Further investigations are needed to determine more effective permanent eradication of *C. pylori* from the gastric mucosa.

References

1. Warren JR, Marshall BJ (1983) Unidentified curved bacilli on gastric epithelium in active chronic gastritis. Lancet I: 1273 – 1275
2. Marshall BJ, Warren JR (1984) Unidentified curved bacilli in the stomach of patients with gastritis and peptic ulceration. Lancet I: 1311 – 1315

3. Meyrick Thomas J, Poynter D, Gooding C et al. (1984) Gastric spiral bacteria. Lancet II:100

4. McNulty CAM, Watson DM (1984) Spiral bacteria of the gastric antrum. Lancet I:1068−1069

5. Buck GE, Gourley WK, Lee WK et al. (1986) Relation of *Campylobacter pyloridis* to gastritis and peptic ulcer. J Inf Dis 153:664−669

6. Marshall BJ, McGechie OB, Rogers PA, Glanchy RJ (1985) *Pyloric campylobacter* infection and gastroduodenal disease. Med J Austr 142:439−444

7. Marshall BJ, Armstrong JA, McGechie DB, Glancy RJ (1985) Attempt to fulfil Koch's postulates for *pyloric campylobacter*. Med J Austr 142:436−439

8. Goodwin CS, McCulloch RK, Armstrong JA et al. (1985) Unusual cellular fatty acids and distinctive ultrastructure in a new spiral bacterium (*Campylobacter pyloridis*) from the human gastric mucosa. J Med Microbiol 19:257−267

9. Pearson AD, Bamforth J, Booth L et al. (1984) Polyacrylamide gel electrophoresis of spiral bacteria from the gastric antrum. Lancet I:1349−1350

10. Langenberg ML, Tytgat GNJ, Schipper MEI, Rietra PJGM, Zanen HC (1984) *Campylobacter-like* organisms in the stomach of patients and healthy individuals. Lancet I:1348

11. Slomiany BL, Bilski J, Sarosiek J et al. (1987) *Campylobacter pyloridis* degrades mucin and undermines gastric mucosal integrity. Biochem Biophys Res Commun 144:307−314

12. Marshall BJ, Hislop I, Glancy R, Armstrong J (1984) Histological improvement of active chronic gastritis in patients treated with De-Nol. Aust N Z J Med 14:(Suppl 4) 907

13. Jones DM, Eldridge J, Whorwell PJ, Miller JP (1985) The effects of various anti-ulcer regimens and antibiotics on the presence of *Campylobacter pyloridis* and its antibody. In: Pearson AD, Skirrow MB, Lion H (eds) Campylobacter III: Proceedings of the Third International Workshop on Campylobacter Infections. Public Health Laboratory Service, London 161

14. McNulty CAM, Gearty JC, Crump B et al. (1986) *Campylobacter pyloridis* and associated gastritis: investigator blind, placebo controlled trial of bismuth salicylate and erythromycin ethylsuccinate. Br Med J 293:645−649

15. Marshall BJ, Goodwin CS, Warren JR, Blincow ED, Blackborn S et al. (1986) Prospective double-blind study of supplementary antibiotic therapy for duodenal ulcer associated with *Campylobacter pyloridis* infection. Dig Dis Sci vol 31 (suppl no 10) Abstract 590 (150S)

16. Langenberg ML, Rauws EAJ, Schipper MEI et al. (1985) The pathogenic role of gastric *Campylobacter*-like organisms. (GCLO's) in GCLO-associated gastritis, studied by attempts to eliminate these organisms. (Abstract 98). In: Pearson AD, Skirrow MB et al. Campylobacter III: Proceedings of the Third International Workshop on Campylobacter Infections. Public Health Laboratory Service, London, 162−163

17. Lambert T, Mégraud F, Gerbaud G, Courvalin P (1986) Susceptibility of *Campylobacter pyloridis* to 20 antimicrobial agents. Antimicrob Agents Chemother 30:510−511

18. Marshall BJ, McGechie DB, Armstrong JA, Francis G (1985) The antibacterial action of bismuth: early results of antibacterial regimens in the treatment of duodenal ulcer. In: Pearson AD, Skirrow MB et al. (eds) Campylobacter III: Proceedings of the third international workshop on Campylobacter infections. Public Health Laboratory Service, London 165−166

19. Marshall BJ, Goodwin CS, Warren JR et al. (1986) Prospective double blind study of supplementary antibiotic therapy for duodenal ulcer associated with *Campylobacter pyloridis* infection. Am J gastroenterol 81:889 (abstr)

20. Langenberg W, Rauws EAJ, Widjojokusumo A, Tytgat GNJ, Zanen HC (1986) Identification of *Campylobacter pyloridis* Isolates by Restriction Endonuclease DNA Analysis. J Clin Microbiol 414−417

21. Morris A, Nicholson G (1986) *Campylobacter pyloridis* ingestion causing gastritis and hypochlorhydria. Austral Microbiol 7:206

Discussion

Goodwin: Sorry, I did not quite catch when the endoscopy was done?

Rauws: Endoscopy was performed within 48 h of the last treatment dose.

Goodwin: I think that is important. Because what we call eradication can turn out to be suppression in short term follow-up.

Rauws: That is for sure. Often a small number of colonies or no bacteria could be cultured directly after the last medication dose. In our follow-up study recurrence of *C. pylori* proved to be recurrence of the same bacterial subtype.

Goodwin: We should wait one or two weeks after the last medication dose. After that time new biopsies should be taken for culture to differentiate between the suppression or the eradication of *C. pylori*.

O'Moráin: The patients who became *C. pylori* positive developed gastritis. Did any one of them develop ulcers?

Rauws: In contrast to what was said yesterday, in all the over 300 patients with gastritis, 3 patients developed an ulcer during follow-up. One gastric and two duodenal ulcers. But that is out of 345 patients and a lot of these patients are not followed-up for more than a few months at the moment.

Attempts to Eradicate *Campylobacter pylori* – Irish Experiences

C. Ó'Moráin

The aetiology of peptic ulcer remains unknown. Aggressive and host defense mechanisms play a role, and an imbalance in these factors is thought to be important. In duodenal ulcers acid hypersecretion, an aggressive factor, has been implicated, however this is not an invariable feature. The natural history of the disease, characterised by remission and exacerbations, resembles herpes simplex infections and high titres have been found in duodenal ulcer, but this may be non-specific and may reflect a break in the mucosa [1, 2]. A new impetus to study infectious agents emerged with the description by Warren and Marshall of Gram-negative bacilli associated with gastritis [3]. More than half a century ago spiral Gram-negative bacteria were found attached to human gastric mucosa [4, 5]. As early as 1950 Professor Fitzgerald of Dublin noted an association between urease production in the gastric mucous layer and peptic ulcer disease [6] Koch's postulates for *Campylobacter pylori* have been fulfilled in the case of gastritis, in that it is invariably found and has been transmitted [7, 8]. Although data linking *Campylobacter pylori* to gastritis and to ulcer disease is sparse, our group have been involved over the past 3 years in studies which suggest that it is, indeed, an important factor.

Campylobacter and Peptic Disease

In a study of 135 patients with peptic disease, including oesophagitis, gastritis, gastric and duodenal ulcer, we found the incidence of *Campylobacter pylori* in the gastric antrum to be at 70%. The highest incidence found was in duodenal ulcer (90%) and the lowest in oesophagitis (30%). *Campylobacter* was identified by microbiological methods, Gram's stain and culture, or histologically by Warthin-Starry silver stain. There were excellent correlations among the three methods. Furthermore, one biopsy was as likely to yield a positive result as were multiple biopsies. We also observed that the organism was cultured most readily from the antrum, and less likely from the body, the fundus and from the oesophagus. Culture was only positive from the duodenum if gastric metaplasia was present. Age, smoking habits, duration of symptoms showed no correlation with *Campylobacter* status. In non-dyspeptic patients undergoing gastroscopy for biopsy in order to rule out diagnosis of coeliac disease, less than 10% of patients were positive for *Campylobacter*.

Patients were randomised to receive either 400 mg cimetidine b.i.d. or 5 ml colloidal bismuth subcitrate q.i.d. There was no significant difference in healing rates between the two treatment groups. Antral biopsies were obtained before and after treatment. The endoscopist, microbiologist and histologist were blind as to the patients treatment. There was a significant decrease in *Campylobacter* in the patients treated with colloidal bismuth subcitrate (70% to 38%).

In further studies 66 consecutive patients with endoscopically proven duodenal ulcer were randomised to receive either 400 mg cimetidine b.i.d. or 5 ml colloidol bismuth subcitrate q.i.d. for 6 weeks. Biopsies were obtained from the antrum once again and assessed blindly by the microbiologist and the histologist. The endoscopist was unaware of the treatment given when assessing healing at 6 weeks. There was no significant difference in healing rates between the groups (72%). However, the rate of *Campylobacter* infection fell in the colloidal bismuth subcitrate group from 93% to 58%. There was no significant decrease in the cimetidine-treated group.

Gastritis and Duodenal Ulcer

The antral biopsies were assessed for the presence of gastritis. Gastritis was evaluated using the criteria of Warren and Marshall [9] as follows: grade 0, normal; grade 1, mild round cell infiltrate; grade 2, focal neutrophil infiltrate; grade 3, neutrophil infiltrate with glandular distortion. Patients with grades 2 or 3 were considered to have gastritis. Treatment with colloidal bismuth subcitrate reduced the incidence of gastritis from 70% to 33%, whereas no effect was seen with cimetidene. Colloidal bismuth subcitrate was unlikely to heal ulcers in patients from whom *Campylobacter* was not cultured, whereas *Campylobacter* status made no difference in treatment outcome with cimetidene. Therefore, ascertaining a patient's *Campylobacter* status could determine appropriate medical treatment for duodenal ulcer. These results confirmed
a) the in vitro bactericidal effect of colloidal bismuth subcitrate in vivo,
b) the high incidence of the organism in peptic disease,
c) the association of histological gastritis and duodenal ulcer,
d) that colloidal bismuth subcitrate heals gastritis.

Campylobacter and Relapse of Duodenal Ulcer

In further studies we have assessed the relationship of *Campylobacter* and duodenal ulcer relapse. Duodenal ulcer is characterised by frequent relapse and remission. H_2-receptor antagonist has been shown to be effective with over 90% healing rates after 4 weeks treatment. Unfortunately, however, relapse is common. Three studies [10–12] have shown that patients treated with colloidal bismuth subcitrate have a lower relapse rate compared to a H_2-receptor antago-

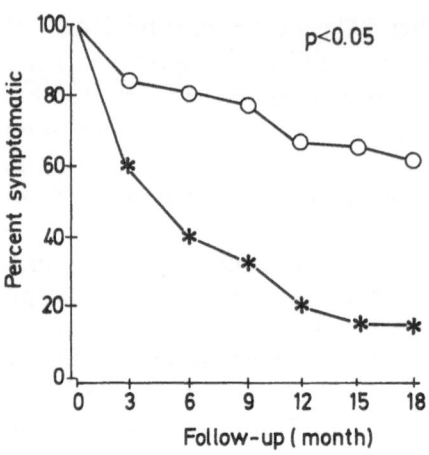

Fig. 1. Rate of symptomatic relapse of duodenal ulcer after treatment with colloidal bismuth subcitrate (*O's*) and with cimetidine (*X's*) (*p* < 0.05)

nist. One study failed to confirm this observation but the number of patients observed in this study was small [13]. We have followed up 40 patients with endoscopically healed duodenal ulcer following a 6-week course of 400 mg cimetidine b.i.d. or 5 ml colloidal bismuth subcitrate q.i.d. for a 1-year period. Patients were reviewed at 3-monthly intervals and were assessed for symptoms of peptic ulcer. Endoscopy was performed at 1 year or sooner if patients were symptomatic. At each endoscopy two antral biopsies were taken. One was placed in formalin for histological evaluation by Warthin-Starry silver stain and by haematoxylin and esoin stain to assess gastritis, and a second biopsy was processed microbiologically by Gram's stain and culture. Twenty-five patients were *Campylobacter*-positive and 15 were *Campylobacter*-negative. Symptomatic and endoscopic relapse was significantly greater in patients who were *Campylobacter*-positive (Fig. 1). Of patients who remained *Campylobacter*-positive following treatment 80% relapsed, while only 27% of patients who were negative for *Campylobacter* relapsed. Patients who were initially *Campylobacter*-positive remained positive, and almost all had histological gastritis on the follow-up. Patients who became *Campylobacter*-negative can be divided into two groups. Those who remained negative did not have any histological evidence of gastritis, and only one had a recurrence of duodenal ulcer. The five patients, on the other hand, who became *Campylobacter*-positive all had histological gastritis and three out of five developed duodenal ulcer. The findings of this study suggest that successful eradication of *Campylobacter* reduces the likelihood of relapse.

Dosage Regimes

In a further study 60 patients with duodenal ulcer were randomised to receive either 240 mg colloidal bismuth subcitrate b.i.d. or 120 mg q.i.d. Endoscopy was performed at 4 and 8 weeks, and antral biopsies were again obtained for

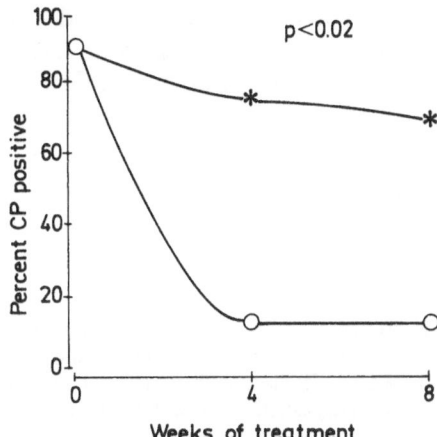

Fig. 2. *Campylobacter pylori* (CP) infection rate in healed duodenal ulcers after treatment with colloidal bismuth subcitrate at 120 mg q.i.d. (*O's*) and at 240 mg b.i.d. ($p < 0.02$)

assessment of gastritis and *Campylobacter* status as outlined above. At the beginning of the study 93% of patients were culture-positive. There was no difference in the healing rates between the two different regimes (Fig. 2). However, there was a significant reduction in the *Campylobacter* status of patients treated with the q.i.d. regime. The reason for this remains unclear, as the colloidal bismuth subcitrate is thought to exert its effect locally by penetrating the mucus layer and then being incorporated into the bacterial wall. Follow-up studies in these patients should prove interesting.

In recent studies we have used antibiotics in association with colloidal bismuth subcitrate and have compared the results to those obtained with colloidal bismuth subcitrate alone. We chose amoxicillin, as this is effective in vitro and is secreted in the gastric juice [14]. Preliminary results suggest that the combination therapy does not affect healing rates of duodenal ulcer but does improve *Campylobacter* clearance rates. Follow-up studies will indicate whether remission is maintained when *Campylobacter* is eradicated.

Other studies in progress seek to ascertain whether long-term maintenance therapy with colloidal bismuth subcitrate is more effective in preventing *Campylobacter* re-infection and duodenal ulcer relapse. We are currently investigating virulence factors of the organism and genetic probes to diagnose the presence of *Campylobacter* in tissue.

Conclusion

We confirm the association of *Campylobacter* and peptic disease and the frequent association of gastritis with duodenal ulcer. Colloidal bismuth subcitrate significantly reduces *Campylobacter* infection. Patients whose ulcers healed and were rendered *Campylobacter*-negative proved less likely to relapse, compared to those in whom the infection persisted. Different dosage regimes may be effective in reducing *Campylobacter* infection. Preliminary results show that a

224   C. Ó'Moráin

combination of antibiotics and colloidal bismuth subcitrate decrease *Campylobacter* infection. The most exciting development seems to be the strong association of *Campylobacter* and relapse of duodenal ulcer.

References

1. Rand KH, Jacobson DG, Cottrell CR, Guild RT, Koch K, McGuigan JE (1982) Relationship of herpes virus type 1 (HSV-1) Infection to duodenal ulcer. Gastroenterology (82) 1154
2. Vestergaard PF, Rine ST (1980) Type specific herpes simplex virus antibodies in patients with recurrent duodenal ulcer. Lancet I: 1273 – 1274
3. Warren JR, Marshall B (1983) Unidentified curved bacilli in gastric epithelium in active chronic gastritis. Lancet I: 1273 – 1275
4. Doenges JL (1938) Spirochaetes in gastric glands of Macaeus rhesus and humans without definite history of related disease. Proc Soc Exp Biol Med 38: 536 – 538
5. Freedberg AS, Barron LE (1940) The presence of spirochaetes in human gastric mucosa. Am J Dig Dis 7: 443 – 445
6. Fitzgerald O, Murphy P (1950) Studies on the physiological chemistry and clinical significance of urease and urea with special reference to stomach. Irish J of Med Science 292: 97 – 112
7. Marshall BJ, Armstrong JA, McGeechie DB, Glancy RJ (1985) An attempt to fulfill Koch's postulates for campylobacter. M J Aust 142: 436 – 439
8. Ramsey EJ, Carey KU, Peterson WL et al. (1979) Epidemic gastritis with hypochlorhydria. Gastroenterology 76: 1449 – 1457
9. Marshall BJ, Warren JR (1984) Unidentified curved bacilli in the stomach of patients with gastritis and peptic ulcer. Lancet I: 1311 – 1315
10. Martin DF, Hollanders D, May SJ, Ravenscroft MM, Tweedle DEF, Millar JP (1981) Difference in relapse rates of duodenal ulcer after healing with cimetidine or tripotassium dicatrate bismuthate. Lancet I: 7 – 10
11. Lee FI, Samloff IM, Hardman M (1980) Comparison of tri-potassium di-citro bismuthate tablets with ramitidine in healing and relapse of duodenal ulcers. Lancet I: 1299 – 1301
12. Hamilton I, O'Connor HJ, Wood HC, Bradbury I, Axon AH (1986) Healing and recurrance of duodenal ulcer after treatment with tri-potassium dicitrate tablets or cimetidine. Gut 27: 106 – 110
13. Kang JV, Piper DW (1982) Cimetidine and colloidal bismuth subcitrate comparison of initial healing and recurrence after healing. Digestion 23: 73 – 79
14. McNulty CA, Dent J, Wise R (1985) Susceptibility of clinical isolates of campylobacter pyloridis to 11 antimicrobial agents. Antimicrobial Agents and Chemotherapy 28: 857 – 858

Discussion

McNulty: Your study will obviously change the treatment of peptic ulceration in the future. Do you think you could hypothesize why the four times daily treatment was better than the twice daily treatment?

O'Moráin: We think people should stand back and try and reason this out. We heard yesterday about triple therapy and before long we might even hear of gastrectomies for the treatment of *C. pylori!* I mentioned that formulation is very important. Now there are different formulations. In our initial studies we used the liquid form of CBS which reduced the incidence of *C. pylori* from 93% down to 58%. When we used the tablet, one T.Q.I.D. (for swallowing), we achieved much better clearance rates from 93% down to 27%. We feel that probably the reason for this is the continuous exposure of *C. pylori* to the bismuth preparation.

Tytgat: At which time of the day did you advise the patients to take bismuth? What was the relationship to the meals?

O'Moráin: We advised our patients to take the bismuth preparation half an hour before meals. We hope that they did comply with that.

Börsch: Your data were beautiful, but I have some reservations about your last slide where you implicated *C. pylori* directly into the genesis of peptic ulcer disease. This concerns a very important question which has not been discussed at the meeting, and there are two sets of data which are controversial. Marshall has shown that the eradication of *C. pylori* improves ulcer healing rates. Your data and also those of Lambert in the *Gastroenterology* abstract issue of May 1987 (92:1489) show that there is a very good healing rate despite the persistance of the campylobacter. And I conclude from all the data I have heard that the only direct implication of campylobacter with ulcer disease is via gastritis and that via this gastritis, campylobacter becomes a risk factor for peptic ulcer disease. The Dutch group said the same thing yesterday. If this is so, logic merely leads us to expect a reduction of the recurrence rate, but does not justify us in expecting an acceleration of the healing process. This is a critical issue. With prostaglandins the same unsound thinking occurred when it was postulated that "cytoprotection" improved healing rates. From a theoretical point of view, this is nonsense. If cytoprotection does anything at all, it might have an effect on recurrences. But with prostaglandins, that has not worked so far either.

McNulty: Maybe Dr. Wyatt would like to comment on her theory of gastric metaplasia in the duodenum related to the etiology of duodenal ulceration.

Wyatt: I am not sure that our work answers the question that has been posed. In a big series of patients with duodenal ulcer and nonulcer dyspepsia we found that the concurrence of gastric metaplasia in the duodenum and *C. pylori* in the stomach — these two factors — identified those patients who had duodenitis (whether there is another factor is not answered).

O'Moráin: May I answer the question. I did not mean to imply that there was a direct relationship between *C. pylori* and duodenal ulcer. I wanted to emphasize, as my Dutch colleagues have also shown, that almost 100% of patients with duodenal ulcer had gastritis. And gastritis is linked with *C. pylori* and *C. pylori* is cleared particularly when we use bismuth.

Marshall: I do not think my study and Dr. O'Morain's really show different ulcer healing rates. We endoscoped the patients 2 weeks after they ceased therapy because we wanted to get an accurate microbiological diagnosis at that point. But you can imagine patients given eight weeks of therapy with cimetidine who still have the ulcer diathesis. And who then cease all therapy for two weeks. Some of those patients relapse in two weeks. In our study, some early ulcer relapses in the Campylobacter positive group are detected as unhealed ulcers. So we have an unusually low healing rate of 60% after eight weeks of cimetidine therapy. The opposite applies to Campylobacter negative patients who have had the ulcer diathesis improved or removed. At eight weeks, even if a small ulcer is present, it may have healed two weeks later when gastroscopy is performed because the ulcer diathesis is no longer present. So you have an artificially improved healing rate in the *C. pylori* negative group. This would accentuate the difference between bismuth or an anti-bacterial agent and an H_2 receptor blocker.

Goodwin: I think as we are coming to the end of our time here, it would be worth emphasizing again the fact that acid is not the main cause of ulcers. Acid causes gastric metaplasia. And if you did not have *C. pylori*, you wouldn't get an ulcer. This has still got to be proven, but this is where we are heading.

Tytgat: I really disagree with that to some extent. I think from the studies on refractory ulcers it has been proven that if you can cut down acid completely, any ulcer will heal. And therefore it appears to have some importance. If I may come back to the problem of bismuth administration, I think the timing is very important indeed — suppose you give the drug, with the meals or right after meals, do you think you might have the same effect as you have shown because your results are better than those we saw in Amsterdam.

O'Moráin: Well, if we gave bismuth with meals or after meals, this would bind with food. And that is why we left ample time so that it would bind with the mucosa and interact with the campylobacter in the mucosa and not interact with food.

Börsch: One final word on the question of ulcer pathogenesis. I think that the best way to sum it up in one or two sentences is to call both acid/pepsin and campylobacter necessary, but by themselves not sufficient conditions for the genesis of peptic ulcer disease. If you put it this way you can reconcile previous with current thinking. All the known data fit into this concept.

Attempts to Eradicate *Campylobacter pylori* – German Experiences

H. MENGE, J. HOFMANN, U. BOENIGK, and M. GREGOR

The strong correlation between the presence of *Campylobacter pylori* on the gastric mucosa and gastritis, with or without peptic ulcers, gave rise to several studies aiming to find a therapy for the eradication of this bacterium from the human stomach (Lanza et al. 1986; Marshall et al. 1986; McNulty et al. 1986). It was a further aim of these studies to investigate whether its disappearance is paralleled by the healing of gastritis or of gastroduodenal ulcers. Two groups of drugs were used in these studies, namely antibiotics and the bismuth salts tripotassium dicitrato bismuthate and bismuth subsalicylate.

For our investigations we chose bismuth subsalicylate as the therapeutic drug. There were 3 reasons for this choice. Firstly, we did not wish to treat gastritis or peptic ulcers with antibiotics considering their multiple side effects and the development of bacterial resistance against them. Secondly, bismuth subsalicylate was selected instead of tripotassium dicitrato bismuthate since the latter drug is not on the German market; thirdly, the hitherto published studies dealing with the eradication of *C. pylori* in patients with gastritis were performed with bismuth subsalicylate (Lanza et al. 1986; McNulty et al. 1986; see discussion).

After the decision to treat *C. pylori* colonization with bismuth subsalicylate, we had to decide whether to take the suspension or the chewable tablets, both being on the market. Up to now only the suspension has been shown to be effective in eradicating *C. pylori,* whereas no comparable investigations using the chewable tablets are available. On the other hand, however, we preferred the idea of chewable tablets, since we thought it much more convenient for the patients to carry tablets rather than a bottle of the suspension and a measuring cup. For these reasons we first of all initiated a prospective multicenter study to compare the effectiveness of the bismuth suspension and the bismuth chewable tablets, both of which contain bismuth subsalicylate, in eradicating *C. pylori.* This investigation has not yet been finished. To date, 97 patients have been included in this study. The CLO test was positive in all cases. Fifty patients were treated with the bismuth suspension, and *C. pylori* was eradicated in 33 of them; 47 persons were treated with bismuth chewable tablets, and the bacterium was eradicated in 36 of them. Obviously, a final statistical analysis can be made only when this study has been completed. So far, however, there are no significant differences between the two groups of patients, showing that the chewable tablets are very probably as effective as the bismuth suspension in eradicating *C. pylori* from the human antral mucosa.

After obtaining the preliminary data of this study, we will be able to start our attempts to eradicate *C. pylori* by using bismuth subsalicylate chewable tablets, based on already published data. If one carefully reads these studies in which the *C. pylori* associated gastritis is treated with bismuth salts (Table 1), one main aspect emerges. McNulty et al. (1986) treated 18 patients, whose CLO test was positive with Pepto Bismol at a dosage of 4×30 ml daily for 3 weeks. *C. pylori* was eradicated in 14 out of the 18 patients. This means giving 4×314 mg Bi^{3+} per day for 3 weeks does not always result in the eradication of the bacterium. Lanza et al. (1986) obtained similar data. These authors treated ten patients with the same regimen. After 2 weeks seven patients were *C. pylori* negative and after a further week, only six out of the ten patients were *C. pylori* negative. Again, giving 1256 mg Bi^{3+} per day does not always result in the eradication of the bacterium. Based on these studies, we decided to increase the daily dosage of Bi^{3+}, and conducted an investigation in which 24 patients with a positive CLO test were treated with 3×3 chewable tablets per day. We assumed that this higher dosage might lead to an earlier elimination of *C. pylori* from the antral mucosa, and therefore reinvestigated the patients after only 5 days treatment.

The following results were obtained. After 5 days treatment, 20 of the 24 patients no longer exhibited any presence of *C. pylori*. Merging these data with the results of McNulty et al. (1986) and Lanza et al. (1986), it is clear that short-term treatment using a higher dosage is as effective as treatment over a longer period with a lower dosage (Table 2).

Our second step was to evaluate the histological sections of the antral mucosa before and after our new therapy schedule. In five of the 24 persons, the biopsies were inadequate for the histological procedure, so we had 19 patients in all, of whom 15 were rid of the bacterium. These 15 persons exhibited histologically confirmed chronic gastritis before starting therapy; after elimination of *C. pylori*, the gastritis had improved or the antral mucosa was normalized in 11 of them, whereas in four no such changes could be discovered.

These results are not as good as those of McNulty et al. (1986) but similar to those obtained by Lanza et al. (1986); so our data lie between those of the two papers published on this subject to date (Table 3).

Table 1. Eradication of *Campylobacter pylori* (C.p.) in patients with gastritis using bismuth subsalicylate

Lanza et al. (1986):	10 patients
Pepto Bismol:	$4 \times$ 30 ml daily
After 14-day treatment	4×314 mg Bi^{3+}
7 patients C.p. neg. – 3 patients C.p. pos.	
After 21-day treatment	
6 patients C.p. neg. – 4 patients C.p. pos.	
McNulty et al. (1986):	18 patients
Pepto Bismol:	$4 \times$ 30 ml daily
After 21-day treatment 14 patients C.p. neg. – 4 patients C.p. pos.	4×314 mg Bi^{3+}

Table 2. Eradication of *Campylobacter pylori* (C.p.) using different dosages of bismuth subsalicylate and different treatment periods

Lanza et al. (1986):	1256 mg Bi^{3+} daily (14 days) 70.0% C.p. negative
McNulty et al. (1986):	1256 mg Bi^{3+} daily (21 days) 77.7% C.p. negative
Menge et al. (1987):	1566 mg Bi^{3+} daily (5 days) 83.3% C.p. negative

Table 3. Improvement of gastritis in *Campylobacter pylori* positive patients using different dosages of bismuth subsalicylate and different treatment periods

Lanza et al. (1986):	1256 mg Bi^{3+} daily (14 days) 70% improvement of gastritis
McNulty et al. (1986):	1256 mg Bi^{3+} daily (21 days) 92.3% improvement of gastritis
Menge et al. (1987):	1566 mg Bi^{3+} daily (5 days) 73.3% improvement of gastritis

In conclusion, we believe that the increased dosage used in this study is more effective in attacking *C. pylori* in the human antral mucosa in a shorter period of time.

References

1. Lanza FL, Rack MF, Peterson DF (1986) Eradication of *Campylobacter pyloridis* with bismuth subsalicylate. Am J Gastroenterol 81:853
2. Marshall BJ, Goodwin CS, Warren JR, Blincow ED, Blackbourn S, Phillips M, Waters TE, Sanderson CR (1986) Prospective double-blind study of supplementary antibiotic therapy for duodenal ulcer associated with *Campylobacter pyloridis* infection. Am J Gastroenterol 81:889
3. McNulty CAM, Gearty JC, Crump B, Davis M, Donovan JA, Melikian V, Lister DM, Wise R (1986) *Campylobacter pyloridis* and associated gastritis: investigator blind, placebo controlled trial of bismuth salicylate and erythromycin ethylsuccinate. Br Med J 239:645–649

Discussion

McNulty: From the data so far we can see that bismuth used on its own is not totally effective. Do you not think that combination therapy is really the way forward?

Menge: No, not yet, because it is not yet clear whether the combination therapy really is superior to the bismuth therapy alone.

Tytgat: Can we really speak about eradication if you take the control biopsies within a few days of the end of therapy? Shouldn't we all agree here that at least 2–3 months should elapse after the therapy, before you can speak of eradication? What we achieve in the vast majority of the patients is suppression, and I think that the word eradication is really misleading.

Menge: I agree with you. It should be changed in the manuscript.

O'Moráin: You did not mention the patients' symptoms.

Menge: We did not investigate them. It is only a pilot study so far.

Rathbone: On a slightly different tack, I just wonder if there is anybody here who has any experience in using furazolidone. It is used in treating Giardia, it is a very cheap drug and there are some reports from China on its use in treating ulcers.

McNulty: I believe that furazolidone is not registered in Europe because of side effects and toxicity.

Tytgat: It has been taken off the market. In the old days we had to warn patients that they might have some epigastric discomfort after taking bismuth. Initially it was even considered that we had to give antacids together with bismuth to get around these annoying effects. Did the patients to whom you gave a high dose of bismuth complain of a burning epigastric sensation?

Menge: No, they did not. I am sure of that. And we gave it – this may be your next question – half an hour before meals.

Börsch: Professor Menge inspired me to do the same kind of study he did, with the same dose of bismuth, but I did it in peptic ulcer patients. Like him, I only have preliminary data. The negative — and I do not say eradication — but the rate for *Campylobacter pylori* negative ulcer patients after 5 days of treatment is only 30%, and he had 84%. There is, as yet, no explanation for these differences, and we did not make a statistical analysis. But these data may be an indication (and we talked about this yesterday) that there could be differences between those strains that are associated with ulcers and those that are not; or it may be that ulceration may predispose patients to prolonged colonization.

Goodwin: The other thing is — we are trying to get the right criteria for trials and taking biopsies in order to be able to assess the results correctly. I would like to suggest that we take biopsies from the fundus as well as the antrum, and check whether *C. pylori* is cleared from both sides.

Menge: The biopsies were taken only from the antrum, and we took four biopsies from each patient.

Goodwin: I am making this suggestion with future workers in mind.

Ober: I would like some clarification on this eradication and suppression business. Why do you say that if the cultures are negative? I agree that they should be taken sufficiently long after the last dose was administered — otherwise the bacterium has not been eradicated and only suppressed. Is this based on the fact (as Dr. Langenberg showed this morning) that you find the same type of *C. pylori* several months later, or what is the reason?

Tytgat: That's the main reason.

Goodwin: Just to answer the last question, *C. pylori* is a very "friendly' organism and likes lots of bugs next to it to grow best. You cannot culture it on a plate with just a few organisms from one colony. You need to have a small drop which you then spread out later on. And almost certainly, our culture techniques are not good enough to recognize very small numbers of the bacterium.

McNulty: Would anyone else like to discuss possible future treatment regimen that they consider might be appropriate in future trials?

Tytgat: Perhaps the chairman can give us some advice on how to proceed from here.

McNulty: Well, I do not think the ideal treatment has yet been decided upon, but I think the two chairmen here obviously disagree, because I consider that the combination treatment has obviously proven to be better than bismuth alone. The antimicrobial chosen is very difficult to decide on. The quinolones looked exciting in vitro but do not work in vivo. Amoxicillin so far looks very good, and possibly nitrofurantoin. Yesterday, Professor Goodwin was suggesting triple therapy. I do not know what other people feel about this, but with triple therapy you may get more side effects from all the antibiotics than you would from the symptoms you are trying to treat!

Section 6

State of the Art Lecture

Campylobacter pylori: Addressing the Controversies

B. J. MARSHALL

Campylobacter pylori (CP) colonization of the gastroduodenal mucosa is associated with peptic ulcer disease, particularly with duodenal ulcer. The bacterium appears to induce cytopathic changes in epithelial cells lining the stomach, is actively phagocytosed by polymorphonuclear leukocytes, and probably causes the histologic changes of active chronic gastritis. Wheras acid hypersecretion affects only a small proportion of ulcer patients, this type of gastritis affects 95% of duodenal ulcer patients and about 70% of persons with gastric ulcer. This association suggests that the current emphasis on acid reducing therapy for ulcer disease may be replaced by therapy directed at the repair of the mucosal defect present in ulcer patients.

Before *C. pylori* is universally accepted as a serious pathogen, the controversies surrounding gastric colonization by the bacterium need to be addressed. While there is much histological data to indicate a pathogenic role for *C. pylori,* the epidemiology of type B gastritis suggests that the bacterium is a harmless commensal, or at worst, a saprophyte which colonizes damaged gastric mucosa.

The Epidemiology of Type B Gastritis

The epidemiology of Type B gastritis was defined by Scandinavian studies in the 1960s (Kekki et al. 1977), before direct-vision biopsy of the antrum was made possible by the modern fiberoptic gastroduodenoscope. As a result, knowledge of gastritis was based on the examination of biopsy specimens taken from the greater curve of the stomach in acid secreting type mucosa. The antrum was rarely sampled. Moreover, the investigators were more often impressed with the chronic inflammation present, i.e., lymphocytes and plasma cells. The polymorphonuclear leukocytes were less obvious to the researchers, and the epithelial cell changes we now associate with *C. pylori* (Tricottet et al. 1986) passed largely unnoticed.

It is reasonable to assume, nevertheless, that the earlier studies were referring to the same type of gastritis we now associate with *C. pylori,* as expressed in a milder form in body type mucosa. It was found that gastritis was present in about 20% of young adults, and increased with age to affect at least 50% of the population by the age of 60 (Kekki et al. 1977). From these earlier studies we

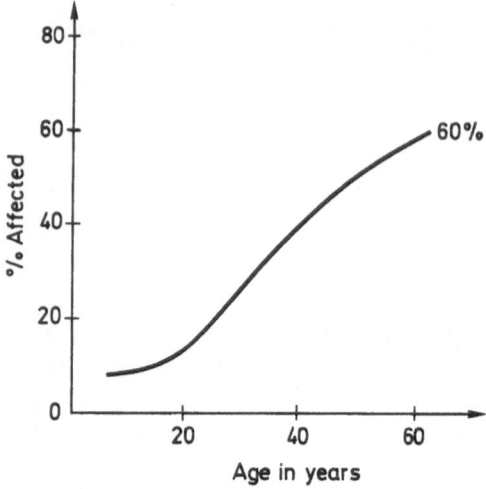

Fig. 1. Epidemiology of type B gastritis (*C. pylori* infection) (Data from Kekki et al. 1977)

can conclude that chronic gastritis is common, increases in frequency with age, and is often asymptomatic (Fig. 1).

Unfortunately, some authors interpreted these findings to mean that chronic gastritis was an inevitable asymptomatic accompaniment of aging and that its association with ulcer disease was mere coincidence. In support of this view were studies such as that of Steer and Colin Jones (1975), which showed that carbenoxolone healed gastric ulcer, while not affecting gastritis. Later it was discovered that cimetidine, a far more effective ulcer healing agent, also healed ulcers without healing the gastritis (McIntyre et al. 1982). The ulcer thus appeared to be a direct consequence of gastric acid secretion rather than of the mucosal inflammation. In addition, there were many asymptomatic persons with type B gastritis who never developed ulcer disease.

Are Type B Gastritis and *C. pylori* Infection the Same Disease?

Recently, *C. pylori* has been added to our evaluation of gastric mucosal histology as a new variable. The bacterium (and/or gastritis) is present in 10% − 25% of normal subjects and most of those without *C. pylori* have histologically normal mucosa (Langenberg et al. 1984; Barthel et al. 1986). In my own experience, patients above the age of 70 have normal gastric mucosa unless this infection is present. Furthermore, when elderly persons with *C. pylori*-associated gastritis are treated, the histological changes reverse once the bacterium is eradicated. These observations suggest that chronic gastritis and *C. pylori* infection are very closely related. Type B chronic gastritis is age related only because this infection is more common in elderly persons (Fig. 2).

Epidemiology and Disease Associations of *C. pylori*

In endoscopy populations, the presence of *C. pylori* is almost always accompanied by active chronic gastritis (Hui et al. 1986; Marshall et al. 1987).

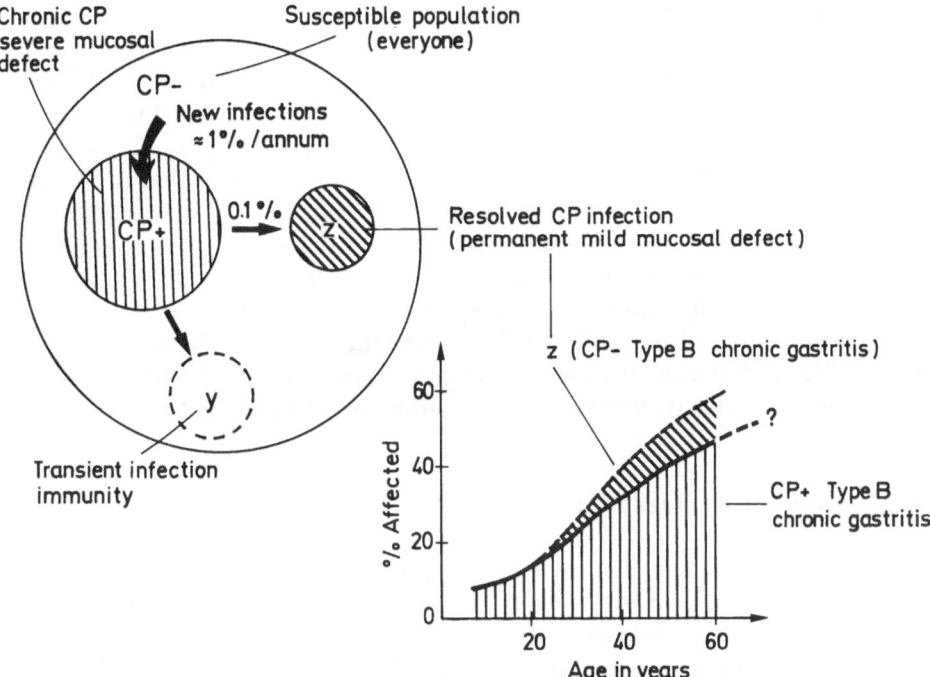

Fig. 2. Type B gastritis explained as *C. pylori* infection. With age, the chance of acquiring chronic *C. pylori* (and of having chronic gastritis) increases. About half the persons who contract the acute infection have a transient episode and may develop immunity (y), the others enter an enlarging pool of persons with chronic gastritis. A small number of persons with chronic infection lose the bacterium, of whom some do not regain a histologically normal mucosa, and remain susceptible to peptic ulcer disease (z)

Tests which detect *C. pylori* may therefore be used to determine the frequency of gastritis in the population. Serological evidence of *C. pylori* infection is present in about 20% of adult blood donors, its occurrence increasing with age. The bacterium, more common in males, is present in 10% – 20% of 20 year olds, and infects 40% – 50% of persons by age 60. Thus the epidemiology of CP infection corresponds to the known epidemiology of chronic gastritis. Infection appears to be less common than histological gastritis (45% at age 60 vs 55% – 60% at age 60), but this could be due to the lower sensitivity of the serological methods. It seems therefore that *C. pylori* infection and type B chronic gastritis affect approximately half of the "normal" population by age 50.

Although reliable data are not available on comparable groups in third world countries, there is evidence to suggest that *C. pylori* infection is widespread there. In India, for example, gastric mucosal urease (a marker for *C. pylori*) was universally present in a series of persons without ulcer disease (Narang et al. 1980). In endoscopy series from Peru (Ramirez-Ramos et al. 1987) and Rwanda (T. Mets, personal communication), the infection was found to be far more common than in equivalent studies in western countries (70% and 93% respectively).

Various Interpretations of the Epidemiological Data

The epidemiological data we have could be explained in two ways. *C. pylori* may have a propensity to affect certain ethnic groups and persons older than 30 years. Alternatively, the infection may be acquired mainly in childhood by fecal-oral spread, in much the same way that *Campylobacter jejuni* is acquired. If the latter hypothesis is correct, then the commonness of the infection in third world countries could be explained as being a result of the poor standards of public hygiene. Similarly, the commonness of the infection in middle aged persons in western countries may be the result of a cohort effect, perhaps from a widespread source of exposure to the bacterium, prevalent 40 years ago. The Second World War caused widespread deterioration in public health standards, soldiers in particular being very common hosts for infectious enteric organisms.

Is *C. pylori* a Public Health Concern?

At this point in time, with so many apparently healthy elderly persons infected, it is difficult to accept that *C. pylori* is a significant pathogen. If aging were the cause of gastritis we would expect to see a gradual transition with age from unchanged to inflamed gastric mucosa. Instead we find only two groups; a group with normal histology and a group with gastritis.

A better appreciation of *C. pylori* as a pathogen may be obtained if we draw the analogy of a tribe of primitive natives 50% of whom have malaria. This could mean that the malaria parasite is a normal commensal, or that malaria is endemic and a major public health problem. In such a population many colonized individuals will be in a state of symbiosis with the parasite. However, the number of such individuals who develop anemia and fever will be greater than in the noninfected persons. In this case asymptomatic persons with malaria are not in an ideal state of health, because statistically, they are at risk of developing the overt disease. Similarly, persons with *C. pylori* infection are not in a state of optimal health, since they are at risk of developing peptic ulcer disease.

C. pylori as a Risk Factor

C. pylori colonization of the stomach is associated with a spectrum of disease ranging from asymptomatic gastritis to peptic ulceration. We can estimate the epidemiology of *C. pylori* associated disease by examining data from both endoscopy studies and serological studies. Serological studies indicate that 20%−25% of the total population has *C. pylori* infection (Marshall et al. 1985a; Eldridge et al. 1985). From postmortem data we know that peptic ulcer occurs in about 8% of persons during their lifetime (Boyd and Wormsley 1985), most of whom can be presumed to have the infection. From endoscopy studies we know that persons who have gastritis but not ulcer (nonulcer dyspepsia [NUD]) are as common as those who have gastritis (*C. pylori*) with ulcer.

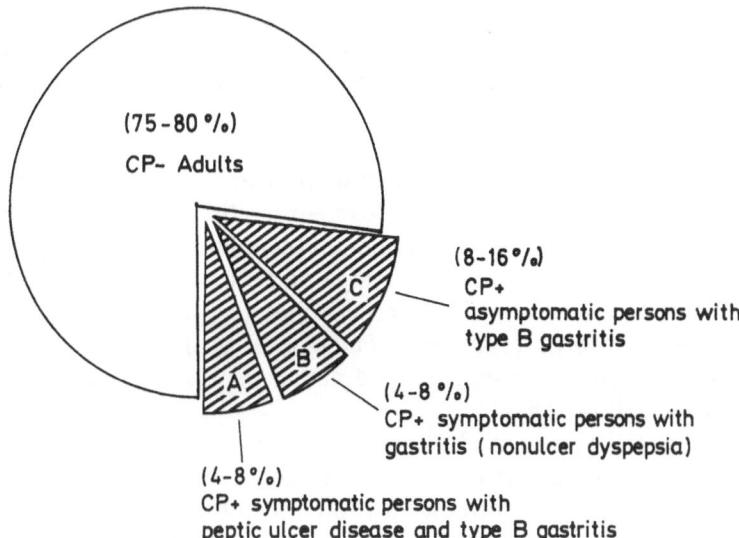

Fig. 3. Epidemiology of *C. pylori:* 20% – 25% of adults have *C. pylori* infection and chronic gastritis (estimated from serological and bioptic studies of persons in the normal group). Group A: 8% of the population develops peptic ulcer disease and most of these persons have *C. pylori,* Group B: An equal number of persons (as determined by endoscopy studies of patients) have *C. pylori* but no ulcer (non ulcer dyspepsia). Group C: This leaves 8 – 12% of the population as persons with asymptomatic *C. pylori* associated gastritis

Combined, all these data show that 25% of adults have *C. pylori* associated gastritis, of which approximately one-third are asymptomatic, one-third have dyspepsia but no ulcer, and one- third have peptic ulcer disease (Fig. 3).

Nearly all cases of peptic ulcer disease occur in the 25% of persons with *C. pylori* infection. This infection thus confers a 20-fold risk of developing peptic ulcer. The risk is acquired with the infection, so that a person with asymptomatic infection presens a threat to noninfected contacts and may be regarded as being a carrier (Goodwin and Armstrong 1986). As the infection is commoner in older persons, grandparents are a potential source of infection.

The Definition of Normality

The presence of *C. pylori* gastritis in about half the population over the age of 60 challenges our concept of gastrointestinal normality in this group. Everyone suffers dyspeptic symptoms at some time, and most people take antacid on occasions, so the definition of normality is an arbitrary one. Two studies have recently addressed this issue. In one study of 292 blood donors who had never been diagnosed as having ulcer disease, normality was defined as corresponding to a person who had not taken antacid in the preceding seven days, and who had never been investigated for dyspepsia with a barium meal or endoscopy. Using a passive hemagglutination test it was found that only 14% of normal donors had serologic evidence of *C. pylori* infection, compared with 28% of the symptomatic donors ($P = 0.008$) (Marshall et al. 1985a). Recently, Skoglund et al. (1987) reported a similar study of workers at the Procter and Gamble company in Cincinnati, Ohio. In that study a sensitive ELISA method detected *C. pylori* antibody in 46% of the workers who consumed antacids but in only 14% of those who did not. These data suggest that "healthy normal" persons with *C. pylori* infection have more dyspepsia than persons without it. *C. pylori* appears to be a risk factor for dyspepsia. In future gastroenterologic surveys, therefore, control subjects should not include those with *C. pylori* infection.

At recent international meetings, and elsewhere in this publication, evidence has been presented which confirms that *C. pylori* causes gastritis (Marshall et al. 1985b; Morris et al. 1985; Peterson et al. 1987; Lambert et al. 1987). The connection between gastritis and actual peptic ulceration has not yet been established, however.

The pathogenic mechanism whereby *C. pylori* damages the gastric epithelial cells is poorly understood. Recently, Leunk et al. (1987) noted that about 60% of *C. pylori* isolates produce a protein cytotoxin which can be shown to cause vacuolation of intestinal cell lines in vitro. If this toxin is important in vivo, then the ultimate clinical syndrome associated with the bacterium may be more severe when a toxin producing organism is present. Presence or absence of cytotoxin could explain why one person with gastritis is asymptomatic wheras another develops gastric ulcer.

Another finding has been that urease generates ammonia from urea present in the extracellular fluid. Ammonia combines with alphaketoglutarate, and removes this essential substrate from the TCA cycle (Lehninger 1978). For this reason ammonia is toxic to aerobic mammalian cells. Each mole of ammonia produced then requires two moles of ATP to be re-entered into the liver's urea cycle. This urea recycling is a normal gastrointestinal function in ruminants who cannot afford to lose their sparse nitrogen stores in the urine as urea (Cheng et al. 1979). In man, however, dietary nitrogen is plentiful and ammonia generation is a wasteful and sometimes harmful metabolic event. In patients with both uremia and *C. pylori* infection, ammonia generation is likely to be greatly increased, and this would be especially harmful to patients with hepatic impairment.

Gastroenterologists now wonder how common *C. pylori* infection is, and how clinically significant it is. If the bacterium is a pathogen in the subgroup who develop duodenal ulcer (DU) disease (Fig. 4b), then can it be a commensal in a patient with asymptomatic gastritis? Common sense would suggest that it could not be both, yet asymptomatic gastritis is very common and apparently harmless. We do not yet have enough information to answer these questions.

If the benefit of eradicating the bacterium in dyspeptic disease can be shown, study of *C. pylori* infection will become more important. The possibility of reinfection from untreated asymptomatic family members will have to be considered. In addition, the syndromes of acute and chronic *C. pylori* associated gastritis will have to be accurately defined. Unless this is done, inappropriate antibacterial therapy will be used in patients with asymptomatic *C. pylori* infection who in fact have more serious gastrointestinal problems.

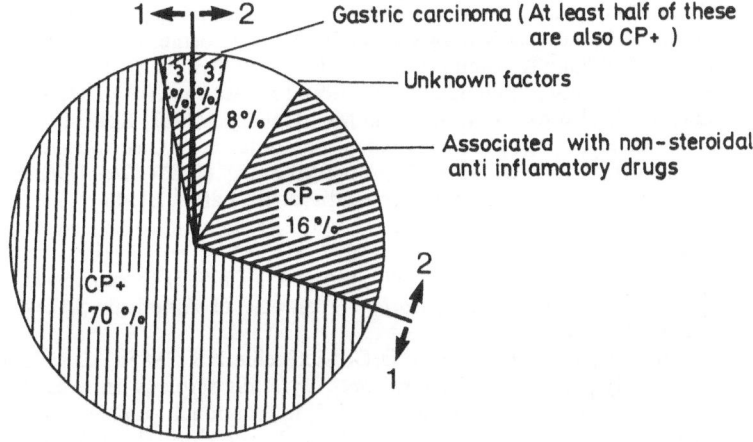

1 : These patients do have type B gastritis

a   2 : These patients do not have gastritis histologically

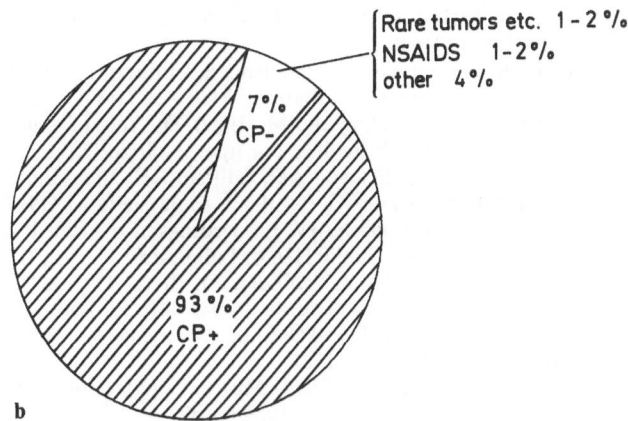

Fig. 4. Disease association with *C. pylori.* **a** Gastric ulcer; **b** duodenal ulcer   **b**

References

1. Barthel J, Westblom U, Gonzalez F et al. (1986) The predictive value of a simple rapid urease test for *C. pyloridis* in asymptomatic volunteers. Am J Gastroenterol 81:852
2. Boyd EJS, Wormsley KG (1985) Etiology and pathogenesis of peptic ulcer. In: Berk JE (ed) Bockus Gastroenterology, 4th edn. Saunders, Philadelphia, p 1015
3. Cheng K-J, McCowan RP, Costerton JW (1979) Adherent epithelial bacteria in ruminants and their roles in digestive tract function. Am J Clin Nutr 32:139–148
4. Eldridge J, Jones DM, Sethi P (1985) The occurrence of antibody to *Campylobacter pyloridis* in various groups of individuals. Campylobacter III. Proc third international workshop on *Campylobacter* infections. Public Health Laboratory Service, London, pp 183–184 (abstract 111)
5. Goodwin CS, Armstrong JA, Marshall BJ (1986) *Campylobacter pyloridis,* gastritis, and peptic ulceration. J Clin Pathol 39:353–365

6. Hui WM, Lam SK, Ho J et al. (1986) Chronic antral gastritis in duodenal ulcer. Natural history and treatment with prostaglandin E1. Gastroenterology 91:1095–1101

7. Kekki M, Villako K, Tamm A, Siurala M (1977) Dynamics of antral and *fundal* gastritis in an Estonian rural population sample. Scand J Gastroenterol 12:321–324

8. Lambert JR, Borromeo M, Korman MG, Hansky J (1987) Role of *Campylobacter pyloridis* in non-ulcer dyspepsia – a randomized controlled trial. Gastroenterology 92 (abstract)

9. Langenberg ML, Tytgat GNJ, Schipper MEI et al. (1984) *Campylobacter*-like organisms in the stomach of patients and healthy individuals. Lancet I:1348

10. Lehninger AL (1978) Ammonia excretion. In: Lehninger AL (ed) Biochemistry. Worth, New York, p 583

11. Leunk RD, Johnson PT, Kraft WG, Morgan DR (1987) Cytotoxic activity in broth culture filtrates of *Campylobacter pyloridis*. Abstracts of American Society for Microbiology, March 1987, No 168

12. Marshall BJ, Whisson M, Francis G, McGechie DB (1985a) Correlation between symptoms of dyspepsia and *Campylobacter pyloridis* serology in Western Australian blood donors. Campylobacter III. Proc third international workshop on *Campylobacter* infections. Public Health Laboratory Service, London, pp 188–189 (abstract 114)

13. Marshall BJ, Armstrong JA, McGechie DB, Glancy RJ (1985b) Attempt to fulfill Koch's postulates for pyloric *Campylobacter*. Med J Aust 142:436–439

14. Marshall BJ, Francis G, Langton S et al. (1987) Rapid urease test in the management of *Campylobacter pyloridis* associated gastritis. Am J Gastroenterol 3:200–210

15. McIntyre RLE, Piris J, Truelove SC (1982) Effect of cimetidine on chronic gastritis in gastric ulcer patients. Aust NZ J Med 12:106 (abstract)

16. Morris A, McIntyre D, Rose T (1985) Rapid diagnosis of *Campylobacter pyloridis* infection. Lancet 1:149

17. Narang APS, Agarwalla ML, Sharma S, Chuttani PN, Datta DV (1980) Presence of urease in the gastrointestinal tract. Indian J Med Res 71:325–328

18. Peterson W, Lee E, Skoglund M (1987) The role of *Campylobacter pyloridis* in epidemic gastritis with hypochlorhydria. Gastroenterology 92:(abstract 564)

19. Ramirez-Ramos A, Pearson AD, Gilman RH, Leon-Barua R, Spira WM, Recavarren S, Watanabe P, Rodriguez C, Bonilla J, Montebette M (1987) Epidemiology of *C. pylori* in Lima, Peru. *Campylobacter* IV. Proceedings of the fourth international workshop on *Campylobacter* infections, Public Health Laboratory Service, London (abstract 134)

20. Skoglund ML, Whalen J, Schindler D, Bierer D (1987) Prevalence of serum IgG antibodies to *Campylobacter pyloridis* among antacid users. Campylobacter IV. Proceedings of the fourth international workshop on *Campylobacter* infections, Public Health Laboratory Service, London (abstract 152)

21. Steer H, Colin Jones DG (1975) Mucosal changes in gastric ulceration and their response to carbenoxolone sodium. Gut 16:590–597

22. Tricottet V, Bruneval P, Vire O, Camilleri JP, Bloch F, Bonte N, Roge J (1986) *Campylobacter*-like organisms and surface epithelium abnormalities in active, chronic gastritis in humans: an ultrastructural study. Ultrastruct Pathol 10 (2)

Discussion

McNulty: Is there any evidence that the incidence of gastritis and peptic ulcer disease in the population has decreased over the past years since the introduction of antimicrobials?

Marshall: I do not know of any evidence. Some interesting things have happened. The duodenal ulcer is supposedly becoming less common. Maybe the high incidence of gastritis in older persons is a cohort effect: in Europe especially. I think that the conditions present in Europe in the 1940s during and after the war certainly could have been factors which encouraged the spread of an enteric organism. I have seen veterans from World War II with CP gastritis who were in New Guinea and the Pacific Islands. They receive a disability pension for "nervous stomach" − a post-war functional dyspepsia syndrome − this being a psychiatric diagnosis.

Tytgat: Barry, do you have any idea what the natural sources of CP are?

Marshall: I was looking at Dr. Mégraud's enzyme profile yesterday. This organism taxonomically resembles Wollinella, which is apparently related to rumen bacteria. *C. pylori* utilizes the substrates which are found in the rumen, and, if you study the physiology of the cow, or of any other ruminant, you will learn that the rumen is lined with a urease-producing flora which generates ammonia from the digestion of urea in the saliva. This ammonia then acts as a nitrogen source; for example, you can feed a cow sawdust and urea, and it will put on muscle bulk. This is because anaerobic rumen bacteria manufacture protein out of ammonia plus carbohydrate and the cow then digests the protein in the bacterial cells. *C. pylori* is similar to the type of organism you would expect to find lining the rumen − or within the rumen − of the cow. These organisms have another purpose: they are micro-aerophilic and they remove the final remnant of oxygen befoe it diffuses from the rumen wall into the anaerobic cell culture found in the rumen. Organisms similar to *C. pylori* have been described by scanning electron microscopy by Cheng and co-workers, who have even outlined a spiral urease-positive organism attached to the mucus-secreting epithelial cells of the abomasum. (The abomasum is the final stomach of the cow and is an acid-secreting stomach.) I think a ruminant is the original source of this organism, and that it was spread to man through unpasteurized milk. There is so much *C. pylori* in the population at present that animals are no longer the main source of infection.

Flemström: Is the concentration of urea in the gastric juice about the same in gastritis patients as in normals?

Marshall: Once the patient develops gastritis, urea is often absent from the gastric juice, and, on average, it is about 10% of the level in the blood, whereas in normal gastric juice it is approximately 60% or 70% of the blood level.

Flemström: What is it that makes the bacterium stick specifically to the gastric surface?

Marshall: The gastric epithelial cell probably has a specific receptor protein to which *C. pylori* binds. This is nothing new: a similar binding mechanism was found in enteropathogenic *E. coli* infection. *C. pylori* does not bind to the intestinal cell, the goblet cell or the squamous cell in the esophagus. Stewart Goodwin and I have observed that cat stomachs have a similar organism, which is found attached only to the mucus-secreting epithelial cells of the stomach.

Börsch: I have tried to think of a direct parallel to *C. pylori* infection in humans and I may have found one. This direct parallel is also very prevalent. Like *C. pylori* gastritis it affects the gastrointestinal tract in its widest sense. It also causes holes or predisposes to their development and is very difficult to treat; it is infective, although this fact is very difficult to prove. This direct parallel is dental caries. Possible solutions concerning therapy of dental caries right now include active immunization. Could you speculate on the role of active immunization against CP in the future treatment of peptic ulcer disease?

Marshall: It appears that the reinfection rate is not high, so immunization seems possible with *C. pylori*. But I do not think I am knowledgeable enough on the immunology of the organism to comment on that. Perhaps Stewart Goodwin would like to make a comment.

Goodwin: I think we have got a lot of work to do. It is obvious that some antigens detect diagnostic antibodies, other antigens detect protective antibodies. This will be sorted out by immuno-blotting, and when we get the right antigens relevant to the protective antibody, then we can make a vaccine.

Marshall: I think a vaccine or some sort of other type of immunization will be necessary to control *C. pylori*. The disease will be recognized as a public health problem which cannot be eradicated completely with antibiotics. I think we will have to immunize a cohort of children so that they do not develop gastritis.

Deltenre: If the concept that *C. pylori* would reduce the resistence of gastric mucosa to acid is true, would not the *C. pylori* gastritis be a self-limiting disease since the *C. pylori* is very sensitive and susceptible to acid?

Marshall: The organism is not susceptible to acid providing urea is present. Whereas in an acute infection urea is present, once the chronic infection has developped there is no urea in the gastric juice. However, there is still urea diffusing towards the organism within the mucus and between the cells. The absence of urea from gastric juice of infected patients may explain why viable *C. pylori* organisms are not usually found in the gastric aspirate.

Deltenre: Excuse me. If *C. pylori* is aggressive enough to reduce the resistence of gastric mucosa by modifying the mucus it is very kind to itself because it is still protected. There is something I do not really understand, conceptually in that situation.

Marshall: It may be that the inflammatory process is the main factor which precedes the formation of an ulcer rather that actual presence of *C. pylori*.

Goodwin: Could I come back to Dr. Engstrands question and your comment on the binding of the organism. What is the evidence that there is a receptor binding? Have there been binding studies?

Engstrand: There is a paper to be presented in Milan in a week, looking at lections on gastric epithelial cells, and I have not yet heard about it, but there will be some data on this.

Goodwin: There was also the report of Rathbone and Gregor in Berlin who found a common epithelial antigen, revealed by monoclonal antibody to *C. pylori*, which reacted with gastric enterocytes. This will be also important.

McNulty: What treatment, trials or research do you think we should be going away to do now?

Marshall: It is difficult to say. I think we should do pilot studies with different antibiotic regimens. Once we have an effective regimen, then we can design a study and predict the number of patients who will be in the effectively treated group, in other words, cleared of *C. pylori* after therapy. In these studies the definition of eradication of the organism should be taken as: a negative biopsy one month after ceasing therapy. Recurrence after that time is probably reinfection. Secondly, I think you must biopsy both the antrum and body of the stomach.

Flemström: What is known about the bacterium and the transport properties of its membrane? Is it sensitive to bismuth − because it transports bismuth − and does it transport other ions too?

Marshall: There are some data which indicate that this organism is sensitive to heavy metals including cadmium, mercury and arsenic. It appears that the soluble component of the bismuth complex enters the cell, the cell dies and then the bismuth becomes insoluble. That may be why we see bismuth precipitating around the cells.

Subject Index